The Liver in Systemic Disease

The Liver in Systemic Disease

A Clinician's Guide to Abnormal Liver Tests

Edited by

Gideon M. Hirschfield
University of Toronto
Canada

Paramjit Gill
University of Warwick
Coventry
UK

James Neuberger
University Hospital Birmingham
Birmingham
UK

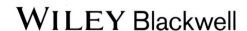

Registered Offices
John Wiley & Sons, Inc., 111 River Street, Hoboken, NJ 07030, USA
John Wiley & Sons Ltd, The Atrium, Southern Gate, Chichester, West Sussex, PO19 8SQ, UK

Editorial Office
9600 Garsington Road, Oxford, OX4 2DQ, UK

For details of our global editorial offices, customer services, and more information about Wiley products visit us at www.wiley.com.

Wiley also publishes its books in a variety of electronic formats and by print-on-demand. Some content that appears in standard print versions of this book may not be available in other formats.

Library of Congress Cataloging-in-Publication Data
Names: Hirschfield, Gideon M., author. | Gill, Paramjit, author. | Neuberger, James, author.
Title: The liver in systemic disease : a clinician's guide to abnormal liver tests / Gideon M. Hirschfield, Paramjit Gill, James Neuberger.
Description: Hoboken, NJ : Wiley, 2023. | Includes bibliographical references and index.
Identifiers: LCCN 2022032482 (print) | LCCN 2022032483 (ebook) | ISBN 9781119802136 (hardback) | ISBN 9781119802167 (adobe pdf) | ISBN 9781119802174 (epub)
Subjects: MESH: Liver Function Tests | Liver Diseases–diagnosis
Classification: LCC RC845 (print) | LCC RC845 (ebook) | NLM QY 140 | DDC 616.3/62–dc23/eng/20220912
LC record available at https://lccn.loc.gov/2022032482
LC ebook record available at https://lccn.loc.gov/2022032483

Cover Design: Wiley
Cover Image: © yodiyim/Adobe Stock Photos

Set in 9.5/12.5pt STIXTwoText by Straive, Pondicherry, India

Printed in Singapore
M116491_111022

Contents

List of Contributors *vii*
Preface *ix*

Section 1   Introduction   *1*

1 **Liver Tests**   *3*
James Neuberger

Section 2   Take-Home Primers: Managing Unexplained Abnormal Liver Tests   *19*

2 **Primary Care**   *21*
Jeetesh V. Patel and Paramjit Gill

3 **Global Perspective**   *31*
Arulraj Ramakrishnan, Grace L.-H. Wong, and Innocent K. Besigye

**Section 3   Take-Home Primers: Managing Unexplained Abnormal Serum
Liver Tests in Secondary Care**   *49*

4 **Intensive Care**   *51*
William Bernal and Sheital Chand

5 **Infections Affecting the Liver in the Immunosuppressed**   *63*
Dinesh Jothimani, Radhika Venugopal, Srividya Manjunath, and Mohamed Rela

6 **The Postoperative Patient**   *75*
Louise China and Douglas Thorburn

7 **Pregnancy**   *85*
Francesca E.M. Neuberger

8 Endocrinology and Metabolic Diseases (Including Diabetes) *99*
Laura Cristoferi, Stefano Ciardullo, Pietro Invernizzi, Gianluca Perseghin, and Marco Carbone

9 Abnormal Serum Liver Tests in Cardiac Disease *111*
James Neuberger

10 Respiratory Disease *121*
Michael J. Krowka and Michael D. Leise

11 Gastroenterology *133*
Kathleen Rooney and Gerry MacQuillan

12 Renal Medicine *145*
Javeria Peracha and Graham Lipkin

13 Dermatology *169*
Jennifer A. Scott and Peter C. Hayes

14 Oncology *179*
Mai Kilany and Morven Cunningham

15 Hematology *191*
Navjyot K. Hansi and Abid R. Suddle

16 Mental Health and Neurology *201*
Fiona M. Thompson

17 Non-Alcoholic Fatty Liver Disease *209*
Matthew Collins and Keyur Patel

Section 4 Practical Issues in Patients with Liver Abnormalities *223*

18 Prescribing in Patients with Abnormal Liver Tests or Liver Disease: A Pragmatic Approach *225*
Paul Selby

19 Invasive Procedures in Patients with Liver Disease *237*
Will Lester

20 Diagnosing Drug-Induced Liver Injury *243*
Guruprasad P. Aithal

Index *255*

List of Contributors

Guruprasad P. Aithal
Nottingham University Hospitals NHS Trust, Nottingham, UK
University of Nottingham, Nottingham UK

William Bernal
Institute of Liver Studies, Kings College Hospital, London, UK

Innocent K. Besigye
College of Health Sciences, Makerere University, Kampala, Uganda

Marco Carbone
University of Milano-Bicocca, Monza, Italy
European Reference Network on Hepatological Diseases, San Gerardo Hospital, Monza, Italy

Sheital Chand
Institute of Liver Studies, Kings College Hospital, London, UK

Louise China
Royal Free London NHS Foundation Trust, London, UK

Stefano Ciardullo
Policlinico di Monza, Monza, Italy
Division of Endocrinology, Department of Medicine and Surgery, University of Milano-Bicocca, Italy

Matthew Collins
McMaster University, Hamilton, Ontario, Canada
Liver Care Canada, Hamilton, Ontario, Canada

Laura Cristoferi
University of Milano-Bicocca, Monza, Italy
European Reference Network on Hepatological Diseases, San Gerardo Hospital, Monza, Italy

Morven Cunningham
Toronto General Hospital, Toronto, Ontario, Canada

Paramjit Gill
University of Warwick, Coventry, UK

Navjyot K. Hansi
Addenbrooke's Hospital, Cambridge, UK

Peter C. Hayes
Royal Infirmary of Edinburgh, Edinburgh, UK

Pietro Invernizzi
University of Milano-Bicocca, Monza, Italy
European Reference Network on Hepatological Diseases, San Gerardo Hospital, Monza, Italy

Dinesh Jothimani
Dr. Rela Institute and Medical Centre,
Chromepet, Chennai, India

Mai Kilany
Toronto General Hospital, Toronto,
Ontario, Canada

Michael J. Krowka
Mayo Clinic, Rochester, MN, USA

Michael D. Leise
Mayo Clinic, Rochester, MN, USA

Will Lester
University Hospitals Birmingham,
Birmingham, UK

Graham Lipkin
Queen Elizabeth Hospital, Birmingham, UK

Gerry MacQuillan
UWA Medical School, University of Western
Australia, Nedlands, Australia

Srividya Manjunath
Dr. Rela Institute and Medical Centre,
Chromepet, Chennai, India

Francesca E.M. Neuberger
North Bristol NHS Trust, Bristol, UK

James Neuberger
Queen Elizabeth Hospital, Birmingham, UK

Jeetesh V. Patel
Dartmouth Medical Centre, West
Bromwich, UK

Keyur Patel
Toronto General Hospital, Toronto,
Ontario, Canada

Javeria Peracha
Queen Elizabeth Hospital, Birmingham, UK

Gianluca Perseghin
Policlinico di Monza, Italy
University of Milano-Bicocca, Italy

Arulraj Ramakrishnan
Kovai Medical Center and Hospital,
Coimbatore, Tamil Nadu, India
Chinese University of Hong Kong, Hong
Kong SAR, China

Mohamed Rela
Dr. Rela Institute and Medical Centre,
Chromepet, Chennai, India

Kathleen Rooney
Department of Hepatology, Sir Charles
Gairdner Hospital, Nedlands, Australia

Jennifer A. Scott
Royal Infirmary of Edinburgh,
Edinburgh, UK

Paul Selby
Cambridge University Hospitals NHS
Foundation Trust, Cambridge, UK

Abid R. Suddle
Institute of Liver Studies, King's College
Hospital, London, UK

Fiona M. Thompson
Institute for Translational Medicine,
University Hospitals Birmingham,
Birmingham, UK

Douglas Thorburn
Royal Free London NHS Foundation Trust,
London, UK

Radhika Venugopal
Dr. Rela Institute and Medical Centre,
Chromepet, Chennai, India

Grace L.-H. Wong
Chinese University of Hong Kong, Hong
Kong SAR, China

Preface

There is no doubt that the prevalence of liver disease is rising globally and has a profound impact on patients, their family, and well as wider society. Liver diseases spans common problems (such as alcohol use disorders, metabolic syndrome, and viral hepatitis) as well as less frequent conditions such as autoimmune and inherited diseases. This parallels a reality that the delivery of modern health care is increasingly complex, with different professionals intervening to manage care. Patients, the public, as well as professionals, are now involved in increasing awareness and prevention by addressing the wider determinants of health.

UK data from the Royal College of Pathologists suggest that around 95% of clinical pathways rely on patients having access to pathology services. Each year in England and Wales (population around 55 million) there are 500 million biochemistry and 130 million hematology tests completed. 300 000 investigations are done each working day with around 50 million reports sent to primary care doctors, meaning that an average of 14 tests are performed annually for each person in England and Wales [1]. Such a pattern of investigation is not exclusive to the UK but is mirrored globally. Of course, there are many types of blood tests and only a proportion will be liver tests. While liver tests are often requested in the knowledge of known liver disease, often abnormalities in liver tests are unexpected (and indeed sometimes unwanted).

This book brings together our experiences of managing liver disorders in primary, secondary, and tertiary care. Clinicians are faced with deciding whether abnormal liver tests are expected abnormalities as part of the patient's condition or whether these abnormalities require further investigation. Further investigation will have possible benefit, and has the potential to harm the patient, as well as increasing costs to health care services.

The purpose of this collection of contributions is to provide a practical and helpful guide to the non-liver specialist. We have focused on when to expect abnormal blood tests and what, if anything, needs to be done, including guidance on further investigations and referral. We appreciate that there is some redundancy and occasional contradiction. This is intentional. With an international, expert, and a specialized team of authors, there will be some variation in view when evidence is lacking: we feel that the reader should be aware that many decisions in medicine are not as clear cut as we would like. We also realize that few if any readers will read the book from cover to cover, so each chapter is designed to be self-contained.

We would like to thank our authors who have devoted time to write their chapters and respond to editorial demands, especially during the many challenges caused by the COVID-19 pandemic. We are grateful to those at Wiley for their help and support and patience, and especial thanks are due to our families who have put up with us and tolerated the multiple phone calls and teleconferences.

Finally, thanks to the readers. We hope you will find the volume helpful and a useful reference.

Gideon Hirschfield, Toronto, Canada
Paramjit Gill, Coventry, UK
James Neuberger, Birmingham, UK
https://www.rcpath.org/discover-pathology/news/
fact-sheets/pathology-facts-and-figures-.html

Section 1

Introduction

1

Liver Tests

James Neuberger

Queen Elizabeth Hospital, Birmingham, UK

KEY POINTS

- The standard liver tests do not measure liver function and none of the analytes measured are specific for the liver.
- The normal range of analytes may vary according to age, sex, ethnicity.
- Normal liver tests do not exclude liver disease.
- Unexpected or unexplained liver tests indicate the need for further investigation.
- Investigation of unexpected abnormal liver tests usually require a full history (including use of drugs and alcohol), examination and usually further serology and imaging.

Introduction

The term "liver function test" (LFT) has become established in health care, but the term is misleading as the blood analytes measured may not accurately reflect the extent or nature of liver disease (Box 1.1). Although a more appropriate term is "liver blood tests," this term is not used in this chapter, as the old term of LFTs has become enshrined in medical use. In addition, other commonly measured analytes give useful guidance on the presence and extent of liver disease (such as full blood count, prothrombin count).

The Reference Range

The term "normal range" has also become established, although it is preferable to use the term "reference range." This range should ideally be determined for each laboratory and each piece of equipment. Factors that may affect the reference range include the selection of healthy people for determination of the reference range and the patient population; other factors that may affect the reference range include sex, age, and ethnic factors, time of day or season when samples are collected, variation in venipuncture technique, preparation,

The Liver in Systemic Disease: A Clinician's Guide to Abnormal Liver Tests, First Edition.
Edited by Gideon M. Hirschfield, Paramjit Gill, and James Neuberger.
© 2023 John Wiley & Sons Ltd. Published 2023 by John Wiley & Sons Ltd.

Box 1.1   Characteristics of Liver Blood Tests

- Not liver specific
- Do not measure function
- Not tests
- May be within normal limits when there is severe liver disease
- May be abnormal when the liver is structurally or functionally normal
- Normal ranges will vary:
  - between laboratories
  - with age
  - with sex
  - with ethnicity
  - with normal physiology (such as pregnancy).
- Not diagnostic for any specific liver disease
- Results in the high normal range may be associated with an increased risk of death

---

storage, and analysis of samples. The reference range should be established by testing at least 120 samples (although many regulatory bodies suggest a higher number) and clear outliers are usually excluded. The reference range may be determined by one of two approaches:

1) *The parametric approach* can be used only when the distribution of values falls within a normal distribution; the reference range lies within the 95% confidence interval.
2) *The non-parametric approach* defines the reference range as lying between the 2.5 and 97.5 percentiles of the population.

Whichever approach is adopted, the implication is that, for healthy individuals, around 5% samples will have values lying outside the reference range. In some cases, such as blood sugar or triglycerides, the reference range is determined more by consensus than the process outlined above.

When abnormal tests are reported, further investigations should be undertaken, the nature and extent will depend on the clinical situation. A guide to further management of abnormal liver tests is given in Box 1.2. This will help to define the presence (if any) of liver disease, the extent of liver damage, and the cause of the abnormal liver tests and, where appropriate, the response to treatment. A clinician needs to understand the several tests available to assess liver function and causes of liver disease and the limitation of these tests.

The Standard Liver Function Tests

Analytes measured in the battery of LFTs include:

- albumin
- aspartate amino transferase (AST)
- alanine amino transferase (ALT)
- alkaline phosphatase (AP)
- gamma-glutamyl transferase (GGT).

Box 1.2 Guidelines for Management of Abnormal Liver Tests

- Initial investigation for potential liver disease should include full blood count, bilirubin, albumin, alanine amino transferase, alkaline phosphatase and gamma-glutamyl transferase.
- Abnormal liver blood test results should be interpreted after review of the previous results, past medical history and current medical condition, review of alcohol and drug history and clinical state.
- The extent of liver blood test abnormality is not necessarily a guide to clinical significance. The clinical significance is determined by the specific analyte which is outside the reference range and the clinical context.
- Patients with abnormal liver blood tests should be considered for investigation with a liver etiology screen, irrespective of level and duration of abnormality.
- In adults, a standard liver etiology screen may include, as clinically appropriate:
  - abdominal ultrasound
  - testing for virus:
    - hepatitis B
    - hepatitis C
    - hepatitis E in those who are immunosuppressed
  - Autoantibodies, including
    - anti-mitochondrial antibody
    - anti-smooth muscle antibody
    - antinuclear antibody
    - anti-liver/kidney microsomal
    - celiac antibodies
  - Serum immunoglobulins
  - Serum ferritin and transferrin saturation
  - Serum caeruloplasmin if under 45-years of age

Source: Adapted from Newsome et al. [1].

Interpretation of liver tests must always be made in the clinical context, and the extent, pattern of liver abnormality, and time course must be considered. For example, a falling high value for ALT may indicate improvement in the extent of hepatitis, but in the case of severe hepatitis, a return to normal values may indicate a failing liver (ALT predominantly coming from hepatocytes). Conversely, a serum ALT in the normal range may be misleading: cirrhosis may be present in the presence of an established cirrhosis and serum ALT in the upper part of the normal range is associated with an increased risk of death.

Albumin

Decreased circulating concentrations of albumin may be the result of either decreased production or increased loss. Levels are normally lower in the second and third trimesters of pregnancy because of increased plasma volume.

Decreased Production of Albumin

Liver disease: the liver synthetizes about 12–15 g albumin daily. Its long half-life (around 21 days) means that low levels from liver disease is not a robust marker of acute liver disease. In advanced liver disease from any cause, low albumin is a consequence of both decreased synthesis and increased catabolism. In those with ascites, loss of albumin to the ascites may contribute to the low serum albumin.

Nutritional deficiency: the synthesis of albumin is dependent on the availability of amino acids (especially tryptophane), iron, and zinc, so nutritional causes may be associated with low serum albumin.

Renal loss: normal loss of albumin through the kidney is normally very low but may increase with fever or exercise. Glomerular disease will lead to increased loss of albumin and may result in nephrotic syndrome.

Gut loss: Protein-losing enteropathy is characterized by loss of proteins including albumin via the gastrointestinal tract that exceeds synthesis. Protein loss through the gut may be due to mucosal disease without erosion (such as celiac disease), gut disease with mucosal erosions (such as Crohn's disease) or increased lymphatic pressure (such as lymphangiectasis).

Extravascular loss: albumin may leak from the vascular to extravascular compartments. For example, in burns, there is increased vascular permeability which, combined with an acute phase response, leads to inhibition of protein synthesis, with a resulting low serum albumin. Similar mechanisms account for low albumin levels in sepsis which is also associated with increased catabolism of albumin.

Multifactorial causes of low albumin: low serum albumin may be seen in a variety of conditions which are associated with a combination of decreased albumin synthesis (which may be induced by inflammatory cytokines switching protein production from albumin to acute phase proteins), leakage from the vascular compartment, and increased catabolism. This may be seen in critical illnesses, for example. In advanced cardiac failure low serum albumin is also due to combinations of poor intake, poor adsorption, decreased synthesis, leakage form vascular compartments, and increased catabolism.

Analbuminemia (with concentration of < 1 g/l) is a very rare cause of low albumin levels.

Increased Loss of Albumin

High levels of albumin are uncommon and are not related to liver disease. Causes include some respiratory disorders such as tuberculosis, dehydration, vitamin A deficiency, excess corticosteroids, and some leukemias. Samples not processed immediately can also give artificial high concentrations of albumin.

Aspartate and Alanine Amino Transferase

The enzymes AST and ALT catalyze the transfer of the α-amino groups of alanine and aspartate to the α-keto-group of ketoglutaric acid, forming pyruvic and oxaloacetic acid, respectively. Whereas ALT is located primarily in the hepatocytes, AST is more widely distributed, including skeletal and cardiac muscle, red and white blood cells, brain, pancreas, and kidney. Within the hepatocyte, ALT is located primarily in the cytosol, whereas AST is located in the mitochondria (80%) and, to a lesser degree, in the cytosol. The reference ranges will vary between laboratories but the upper limit of normal is higher in males than females and should be considered in the light of body weight.

In most cases of liver damage, both AST and ALT are elevated. Very high levels (> 500 iu/l) are seen in fulminant hepatic failure, ischemic hepatitis, acute Budd–Chiari syndrome, hepatic necrosis from drugs or hepatic artery ligation.

Historically, there was much emphasis placed on the ratio of AST to ALT. In general, serum ALT levels are higher than serum AST in liver diseases, while AST is greater in some cases of alcohol-related injury, steatosis, myopathy, ischemic hepatitis, hemolysis, thyroid disease, after strenuous exercise, and sepsis. In some instances, this increase is due to AST from non-hepatic sources (such as muscle) or hepatic mitochondrial damage leading to a rise in mitochondrial AST (mAST). Although the ratio of AST to mAST may be helpful in defining liver causes of raised transaminases, mAST is rarely measured in clinical practice. Rarely, AST may bind to immunoglobulin A, leading to elevated measured levels; this is seen occasionally in association with liver malignancy.

Low levels of ALT and AST may be seen in patients on long-term hemodialysis, and this may be due, in part, to pyridoxine deficiency. In those in the very advanced stage of fulminant hepatic failure, serum transaminase activity falls; this may be a sign of necrotic liver rather than improvement in liver function.

Alkaline Phosphatase

Alkaline phosphatases (ALPs) are in a family of enzymes that hydrolyze phosphate esters. There are several isoenzymes which differ in distribution and substrate. Isoenzymes are found in the liver, bone, intestine, placenta, leukocytes, and kidney. Within the liver, where are two isoenzymes, the ALP is distributed in sinusoidal and canalicular membranes, as well as the cytosol.

There are several different approaches to the measurement of ALP and laboratory values and normal ranges vary according to methodology. The normal range of ALP is dependent on:

- age: levels are high in the newborn and in puberty and fall in middle age and rise again in the elderly
- sex: levels are higher in men than women
- height and weight: levels correlate directly with weight and inversely with height
- smoking: is associated with increase in levels
- pregnancy: levels tend to rise in pregnancy because of placental ALP.

Elevated levels of ALP are seen in association with:

- liver and biliary disease (see below)
- bone disease where levels are increased where there is increased osteoblastic activity (such as following fractures, Paget's disease of the bone, and some cancers, but not in osteoporosis)
- pregnancy
- chronic renal failure and some renal malignancies
- some malignancies
- congestive heart failure

- some infections
- systemic inflammation
- bowel disease, including celiac disease.

Liver Causes of Raised Alkaline Phosphatase

Raised levels of ALP are seen in most forms of liver disease and include:

- Biliary disease:
  - primary biliary cholangitis (PBC)
  - primary sclerosing cholangitis
  - bile duct obstruction
  - vanishing bile duct syndromes
  - some genetic biliary diseases such as benign recurrent cholestasis
  - chronic liver transplant rejection
  - cholecystitis.
- Drug induced liver injury
- Liver infiltration:
  - sarcoidosis and other granulomatous diseases
  - tuberculosis
  - amyloid
  - lymphoma
  - malignant infiltration.

Other causes such as infection, cirrhosis, hepatitis where elevated ALP is less marked than transaminase levels. Mild elevations in ALP are seen not infrequently in non-alcohol-related fatty liver disease (NAFLD; 10% of patients may have isolated mild ALP rises). Occasionally there is a familial increase in ALP.

It is usually possible to determine whether the raised ALP is due to hepatic or non-hepatic causes by analyzing the isoenzymes, most rely on GGT (see below) as, in general, rises in liver and biliary ALP is mirrored by rises in GGT.

Low levels of ALP are uncommon but may be seen in Wilson's disease, hypothyroidism and iodine deficiency, pernicious anemia, zinc deficiency, achondroplasia, and hypophosphatasia.

Gamma-Glutamyl Transferase

GGT catalyzes the transfer of peptide γ-glutamyl groups to other amino acids, as well as being involved in the metabolism of some glutathione conjugates of drugs, and is also associated with oxidative stress. There are several isoenzymes. The enzyme is widely distributed in membranes including liver, biliary tree and gall bladder, spleen, pancreas, kidney, heart, and lung. Within the liver, GGT is distributed throughout the liver and in the biliary tree but is concentrated in the biliary epithelial cells in the small bile ductules. There is a correlation between higher levels of GGT with heart disease, stroke, and type 2 diabetes. The reference range is dependent on:

- Age: high in newborns and in adults, increases with age.
- Sex: levels are higher in men than women.

Levels of GGT are elevated in several scenarios:

- *Alcohol and drugs*: GGT levels can be induced by alcohol consumption and a number of enzyme-inducing drugs such as phenytoin and barbiturates
- Pancreatic disease
- Lung disease
- Renal failure
- *Liver disease*: in general, levels of GGT parallel those of hepatic ALP and GGT may be a more sensitive indicator of liver disease than ALP. The exception is with some forms of very rare genetic familial intrahepatic cholestasis syndromes. A raised GGT in the presence of excess alcohol consumption is not necessarily a sign of liver disease. Patients with NAFLD will very frequently have GGT elevations.

Bilirubin

Bilirubin is derived primarily from the degradation of hemoglobin. The metabolism of bilirubin and the various mechanisms of hyperbilirubinemia are shown in Figure 1.1.

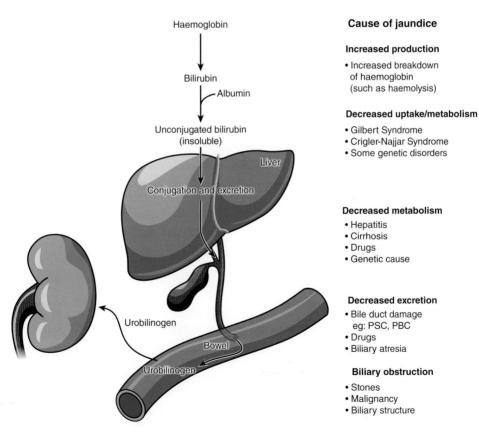

Figure 1.1 Metabolism of bilirubin and causes of jaundice.

The normal range of bilirubin is affected by sex and is higher in men than women. Usually, the laboratories measure total serum bilirubin, although assessment of conjugated and unconjugated bilirubin will help to determine whether there is increased production or decreased excretion. As shown in Figure 1.1, unconjugated bilirubin is not water soluble (it is transported in plasma conjugated primarily to albumin) and therefore it is not seen in the urine in increased amounts.

Causes for elevated levels of serum bilirubin can be seen in Box 1.3. Thus, unless there is a clear cause for the high serum bilirubin, it is helpful to measure direct and total bilirubin to distinguish the "pre-hepatic" causes of hyperbilirubinemia from hepatic and biliary causes. A clinical rule of thumb is that unconjugated hyperbilirubinemia is not associated with dark urine, but the clinical assessment of both clinical jaundice and bilirubinuria are unreliable. Hemolysis is associated with increased unconjugated bilirubin, a reticulocytosis, and low haptoglobin (a protein that binds free bilirubin).

Gilbert's syndrome is a very common and innocent explanation for elevated total bilirubin, with near normal direct bilirubin values. It is an autosomal recessive condition related to variations in the *UGT1A1* gene, which codes for uridine diphosphate glucuronosyltransferase, an enzyme involved in bilirubin conjugation. Thus, the person has higher levels of unconjugated serum bilirubin which may lead to mild jaundice (without dark urine), and levels are greater at times of physical or emotional stress. No treatment or routine follow-up is required. The diagnosis is made on the basis of a raised unconjugated serum bilirubin and

---

Box 1.3   Causes for Elevated Levels of Serum Bilirubin

Unconjugated bilirubin:

- Increased production:
  - Hemolysis
  - Resorption of hematoma
  - Ineffective hematopoiesis
- Decreased clearance:
  - Neonatal jaundice
  - Gilbert's syndrome
  - Crigler–Najjar syndrome
  - Shunt hyperbilirubinemia
- Drugs

Decreased metabolism and excretion:

- Cirrhosis and hepatitis
- Rotor syndrome
- Dubin–Johnson syndrome
- Sepsis
- Lymphoma
- Vanishing bile duct syndrome
- Biliary disease
- Biliary outflow or obstruction

no signs of hemolysis. The diagnosis can, if necessary, be confirmed by mutation analysis of the gene involved, but generally this is not relevant practically. Other mutations may lead to the Crigler–Najjar syndrome, which presents in the newborn. Enzyme levels are much lower than those seen in Gilbert's syndrome. High levels of unconjugated bilirubin may lead to neurological damage in the child and therefore active management by specialists may be indicated.

Prothrombin Time

Although the prothrombin time is not usually considered to be a liver test, it is a useful measure of liver function in that the hepatocytes synthetize most of the clotting factors and, as they are short-lived, the degree of abnormality is a useful guide to liver function, especially in the setting of acute hepatitis and liver failure. In liver disease, the normal balance of clotting is disrupted and so the prothrombin time cannot be taken as a robust marker of clotting. Prolongation of the prothrombin time is also seen in other situations, such as vitamin K deficiency.

Other Analytes in Liver Disease

There are changes in many other analytes that can reflect the presence and severity of liver disease.

Kidney Blood Tests

Serum urea is often low in those with cirrhosis because of the reduced syntheses, and rarely because of fluid overload. This may be counteracted by a rise associated with overuse of diuretics or the onset of hepatorenal syndrome.

Hematologic Analytes

Hypersplenism, often associated with portal hypertension, may be associated with low red cells, white cells, and platelets. Occasionally, thrombocytopenia is the presenting feature of cirrhosis.

Anemia: there are many causes for anemia in those with liver abnormalities: causes include hypersplenism, nutritional deficiency, blood loss secondary to portal hypertensive gastropathy or variceal bleeding, and anemia of chronic disease and cirrhosis-associated reduced erythropoiesis.

Hemolysis: there are many causes for hemolysis, including drug toxicity and spur cell anemia (especially in alcohol-related liver disease), or it may be related to the cause of liver disease, such as autoimmune hemolysis associated with autoimmune liver diseases (autoimmune hepatitis or primary sclerosing cholangitis) or toxicity (such as Wilson's disease).

Leukopenia: leukopenia is usually related to hypersplenism, but other causes such drug toxicity or primary bone marrow disease should be considered.

Thrombocytopenia: low platelets may be seen in association with reduced production because of low levels of thrombopoietin, or increased consumption because of hypersplenism or immune thrombocytopenia.

Markers of Malignancy

Alfa-fetoprotein (AFP) is associated with several malignancies, including primary liver-cell cancer (hepatocellular carcinoma). As with other cancer markers, not all primary liver cancers are associated with increased levels of AFP, and raised levels may be found in other liver conditions, especially when associated with liver-cell regeneration. It should also be noted that some markers used to diagnose malignancy (such as CA19-9 and carcinoembryonic antigen) may be elevated in those with cirrhosis and ascites in the absence of malignancy.

Selected analytes used in the diagnosis of cause of liver disease are shown below. As can be seen, abnormalities are common in a variety of clinical situations and so must be interpreted in the light of clinical and other investigations.

Alpha 1-Antitrypsin Deficiency

There are several phenotypes of alpha 1-antitrypsin deficiency (AAT), characterized by the Pi notation. The common (normal phenotype) is PiMM. PiZZ is associated with very low levels (10%–15%) of AAT and clinical disease. Other phenotypes (Pi MS, SS, MZ) are associated with serum levels of AAT between 40% and 80% and the association with liver disease is less clear, albeit in multiple studies it is accepted as a risk factor for poorer outcomes. AAT is an acute phase protein so, in the acutely ill patient, levels associated with AAT deficiency may be within the normal range. As AAT is synthesized primarily by the liver, low levels are seen also in those with cirrhosis or hepatitis so the possibility of liver disease secondary to AAT should be assessed by phenotyping.

Ceruloplasmin

Ceruloplasmin is measured for the consideration in the diagnosis of Wilson's disease. Very low levels are seen in genetic condition of aceruloplasminemia; around 75% of those with Wilson's disease have low levels, but the diagnosis also requires assessment of serum copper and urinary copper excretion. Low levels may also be seen in association with liver disease, with copper deficiency, nephrotic syndrome, excess zinc levels, and malabsorption in children. Ceruloplasmin is an acute phase protein so may be elevated in sepsis and other inflammatory diseases. High levels can be seen with copper toxicity, and in the third trimester of pregnancy.

Ferritin

High levels of serum ferritin may be due to increased synthesis consequent on iron overload, as a result of cellular damage or as an acute phase protein. Iron accumulation and high serum ferritin may be a result of primary disease (such as genetic hemochromatosis), to secondary overload (such as multiple transfusions), excessive iron intake, hereditary aceruloplasminemia, and ineffective erythropoiesis (such as sideroblastic anemia). High levels are also seen in some malignancies, hereditary hyperferritinemia, acute and chronic infections, and chronic inflammatory disorders, and some autoimmune disorders. Finally, high ferritin levels are also seen in chronic liver diseases and alcohol excess. Thus, there are many causes for a raised serum ferritin. In primary care with a hepatology perspective, the most common cause of elevated ferritin (with usually normal iron saturations) is NAFLD/metabolic syndrome. If associated with a high iron saturation, then consideration should be given to testing to look for genetic hemochromatosis.

Autoantibodies

There are several autoantibodies included in the liver screen. Not all patients being investigated for liver disease need autoantibody testing at the outset, if more common explanations based on clinical history alone provide adequate explanation. This is particularly relevant to investigating patients with NAFLD. Autoantibodies linked to autoimmune hepatitis include some anti-nuclear antibodies (ANA), antibodies to smooth muscle antibody, liver–kidney microsomal type 1, and liver cytosol antigen type 1.

Anti-Nuclear Antibodies

ANA are a family of autoantibodies with a diverse reactivity and diverse implications for the diagnosis of liver disease. ANA are found in NAFLD, autoimmune hepatitis type 1, PBC, primary sclerosing cholangitis, viral hepatitis, and drug induced liver injury. Some of the ANA are diagnostic (for example, anti gp-210 and sp-100 for PBC). Autoimmune hepatitis is associated with homogenous, speckled, and nucleolar patterns of ANA with an immunofluorescence pattern of ANA on HEp-2 cells often homogenous or speckled. The nuclear reactant in AIH is the same as that seen in systemic lupus erythematosus (chromatin). Other patterns of ANA associated with AIH include anticentromere antibodies, multiple nuclear dot, and antinuclear envelope antibodies. Perinuclear antineutrophil cytoplasmic antibodies are also antinuclear antibodies that are associated with ANA and PSCs.

Anti-Mitochondrial Antibodies

Anti-mitochondrial antibodies are virtually diagnostic for PBC when tested in the context of cholestatic (elevated ALP in particular) serum liver tests.

Antibodies for Celiac Disease

Some liver diseases are associated with celiac disease and celiac disease itself may result in liver abnormalities. The presence of anti-tissue transglutaminase antibodies suggests, but does not prove, celiac disease, which should usually be confirmed or refuted by small bowel histology, given a need to recommend life-long gluten-free diets.

Immunoglobulins

The commonly assessed immunoglobulins (Ig) are IgG, IgA, and IgM. Polyclonally increased immunoglobulin levels are seen in chronic infection (such as osteomyelitis and endocarditis), chronic inflammation, autoimmune diseases, and some neoplasms,as well as liver disease. Within the context of liver disease, IgG levels are a useful guide to the activity of autoimmune hepatitis; high IgA levels are seen in alcohol and NAFLD and elevated IgM with PBC, but this is far from specific.

Hepatitis Viral Markers

Hepatitis A virus (HAV): IgM anti-HAV suggests recent infection, and IgG anti-HAV suggests previous infection or immunization.

Hepatitis B (HBV): the common antibodies and antigens measured are to core and surface. HBV DNA measurement has largely replaced testing for e antigen or antibody, as it is more reliable measure of active infection and its level determines the need for treatment. The interpretation of serology is shown in Table 1.1. Occasionally, patients are negative for hepatitis B surface antigen and antibody but positive for antibody to hepatitis B core

Table 1.1 Interpretation of hepatitis B serology.

Serology	Result
Not previously exposed to HBV or susceptible:	
HBsAg	Negative
Anti-HBc	Negative
Anti-HBs	Negative
Recovered from previous HBV infection:	
HBsAg	Negative
Anti-HBc	Positive
Anti-HBs	Positive
Immune following HBV vaccination:	
HBsAg	Negative
Anti-HBc	Negative
Anti-HBs	Positive (titres > 100 suggest successful immunity)
Acute infection:	
HBsAg	Positive
Anti-HBc	Positive
IgM anti-HBc	Positive
Chronic infection:	
Anti-HBs	Negative
HBsAg	Positive
Anti-HBc	Positive
IgM anti-HBc	Negative
Interpretation unclear:[a]	
Anti-HBs	Negative
anti-HBc	Positive
anti-HBs	Negative

anti-HBc, antibody to hepatitis B core antigen; anti-HBs, antibody to hepatitis B surface antibody; HBsAg, hepatitis B surface antigen; IgM, immunoglobulin M.
[a] Resolved infection (most common), false-positive anti-HBc, low level chronic infection, resolving acute infection.
Source: Adapted from Centers for Disease Control and Prevention [2].

antigen. This usually indicates previous infection but may rarely been seen in resolving infection or chronic infection.

Hepatitis C (HCV): HCV antibody shows current or past infection; active disease is shown by the presence of HCV RNA.

Hepatitis E (HEV): IgM antibody indicates recent infection and IgM past infection. Chronic HEV infection is seen primarily in the context of immunosuppression and active infection is shown by HEV RNA.

Assessment of Hepatic Fibrosis

Liver histology is the de facto "gold" standard for the assessment of hepatic fibrosis. Although liver biopsy is very safe, it is an invasive procedure with associated risks, including pain, bleeding, organ puncture, as well as of course sampling error. There are several non-invasive approaches to assess the degree of hepatic fibrosis and a number of models based on clinical and serological measures have been proposed. Many of these models are disease specific. For NAFLD, the National Institute for Health and Care Excellence recommends using a non-invasive scoring system, such as the following:

- ELF™ (Enhanced Liver Fibrosis) test, (Siemens Healthcare, Tarrytown, NY): the result is derived from a composite of hyaluronic acid, aminoterminal propeptide of type III procollagen, and tissue inhibitor of metalloproteinase 1. A score of 10.51 or above, for example, in some studies suggests advanced liver fibrosis.
- NAFLD Fibrosis Score [3] is derived from age, body mass index, blood glucose, platelet count, albumin, and AST : ALT ratio. An intermediate or high score (greater than minus 1.455) suggests advanced liver fibrosis.
- Fibrosis-4 Index for Liver Fibrosis score [4] is derived from age, AST, ALT, and platelet count. A score of greater than 2.67 suggests advanced liver fibrosis.

These models are often applied in other etiologies of liver disease.

Imaging

Ultrasound is an unreliable measure of fibrosis and cirrhosis. Transient elastography (such as with the FibroScan®, Echosens, Paris, France) uses ultrasound to assess the degree of fibrosis and is being used increasingly in clinical practice (Figure 1.2). Other imagining modalities using either magnetic resonance imaging (MRI) or computed tomography (CT) and elastography have been used but, because of the cost and exposure to radiation (for CT), these modalities are not often used in clinical practice but they are of value in research. Most clinical pathways now suggest the use of a non-invasive blood screening test (e.g. FIB-4) and then elastography, if indicated, based on local availability.

Assessment of Liver Fat

While liver ultrasound may show an echobright liver in the presence of hepatic steatosis; this is not a robust marker and is subjective. Other imaging technique, such as CT and MRI may also characterize hepatic steatosis but use of the controlled attenuation parameter (CAP)

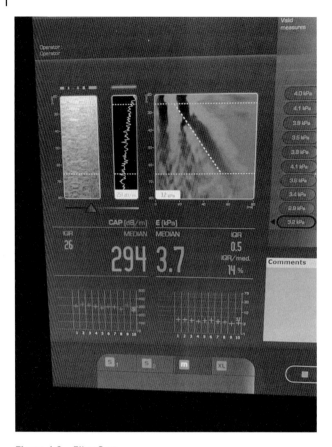

Figure 1.2 FibroScan.

score in a FibroScan will give a quantitative assessment, but the value needs to be interpreted in light of the underlying liver disease. None of these distinguish microvascular and macrovascular steatosis; histology is the gold standard. Radiologic descriptions of severity do not correlate with clinical urgency or impact.

Assessment of Alcohol Use

Traditionally, serum GGT was used as an indirect marker of alcohol use but, as described above, this is not specific or sensitive. Measurement of alcohol in blood, breath, or urine provides clear evidence of recent alcohol consumption. In the last decade, other analytes (mainly metabolites of alcohol) have been used to detect recent alcohol consumption. Urinary ethyl glucuronide and urinary ethyl sulfate are helpful in assessing alcohol use in recent days. Whole blood phosphatidyl ethanol is helpful in the detection of alcohol use in the previous weeks. Scalp hair ethyl glucuronide is helpful in demonstrating chronic excessive alcohol use in the past three to six months. In contrast, serum carbohydrate-deficient transferrin is less robust as a marker.

Functional Tests of Liver Function

There have been several measures of liver function that depend on the ability of the liver to metabolize or clear drugs. These include the aminopyrine clearance test, the aminopyrine breath test, and galactose elimination capacity. These are cumbersome to perform and assess only some aspects of liver function. They rarely used today in clinical practice.

Liver Biopsy

Liver biopsy is indicated when information for diagnosis, management, treatment, or prognostication is not available from non-invasive techniques. There are various approaches to liver biopsy, but the percutaneous approach is the most common and it may be done as a daycase where appropriate. It is most commonly performed in the imaging department under ultrasound guidance.

The risks of percutaneous liver biopsy include bleeding, organ perforation, sepsis, and death. Bleeding occurs in up to 10% with major bleeding occurring in less than 2%. Risk factors for bleeding from percutaneous biopsy include older age, comorbidities, indication for biopsy, and coagulation. Mortality associated with biopsy is less than 1/1000.

Models Assessing Prognosis in Liver Disease

A number of models have been used to assess the overall severity of liver damage in liver disease. Of the general models (which apply to all those with cirrhosis), the Child classification (with the later modification called Child–Pugh) classification depends on albumin, international normalized ratio, bilirubin, ascites, and encephalopathy, and has been the standard for many years, but it is used less now as some of the parameters are subjective [5].

More recently, the MELD (Model for End-stage Liver Disease) score has been used. There are several modifications, but the original MELD score depends on international normalized ratio, bilirubin, and creatinine [6]; the MELD-sodium includes the serum sodium. These scores are useful in predicting outcomes. There are many disease-specific models.

References

1. Newsome, P.N., Cramb, R., Davison, S.M. et al. (2018). Guidelines on the management of abnormal liver blood tests. *Gut* 67 (1): 6–19.
2. Centers for Disease Control and Prevention, Division of Viral Hepatitis. *Interpretation of Hepatitis B Serologic Test Results*. Washington, DC: Department of Health and Human Services. https://www.cdc.gov/hepatitis/hbv/profresourcesb.htm#section1. Accessed 5 May 2022.
3. NAFLD Fibrosis Score Online Calculator. https://nafldscore.com. Accessed 5 May 2022.
4. Fibrosis 4 Score. http://gihep.com/calculators/hepatology/fibrosis-4-score. Accessed 5 May 2022.

5. Child CG. Child-Pugh score for cirrhosis emortality. MD Calc. https://www.mdcalc.com/child-pugh-score-cirrhosis-mortality. Accessed 5 May 2022.
6. Organ Procurement and Transplantation Network. MELD calculator. https://optn.transplant.hrsa.gov/data/allocation-calculators/meld-calculator. Accessed 5 May 2022.

Further Reading

Arnts, J., Vanlerberghe, B.T.K., Roozen, S. et al. (2021). Diagnostic accuracy of biomarkers of alcohol use in patients with liver disease: a systematic review. *Alcohol. Clin. Exp. Res.* 45 (1): 25–37.

Caldwell, S. and Carlini, L.E. (2020). Coagulation homeostasis in liver disease. *Clin. Liver Dis. (Hoboken)* 16 (4): 137–141.

Neuberger, J., Patel, J., Caldwell, H. et al. (2020). Guidelines on the use of liver biopsy in clinical practice from the British Society of Gastroenterology, the Royal College of Radiologists and the Royal College of Pathology. *Gut* 69 (8): 1382–1403.

Oeda, S., Tanaka, K., Oshima, A. et al. (2020). Diagnostic accuracy of FibroScan and factors affecting measurements. *Diagnostics (Basel)* 10 (11): 940.

Schreiner, A.D. and Rockey, D.C. (2018). Evaluation of abnormal liver tests in the adult asymptomatic patient. *Curr. Opin. Gastroenterol.* 34 (4): 272–279.

Schreiner, A.D., Bian, J., Zhang, J. et al. (2019). When do clinicians follow-up abnormal liver tests in primary care? *Am. J. Med. Sci.* 358 (2): 127–133.

Section 2

Take-Home Primers

Managing Unexplained Abnormal Liver Tests

2

Primary Care

Jeetesh V. Patel[1] and Paramjit Gill[2]

[1] *Dartmouth Medical Centre, West Bromwich, UK*
[2] *University of Warwick, Coventry, UK*

KEY POINTS

- Primary care is the first point of contact in many healthcare systems.
- Liver function tests (LFTs) are common, inexpensive tests that are frequently ordered for patients with non-specific symptoms or as part of routine health checks.
- Interpretation of LFTs can be challenging but a comprehensive history and examination will usually allow understanding of these results.

Introduction

Primary care is the cornerstone of most national healthcare systems, providing "front door" access for the greater majority of a country's population. At its heart is general practice – doctors working as a general practitioner (GP) or family physician. GPs provide a broad-based and holistic approach for patients seeking improved health and wellbeing. They are required to diagnose illness and to "filter" serious pathologies or conditions needing specialist hospital intervention and those who can be treated safely within the community setting under their care. Undertaking a full history and examination remains the cornerstone of managing a patient with abnormal LFTs.

Abnormal LFTs can be a challenge and create uncertainty for GPs in primary care. They are responsible for the regular interpretation of these tests for hundreds of patients each week. The reasons for this apprehension and uncertainty is multifactorial and relates in part to: (i) the high burden of mortality and morbidity associated with liver disease; (ii) wide variability in the relationship between LFTs and hepatocellular damage; and (iii) the incidental nature with which LFTs are requested.

The Liver in Systemic Disease: A Clinician's Guide to Abnormal Liver Tests, First Edition.
Edited by Gideon M. Hirschfield, Paramjit Gill, and James Neuberger.
© 2023 John Wiley & Sons Ltd. Published 2023 by John Wiley & Sons Ltd.

Liver Disease in the UK

Liver disease is a key issue for the health of the population in England [1]. In 2020, cirrhosis and other diseases of the liver were the second highest cause of death in those aged 35–49 years, and among the top five causes among adults of other age groups [2]. Tragically, many of these deaths are preventable, where causes are related to lifestyle and unhealthy environments such as alcohol excess, obesity and some medications. As an investigation, LFTs represent a simple investigation for GPs synonymous with a "routine" assessment of general health. Unfortunately, LFTs do not appear to be reliable; they can be normal in the presence of serious liver disease and, conversely, abnormal in other pathologies. Of the liver enzymes common to LFTs, alanine amino transferase (ALT), aspartate amino transferase (AST), alkaline phosphatase (ALP), and gamma-glutamyl transferase (GGT) are released by organs other than the liver. The degree of liver damage is difficult to interpret by absolute circulating levels of these enzymes alone [3]. These LFTs give us more of an appreciation of the possible pattern of a patient's liver disorder, whether hepatocyte damage (AST, ALT), cholestasis (bilirubin, GGT, ALP) or both.

In a UK study of 95 977 primary care patients free of liver disease, abnormal LFTs were seen in some 20% and, on 3.7 year follow-up, 1.15% developed liver disease [4]. There is typically a "reactive" approach when it comes to the management of incidental abnormal LFTs in otherwise healthy patients. We lack a "proactive" approach to screen for liver disease itself. With much of the focus for the GP not to "miss" insidious disease, LFTs are frequently included as a first-line investigation for patients with constitutional symptoms of loss of appetite, malaise and other vague symptoms, such as fatigue, itching, abdominal pain and distension. Signs such as jaundice, dark urine and pale stools appear more specific to the liver. Broadly speaking, the GP will commonly encounter liver disease in the form of neonatal jaundice, congenital and inherited disorders, immune and autoimmune disorders, fatty infiltration, toxicological and pharmacological damage, cholestatic syndromes, chronic infections and cancer. The aim of this chapter is to help primary care professionals to deal with incidental findings of abnormal LFTs, to appreciate when further investigation is warranted, what investigations to arrange in primary care and when to refer to a specialist.

Isolated Raised Liver Transaminase in a Healthy Individuals

It is common place in primary care for an isolated AST or ALT to be seen in an otherwise healthy individual having a "routine" set of bloods taken. A repeat of the LFTs is likely to be the response, but what if it is sustained? What if there is a history of past bloods with similar trends? The likelihood is that the AST or ALT is raised in response to fatty infiltration because this is by far the most common liver disorder encountered in primary care.

Non-alcoholic Fatty Liver Disease

Non-alcoholic fatty liver disease (NAFLD) covers a spectrum of diseases from non-alcoholic fatty liver to non-alcoholic steatohepatitis (NASH) and cirrhosis. NAFLD is a common disorder, with an estimated worldwide prevalence of 25%, associated with type

2 diabetes, obesity, dyslipidemia and the metabolic syndrome [5]. This is typically recognized as a benign condition, although estimates suggest that up to 40% of patients with fatty liver progress to advanced stages of fibrosis [6]. The pathogenesis of NAFLD is complex, involving the interplay of lifestyle factors, microbiota, dyslipidemic metabolism, insulin resistance, and hepatocyte injury and inflammation. The most important factor in the adverse progression of the patient with fatty liver is the presence of fibrosis. While the progression of fibrosis is slow, it is accelerated in states such as NASH. It is important to note that cardiovascular disease remains the main cause of death in patients with NAFLD. Nonetheless, NAFLD is a considerable healthcare challenge in primary care. Given its link with obesity, it is, troublingly, increasingly more common in childhood. In the Avon Longitudinal Study of Parents and Children (ALSPAC), 1 in 5 young people was found to have steatosis and 1 in 40 had fibrosis around the age of 24 years [6].

The diagnosis of NAFLD can be made using ultrasound where steatosis is present in more than 5% of the parenchyma, alcohol intake is within normal limits (< 20 g or 2.5 units/ day for women and < 30 g or 3.75 units/day in men), and in the absence of other secondary causes. It is important to note that NAFLD can be present in the absence of abnormal LFTs. Risk factors associated with the metabolic syndrome should raise a suspicion of NAFLD [7]. If NAFLD is present, it is important to use non-invasive scoring systems to interpret the stage of disease (e.g. the enhanced liver fibrosis test, NAFLD Fibrosis Score, Fibrosis (FIB)-4 score) [8]. Depending on these scores, a decision can be made as to whether to refer the patient who is at high risk of liver fibrosis to secondary care or to continue monitoring in the community.

Alcohol and Liver Disease

Long-term heavy alcohol intake is globally recognized as a key cause for chronic liver disease, and in the UK around 7700 people die each year due to alcohol-related liver disease, mostly between the ages of 40 and 65 years [9]. Heavy alcohol intake damages the liver in the form of alcoholic steatosis, alcoholic hepatitis, cirrhosis and hepatocellular carcinoma [10]. Prolonged abstinence from alcohol represents is the only real option to slow this progression. Interestingly, alcoholic liver disease is not confined to just those with alcohol dependency. The pathophysiology is complex, involving environmental and genetic factors that modulate the toxic effects of alcohol and its metabolites on the liver [8].

The challenge for primary care is to identify patients early and implement lifestyle changes. Many of these patients will be asymptomatic and are unlikely to present with concerns over their drinking habits. Clues to a diagnosis may come from other areas such as the presence of macrocytosis, gout, reduced albumin levels. GGT levels may be useful to decipher a history of heavy alcohol intake. Unfortunately, most patients with cirrhosis are undiagnosed and it is often the later complications of cirrhosis (e.g. ascites) that lead to the presentation of the patient [11].

In summary, patients with persistently elevated AST or ALT are likely to have NAFLD. A repeat set of bloods including GGT, a full blood count (and tests to investigate secondary causes as appropriate) are needed (Box 2.1). Ultrasound can be used to confirm the diagnosis and patients should be stratified with respect to alcohol intake and risk of fibrosis. A referral to secondary care is needed for those with a high risk of fibrosis.

Box 2.1   Investigations for Non-alcoholic Fatty Liver Disease

When to investigate	Persistently raised AST or ALT (3 months)
How to investigate	Repeat LFTs with GGT and full blood count (consider liver screen coagulation, viral serology: cytomegalovirus, Epstein–Barr virus, HIV, viral hepatitis screen, ferritin and ceruloplasmin, autoantibodies, immunoglobulins)
	If isolated AST or ALT rise only, arrange ultrasound of the liver
When to refer	If the diagnosis is unclear or raised risk of fibrosis

---

Chronic Infections of the Liver

Infections with viral infections such as hepatitis B and C are typically asymptomatic. In the acute setting, individuals may present with features of malaise, fever, arthralgia, jaundice and abnormal LFT levels [12]. Patients with chronic hepatitis B virus (HBV) infection can often remain undiagnosed until they develop signs of advanced liver disease [7].

Hepatitis B Virus

Infection with HBV usually follows exposure to infected blood and body fluids, through sexual contact, blood transfer (by the sharing of needles and syringes in drug misuse) and vertical transmission from infected mother to child. During an acute infection, viral surface antigen (HBsAg) and envelope antigen (HBeAg) circulate within the bloodstream. The host immune response results in antibodies (immunoglobulin M and later G), which target the core antigen (anti-HBc) and HBeAg. These antigens clear during the recovery of the patient. In chronic infections, HBsAg persists for more than six months, and this likelihood is greatest in the neonates of mothers with HBV (90%) and lowest in adults (5%) [13]. Immunosuppression can reverse the immunity of those patients who have already mounted a successful immune response to HBV. The complications of chronic HBV infection include fibrosis, cirrhosis, and hepatocellular carcinoma.

There is a huge global variation in rates of HBV, where it is seen to be endemic in China and Pakistan ($\geq$8% as defined by the World Health Organization), raised rates (2–7%) are also seen across South East Asia, sub-Saharan Africa, North Africa, Eastern and Southern Europe, the Eastern Mediterranean, South America, and Alaska [14]. Here, infections are predominately seen in children. Rates in the UK are much lower; chronic HBV has an estimated prevalence of 0.1–0.5% [14]. Hepatitis B prevalence is typically low in Northern and Western Europe, Australia, and North America. Here, infections are predominately seen in adults. Of note, the majority of newly diagnosed chronic HBV infections are among migrant individuals living in the UK who were born in countries with endemic or high HBV prevalence [15].

Hepatitis C Virus

In the UK, chronic hepatitis C virus (HCV) infection has a similar rate of infection to HBV with some 120 000 people affected, some 0.4% of the adult population [16]. Hepatitis C disproportionately affects marginalized and underserved populations in the UK, with

---

Box 2.2 Groups at Risk of Chronic Viral Hepatitis

- People born in high/intermediate prevalence areas and their children
- Household contacts of HBsAg-positive individuals
- People who have ever injected drugs
- Multiple sexual partners
- History of sexually transmitted diseases
- Men who have sex with men
- Prison inmates
- HIV infection
- Pregnant women
- Candidates for blood/tissue/organ donation
- Individuals undergoing immunosuppressive therapy

Box 2.3 Investigations for Hepatitis

When to investigate	Chronic ALT or AST elevation
How to investigate	Screen for hepatitis B/C, hepatitis D, and HIV (co-infection confers a poorer prognosis)
When to refer	Referral all to secondary care (consider hepatocellular carcinoma screening with annual ultrasound)

---

reduced engagement with healthcare and poorer health outcomes. Globally, the UK is considered a low-prevalence country. Similar to HBV, studies suggest that individuals of South Asian origin are among those at increased risk of hepatitis C infection [17]. Unlike HBV, chronic HCV can be treated and cured with antiviral therapy.

In summary, suspect chronic viral hepatitis in those with chronic elevation of transaminases and those in at risk groups (Box 2.2). Screen for viral hepatitis as well at co-infection with HIV, as this confers a poorer outcome. All patients with chronic hepatitis will need referral to secondary care for monitoring of potential complications with fibrosis, cirrhosis, and hepatocellular carcinoma (Box 2.3).

Hyperbilirubinemia

Hyperbilirubinemia and jaundice are hallmarks of liver disease. They can indicate quite serious disease. High circulating levels of bilirubin stem from hepatic metabolic disorders, increased production and reduced clearance. Bilirubin is a byproduct during the normal catabolic breakdown of haem, which is produced during the splenic replacement of aged red blood cells. Bilirubin is then metabolized for the liver for excretion, either through the urine or in bile. Its chemical structure is based on porphyrin, organic ring structures that characteristically afford color. The metabolites of bilirubin give the characteristic straw yellow color of urine and the brown color of feces. The role of the liver in bilirubin metabolism is to conjugate it with glucuronic acid, making it soluble in water for excretion. From the outset, it is often useful to determine whether this is a problem with conjugated or unconjugated bilirubin.

Unconjugated Hyperbilirubinemia

As mentioned, bilirubin is a byproduct of the breakdown of haem. High levels of unconjugated bilirubin are likely to be due to extrahepatic disorders or a defect in conjugation (Box 2.4). Unconjugated bilirubin is insoluble and so *does not* cause signs such as dark urine or pale stools. Typically, raised levels of unconjugated bilirubin are likely to be due to hemolytic anemia or genetic disorders of bilirubin conjugation such as Gilbert or Crigler–Najjar syndrome. Incidental hyperbilirubinemia seen in a healthy individual should warrant a repeat of the LFTs to include GGT, fractionated bilirubin (direct/indirect/spilt bilirubin assays), and a full blood count (with reticulocytes and smear as per local practice). The hematology may reflect the presence of hemolytic disorders, bloodborne disorders, and some cancers. GGT levels would be useful to identify a problem with cholestasis and a possible mixed picture. In the absence of hemolysis, unconjugated hyperbilirubinemia in an otherwise healthy patient can be attributed to Gilbert syndrome without further need for investigation. Gilbert syndrome involves a deficiency in the enzyme that conjugates bilirubin with glucuronic acid. It is essentially a benign condition, and hyperbilirubinemia may present in a healthy individual during times of stress and fasting. Crigler–Najjar syndrome represents a similar metabolic deficiency, although it is more severe and the patient is unlikely to be well.

Conjugated Hyperbilirubinemia

In acquired liver disease, both split fractions of bilirubin will be raised. Damage and necrosis to the parenchyma from infection, drugs, inflammation, autoimmunity, cirrhosis, and malignancy are likely to cause the release of bilirubin through a number of mechanisms. Cholestatic syndromes are a common cause for extrahepatic pathways for jaundice. Patients with biliary obstruction may be asymptomatic or may present with non-specific symptoms including abdominal pain, itching, and dark urine. In severe cholestasis, there are also pale stools and steatorrhoea. Gallstones are a common cause for cholestasis, and identification

---

Box 2.4   Causes of Unconjugated Hyperbilirubinemia

- Autoimmune hemolytic anemia
- Cold reactive
- Drug induced (associated with approximately 150 drugs)
- Mixed type
- Warm reactive
- Hemoglobin disorders
- Sickle cell anemia
- Thalassemia
- Hereditary disorders of conjugation

is usually by radiography and ultrasound. Defects in hepatic excretory function include Dubin–Johnson syndrome, Rotor syndrome, benign intrahepatic cholestasis, and progressive familial intrahepatic cholestasis.

In summary, investigations for jaundice should begin with a fractionated bilirubin together with LFTs, a full blood count and liver ultrasound.

Neonatal Jaundice

Parental concerns of neonatal jaundice are a common need for LFT interpretation for the youngest patients seen in primary care. Neonatal jaundice is a common affliction for newborns and, in the main, it is essentially a harmless condition. It is, however, important to be wary of those babies that need further investigation and work-up with the pediatric department. Neonatal jaundice affects around 50% of term and 80% of preterm babies [18].

Physiological and Prolonged Jaundice

If present at birth, jaundice will *always* be pathological and will be picked up on a postnatal ward and dealt with within secondary care. Non-pathological jaundice (i.e. physiological jaundice) is more likely to be seen in general practice. Manifest after the first few days of life, the transitional change from maternally derived blood in the fetus to the baby's own blood following its birth leads to a substantial flux in red blood cell turnover and metabolism. Haem is catabolized and converted to unconjugated bilirubin for processing (conjugation) within the newborn liver. This increased prehepatic supply may be beyond the metabolic and excretive capacity of a newborn liver, and the resultant accumulation of unconjugated bilirubin presents as jaundice.

Bilirubin levels in the newborn can be measured within the community by the midwife or a health visitor. Some babies may need referral to hospital for assessment and consideration of phototherapy. Physiological jaundice disappears at around two weeks of age, usually without the need for treatment. Although the mechanisms are not fully understood, breast milk is known to exacerbate and to prolong jaundice in the newborn. Jaundice persisting after this time is termed "prolonged jaundice," and the GP should be alert to differentials of liver disease in the newborn that could be mistaken for physiological jaundice (Box 2.5). Referral to pediatrics is necessary for babies with jaundice persisting more than two weeks; further blood tests should be arranged as appropriate to investigate pathological causes. Biliary atresia is a rare cause of jaundice in the newborn but early diagnosis and surgical intervention is essential to prevent long-term liver damage.

Box 2.5	Investigations for Jaundice
When to investigate	Visible jaundice in the newborn
How to investigate	Bloods: split bilirubin, full blood count, C-reactive protein, LFTs, urine dip
When to refer	Referral with bloods? G6PD (Mediterranean, African? Pyruvate kinase? Blood film?)

G6PD, glucose-6-phosphate dehydrogenase.

Box 2.6   Important Considerations for Neonatal Jaundice in Primary Care

- Blood group differences between mother and baby; this leads to more rapid blood cell breakdown causing early and sometimes severe jaundice (Rhesus, ABO incompatibility, DAT antigens)
- Infections (sepsis, urinary tract infections)
- Blockages to bile drainage (biliary atresia)
- Liver problems (Gilbert syndrome, Crigler–Najjar syndrome, autoimmune diseases)
- Blood cell problems (hereditary spherocytosis, G6PD activity, pyruvate kinase deficiency, congenital hemolytic anemia)

Pathological Jaundice

Prolonged jaundice should be assessed in line with the clinical picture. Were there any neonatal concerns? We should know the baby's feeding pattern; is the weight gain pattern normal? What is the color of the baby's urine and stools? Physiological jaundice is due to unconjugated bilirubin, and so dark urine, which is seen with high levels of conjugated bilirubin, would be unexpected. Similarly, jaundice with pale stools or steatorrhoea is seen in cholestasis and conjugated hyperbilirubinemia – is this biliary atresia or a bile duct problem? Pathological causes of unconjugated hyperbilirubinemia jaundice in babies are likely to stem from hemolytic anemias (e.g. mother and baby blood group incompatibility issues or hereditary metabolic disorders with red blood cells). Much rarer causes of unconjugated hyperbilirubinemia include disorders of bilirubin conjugation such as Gilbert or Crigler–Najjar syndrome.

In summary, babies with mild jaundice are likely to present to primary care given that this is typically a physiological condition which resolves after two weeks of birth. Jaundice persisting after this time warrants investigation (Box 2.5), and the consideration of blood tests to confirm that the jaundice is from unconjugated hyperbilirubinemia. Blood tests for other causes of jaundice and unconjugated hyperbilirubinemia should also be considered and a referral made to pediatrics (Box 2.6).

References

1. Davies, S.C. (2011). *Annual Report of the Chief Medical Officer: On the State of the Public's Health*. London: Department of Health.
2. Office for National Statistics (2021). Deaths registered in England and Wales. Table 9a: Leading causes of death by age-group and sex, deaths registered in 2020, England and Wales. Statistical Bulletin. London: ONS.
3. Hall, P. and Cash, J. (2012). What is the real function of the liver 'function' tests? *Ulster Med. J.* 81 (1): 30–36.
4. McLernon, D.J., Donnan, P.T., Ryder, S. et al. (2009). Health outcomes following liver function testing in primary care: a retrospective cohort study. *Fam. Pract.* 26 (4): 251–259.

5. Vernon, G., Baranova, A., and Younossi, Z.M. (2011). Systematic review: the epidemiology and natural history of non-alcoholic fatty liver disease and non-alcoholic steatohepatitis in adults. *Aliment. Pharmacol. Ther.* **34**: 274–285.

6. Abeysekera, K.W.M., Fernandes, G.S., Hammerton, G. et al. (2020). Prevalence of steatosis and fibrosis in young adults in the UK: a population-based study. *Lancet Gastroenterol. Hepatol.* 5 (3): 295–305.

7. Fattovich, G. (2003). Natural history of hepatitis B. *J. Hepatol.* 39 (Suppl 1): S50–S58.

8. Stickel, F., Datz, C., Hampe, J., and Bataller, R. (2017). Pathophysiology and management of alcoholic liver disease: update 2016 [published correction appears in *Gut Liver.* 2017 May 15;11(3):447]. *Gut Liver* 11 (2): 173–188.

9. Office for National Statistics (2016). Number of deaths caused by alcoholic liver disease and other causes associated with the misuse of alcohol, deaths registered in England and Wales. https://www.ons.gov.uk/peoplepopulationandcommunity/ birthsdeathsandmarriages/deaths/adhocs/007370numberofdeathscausedbyalcoholicliver diseaseandothercausesassociatedwiththemisuseofalcoholdeathsregisteredinenglandand wales2016 (accessed 26 April 2022).

10. Morgan, T.R., Mandayam, S., and Jamal, M.M. (2004). Alcohol and hepatocellular carcinoma. *Gastroenterology* 127: S87–S96.

11. Lilford, R.J., Bentham, L., Girling, A. et al. (2013). Birmingham and Lambeth Liver Evaluation Testing Strategies (BALLETS): a prospective cohort study. *Health Technol. Assess.* 17 (28): i–xiv, 1–307.

12. National Institute for Health and Care Excellence. Hepatitis B. Clinical Knowledge Summaries. https://cks.nice.org.uk/topics/hepatitis-b/diagnosis/when-to-test-for-hepatitis-b. Accessed 26 April 2022.

13. Health and Safety Executive. Hepatitis B virus (HBV). https://www.hse.gov.uk/biosafety/ blood-borne-viruses/hepatitis-b.htm Accessed 26 April 2022.

14. World Health Organisation. Heptatits B. Geneva: WHO; 2002. https://apps.who.int/iris/ bitstream/handle/10665/67746/WHO_CDS_CSR_LYO_2002.2_HEPATITIS_B.pdf; jsessionid=F89A0070DDEE2B34F204EC538ECD248D?sequence=1#page=1&zoom= auto,-149,603. Accessed 26 April 2022.

15. Martin, N.K., Vickerman, P., Khakoo, S. et al. (2019). Chronic hepatitis B virus case-finding in UK populations born abroad in intermediate or high endemicity countries: an economic evaluation. *BMJ Open* 9 (6): e030183.

16. UK Health Security Agency. Hepatitis C in the UK 2022: Working to eliminate hepatitis C as a public health problem; full report. London: HSA; 2022. https://www.gov.uk/ government/publications/hepatitis-c-in-the-uk. Accessed 26 April 2022.

17. Office for Health Improvement and Disparities. Hepatitis C Migrant Health Guide. London: DHID; 2014 (updated 2021). https://www.gov.uk/guidance/hepatitis-c-migrant-health-guide. Accessed 26 April 2022.

18. Woodgate, P. and Jardine, L.A. (2011). Neonatal jaundice. *BMJ Clin. Evid.* 2011: 0319.

3

Global Perspective

Arulraj Ramakrishnan[1], Grace L.-H. Wong[2], and Innocent K. Besigye[3]

[1] Kovai Medical Center and Hospital, Coimbatore, Tamil Nadu, India
[2] Chinese University of Hong Kong, Hong Kong SAR, China
[3] College of Health Sciences, Makerere University, Kampala, Uganda

---

KEY POINTS

- Abnormal liver function tests (LFTs) are prevalent universally, but they may related to the prevalence of certain infections/conditions prevalent in that country or region.
- In many healthcare systems, primary care is not developed.
- Globally, liver specialists are scarce and interpretation and management of LFTs are done by hospital generalists.
- History, examination, and awareness of common conditions prevalent locally enables management of abnormal LFTs in a cost-effective manner.
- Alcohol-related liver disease and non-alcoholic fatty liver disease (NAFLD) are on the rise in India, and, together with viral hepatitis, contribute to the majority of abnormal LFTs.
- Drug-induced liver injury in India, particularly the use of complementary and alternative medicine use, needs to be considered during evaluation of LFTs.

Introduction

The commonly used term "liver function tests," is best termed "liver tests" because these tests are markers of liver disease rather than measures of liver function. The standard liver tests include aspartate aminotransferase (AST), alanine amino transferase (ALT), alkaline phosphatase (ALP), bilirubin, gamma glutamyl transferase (GGT) and albumin. Liver tests are inexpensive and are a good predictor of not only mortality from liver disease but also mortality from other cause. ALT has been proved more useful in the evaluation of hepatic disease because it is found in greater concentration in the liver than in other organs. Since they are neither specific nor indicative of any particular

The Liver in Systemic Disease: A Clinician's Guide to Abnormal Liver Tests, First Edition.
Edited by Gideon M. Hirschfield, Paramjit Gill, and James Neuberger.
© 2023 John Wiley & Sons Ltd. Published 2023 by John Wiley & Sons Ltd.

disease, further testing is usually required to define the cause and extent of disease. This can be done either by extensive testing or by using a more focused approach (estimated costs of US$448 vs. US$502/patient, respectively), with both identifying the aetiology in only 55% of cases [1]. An assessment of the patient with suspected or clinically obvious liver disease is not only context dependent but also location and cost dependent. Generic algorithms for the evaluation of liver disease may not be applicable universally because not only does the history and examination aid interpretation of abnormal LFTs but also the country of origin of the patient is essential. As a number of conditions are more prevalent in some parts of the world, this chapter provides an overview from India, the Far East, and Africa. Since abnormal liver tests and their patterns are covered in Chapter 1, the focus in this chapter is on common patterns of abnormal liver tests seen in practice (Figure 3.1):

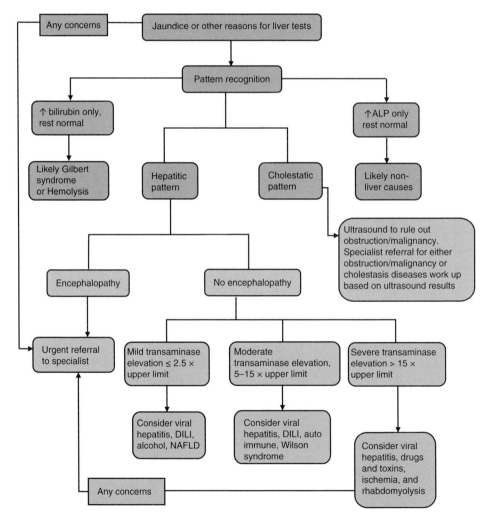

Figure 3.1 Simplified response to abnormal liver tests in India.

- Isolated raised bilirubin (e.g. Gilbert syndrome, hemolysis).
- Cholestatic; predominantly raised ALP and GGT, such as primary biliary cholangitis (PBC), biliary obstruction, hepatic congestion and drug-induced liver injury.
- Hepatitic; predominantly raised ALT and AST, such as viral hepatitis, NAFLD, alcohol-related liver disease (ARLD), autoimmune hepatitis (AIH), and drug-induced liver injury (DILI).
- Infiltrative, such as tuberculosis (TB), malignancy.

Indian Perspective

The burden of liver disease according to etiology and stage is not available, even from the developed-country population-based studies. Studies have tried to define normal values of transaminases for Indian population, but most laboratory values are based upon Western populations and those provided by the manufacturers of kits. Presentation of liver disease in India is often late. It occurs in young people and accounts for one fifth (18.3%) of all cirrhosis deaths globally [2]. Epidemiological data from Indian population-based studies on the prevalence of abnormal liver tests, their etiology, and fibrosis, are also scarce. Hepatitis B (33.3%), is the most common cause of chronic liver disease in India [3], followed by hepatitis C (21.6%), alcohol (17.3%), and NAFLD (12.8%), but alcohol (34.3%) is the most common cause when stratified by the presence of cirrhosis. Significant regional heterogeneity exists between different regions of India, viral hepatitis B and C being more common in northern and eastern regions compared with southern regions, where alcohol is more common.

Patterns of Specific Liver Disorders in the Indian Context

Viral Hepatitis

In India during 2011–2013, 804 782 viral hepatitis cases and 291 outbreaks were reported. Among the outbreaks with known etiology, 48% were caused by hepatitis E virus (HEV), 33% hepatitis A infection (HAV), 12% hepatitis A and E, and 7% hepatitis B or C [4]. Viral hepatitis contributes to 43% of acute liver failure in India, with HEV contributing to 29.5%, hepatitis B virus (HBV) 7.4%, HAV 2%, and dual (HAV and HEV) infection accounting for 3.9% [5]. Viral hepatitis most often produces a hepatic pattern of liver injury (AST and ALT level elevations predominate). Some patients are asymptomatic with normal aminotransferase levels but may still be infected chronically with HBV or hepatitis C virus (HCV). Interpretation of abnormal viral markers is essential in countries with high endemicity like India to avoid confusion between active infection and immunity.

Hepatitis A Infection

HAV is a single-stranded, non-enveloped RNA virus belonging to the family Picornaviridae, classically spread via the fecal–oral route. HAV is defined as an acute illness with a discrete onset of any sign or symptom consistent with acute viral hepatitis (e.g. fever, headache, malaise, anorexia, nausea, vomiting, diarrhea, abdominal pain, or dark urine) with (i)

Table 3.1 Hepatitis A antibody tests and different clinical situations.

Infection state	Total anti-HAV (IgG, IgM)	Anti-HAV IgM
Acute HAV	Positive	Positive
Resolved HAV	Positive	Negative
Immunization	Positive	Negative

HAV, hepatitis A infection; Ig, immunoglobulin.

jaundice or elevated total bilirubin levels ≥ 3.0 mg/dl, *or* (ii) elevated serum ALT levels > 200 iu/l, *and* (iii) the absence of a more likely diagnosis [6]. Acute HAV infection is confirmed by immunoglobulin (Ig) M antibody to hepatitis A virus (anti-HAV) positivity (Table 3.1). Acute HAV infection is generally mild and subclinical but contributes to 2% of acute liver failure [5] in India. Most infections are managed with supportive care. Patients develop lifelong immunity (IgG) to HAV following early childhood asymptomatic HAV infection [7]. HAV vaccination is not recommended in India [7] because of high endemicity, except for patients with decompensated chronic liver disease awaiting transplant and those who are immunosuppressed (inactivated vaccines are preferred).

Hepatitis B Infection

HBV is a double-stranded DNA virus belonging to the family Hepadnaviridae. It has a prevalence of 2% in India. Transmission is predominantly from an infected mother to her child, from inoculation injury, or horizontal transmission at young age, with sexual and parenteral transmission (e.g. via blood transfusions, intravenous drug abuse) contributing to a minority of cases.

Acute HBV infection is diagnosed by the onset of signs or symptom consistent with acute viral hepatitis (e.g. fever, headache, malaise, anorexia, nausea, vomiting, diarrhea, and abdominal pain), and either jaundice, or elevated serum ALT levels above 100 iu/l. It is confirmed by the presence of hepatitis B surface antigen (HBsAg) and positive immunoglobulin M antibody to hepatitis B core antigen (anti-HBc) [6]. The majority of patients with acute infection will remain asymptomatic and only 30% develop icteric hepatitis. Acute HBV infection as a cause of acute liver failure is possibly decreasing over time in India.

Chronic HBV in endemic areas is incidentally found in asymptomatic persons with no evidence of liver disease or may have a spectrum of disease ranging from chronic hepatitis to cirrhosis or liver cancer. Chronic HBV is characterized by persistence of HBsAg for longer than six months with positive anti-HBc (IgG) and negative hepatitis B surface antibody (anti-HBs). Hepatitis B envelope antigen (HBeAg) positivity usually indicates active viral replication and liver injury. HBeAg becoming negative and development of hepatitis B envelope antibody (anti-HBe) over time is associated with lesser viral replication (lower levels of HBV DNA and transaminase values), and less (or no) hepatic inflammation. HBV DNA level and HBeAg status are used to determine the need for treatment and play a crucial role in estimating the response to treatment [6].

HBV reactivation occurs in patients with previously documented resolved HBV, or with the low replicating HBsAg (carrier) state. It is characterized by sudden increase in HBV replication or the reappearance of active inflammatory disease of the liver. Reactivation is usually triggered by immunosuppression or chemotherapy in the host or spontaneously. Clinical manifestations can vary from a transient, clinically silent, disease to liver failure. HBV reactivation diagnosis is dependent on the HBV disease state before activation. In patients with resolved HBV (negative HBsAg and positive anti-HBs), decline in anti-HBs and the reappearance of HBsAg indicates reactivation. In low replicating HBsAg (carrier) state, reactivation is diagnosed by a rise in the serum HBV DNA or a rise in the serum ALT levels.

Table 3.2 summarizes the serological tests used in assessment of hepatitis B infection and its interpretation. Treatment recommendations are beyond the scope of this chapter; suffice to say that newer antiviral drugs (such as entecavir and tenofovir) have a high barrier

Table 3.2 Interpretation of hepatitis B serologic test results.

Interpretation	Test	Result
Susceptible	HBsAg	Negative
	Anti-HBc	Negative
	Anti-HBs	Negative
Immune due to natural infection	HBsAg	Negative
	Anti-HBc	Positive
	Anti-HBs	Positive
Immune due to hepatitis B vaccination	HBsAg	Negative
	Anti-HBc	Negative
	Anti-HBs	Positive
Acutely infected	HBsAg	Positive
	Anti-HBc	Positive
	IgM anti-HBc	Positive
	Anti-HBs	Negative
Chronically infected	HBsAg	Positive
	Anti-HBc	Positive
	IgM anti-HBc	Negative
	Anti-HBs	Negative
Interpretations unclear 4 possibilities:	HBsAg	Negative
1. Resolved infection (most common)	Anti-HBc	Positive
2. False positive	Anti-HBs	Negative
3. "Low level" chronic infection		
4. Resolving acute infection		

anti-HBc, antibody to hepatitis B core antigen; anti-HBs, hepatitis B surface antibody; HBsAg, hepatitis B virus surface antigen; Ig M, immunoglobulin M.
Source: Adapted from US National Notifiable Diseases Surveillance System. Surveillance Case Definitions for Current and Historical Condition [6].

to resistance and decrease morbidity and mortality in HBV infection. The World Health Organization (WHO) recommends HBV vaccination in routine immunization programs because vaccination prevents HBV infection and decreases the incidence of chronic liver disease and hepatocellular carcinoma. Vaccination in India is essential for household contacts of people who are HBsAg-positive and those undergoing dialysis.

Hepatitis C

HCV is an enveloped, single-stranded RNA virus belonging to the family Flaviviridae, which has six genotypes. Genotype 3 is the most common (61.8%) in India, followed by genotype 1 (31.2%). Although the estimated prevalence of HCV is low, at 0.5%, with one fifth of the world's population, India accounts for a large proportion of the worldwide HCV burden. The predominant modes of transmission of HCV in India are unsafe therapeutic injections and blood transfusions. Acute HCV infection is usually asymptomatic, or only produces mild, non-specific, flu-like symptoms, and is infrequently diagnosed in the acute phase, with spontaneous clearance in about 15% of infected patients. Chronic HCV is characterized by presence of one or more of jaundice, peak elevated total bilirubin levels ≥ 3.0 mg/dl, or peak elevated ALT levels greater than 200 iu/l [6]. Three tests are commonly used to define hepatitis C status: anti-HCV antibody, HCV RNA, and HCV genotyping. Anti-HCV is used for screening but, for confirmation, HCV RNA is performed (Table 3.3). Although treatment recommendations are beyond the scope of this chapter, it should be emphasized that newer antiviral drugs will not only decrease the morbidity and mortality due to HCV infection but will also help with eradication.

Hepatitis D

Hepatitis D virus (HDV) is an RNA virus that encodes for a hepatitis D antigen (HDAg). HDV infection requires the presence of HBV infection and can be acquired as either a co-infection (simultaneously with HBV) or a superinfection (on a pre-existing HBV infection). HDV infection is spread via the parenteral route but is infrequent in India. Treatment is predominantly of the superinfection or co-infection of HBV.

Hepatitis E

HEV virus is a positive-stranded non-enveloped RNA virus belonging to the family Hepeviridae. HEV is primarily spread via the fecal–oral route and is the most frequent

Table 3.3 Interpretation of hepatitis C tests.

Test	Interpretation
Anti-HCV antibody	Positive indicates infection, past or present; if positive, confirm with PCR
HCV RNA PCR	Positive indicates current infection; negative indicates cure post-treatment
HCV genotype	Genotypes 1–6; helps to monitor cure rates of individual genotypes

HCV, hepatitis C virus; PCR, polymerase chain reaction.

cause of acute viral hepatitis in India [4]. HEV infection is not only the most common cause of acute liver failure in India [5] but is also the main reason for acute deterioration in patients with compensated chronic liver disease. Chronic HEV infection has been defined as persistence of HEV replication for six months; it occurs in patients who are immunosuppressed failing to clear HEV infection. Acute HEV infection does not usually require antiviral therapy, but ribavirin may be considered in cases of severe acute hepatitis E or acute on chronic liver failure. In immunosuppressed patients with persisting HEV replication three months after detection of HEV RNA, ribavirin monotherapy for 12 weeks is recommended. Although broad adoption of HEV vaccines is difficult, they could be considered in special situations like pregnant women, who are at highest risk of HEV illness during epidemics.

Alcohol-Related Liver Disease

In India, alcohol consumption accounts for 22.2% of all deaths due to cirrhosis and for 19.9% of all deaths due to liver cancer [8]. Patients may present with non-specific digestive symptoms with history of excessive alcohol consumption (> 2–3 units/day). The combination of modestly raised AST, higher than ALT, with a raised mean corpuscular volume and GGT will identify ARLD. Alcoholic hepatitis is a severe form of hepatitis (due to protracted or binge drinking) that may be mild or life threatening. It is characterized by high serum bilirubin and prolonged clotting, and is associated with a dismal prognosis. Chronic ARLD is the most common cause for liver cirrhosis presentation. It occurs at a younger age and associated with higher morbidity and mortality in India [3]. A robust national alcohol policy with interventions aimed at reducing the harmful effects of alcohol is the key with increase in per capita annual alcohol consumption in Indian adults with rising incomes [8]. Abstinence and nutrition remains the main stay of treatment in ARLD.

Non-alcoholic Fatty Liver Disease

In India, NAFLD is usually associated with metabolic syndrome. The prevalence in India of NAFLD on ultrasonography is 30% and it accounts for 10.9% of deaths due to cirrhosis and 9.6% of deaths due to liver cancer [8]. Most patients are asymptomatic, with incidental detection of raised liver enzymes or fatty liver on ultrasound. Liver tests show either normal or mildly elevated AST and ALT, with ALT higher than AST, but tests are unreliable to rule out NAFLD. The spectrum of NAFLD presentations (simple steatosis, non-alcoholic steatohepatitis (NASH), NASH-related cirrhosis, and NASH-related hepatocellular carcinoma) is covered in detail in other chapters. In the Indian context, differentiation between simple steatosis and NASH (higher risk of progression), is based on parameters including female sex, age, AST/ALT ratio, the presence of diabetes mellitus, and other components of metabolic syndrome [9]. Elastography techniques help to ascertain NAFLD fibrosis stage non-invasively [9]. NAFLD pharmacology is evolving but, suffice to say, in India, the mainstay for halting disease progression is lifestyle changes in the form of dietary restrictions and regular exercises.

Autoimmune Hepatitis

Data from a tertiary center show the incidence of AIH to be 7.2%/year among patients with chronic liver disease [10]. AIH is characterized by female sex, elevations of aminotransferases, non-specific or organ-specific autoantibodies, and increased levels of gamma globulins (especially IgG). Organ-specific autoantibodies, particularly high titers of anti-smooth-muscle antibody, antinuclear antibody, liver/kidney microsomal antibody, antibodies to liver-soluble antigen, and anti-liver cytosol type-1 antibody, are suggestive, but on their own do not confirm a diagnosis of AIH. AIH is divided into type 1 (the majority, patients with antinuclear antibody, smooth-muscle antibody positivity) and type 2 (the minority, those with liver/kidney microsomes, liver cytosol type-1 positivity). A minority of patients with types 1 and 2 express anti-liver-soluble antigen, which is highly specific for AIH. The diagnosis of AIH can be difficult at times, but clinical criteria after exclusion of other liver diseases as part of the workup are usually sufficient to make a diagnosis of or to exclude AIH. Simplified diagnostic criteria have higher sensitivity and specificity in Asia and are based on clinical, biochemical, serological, and histological features to determine the probability of AIH and response to immunosuppression [11]. AIH presents rarely as acute liver failure and infrequently as acute hepatitis; however, up to 80% present with chronic hepatitis with 33% having cirrhosis, indicating insidious progression. Immunosuppressive therapy with corticosteroids and/or azathioprine helps to achieve remission in AIH.

Primary Biliary Cholangitis

PBC is an autoimmune liver disease presenting with cholestasis involving the intrahepatic small bile ducts. The presence of raised ALP and positive anti-mitochondrial antibody (AMA, which has high sensitivity and specificity) establishes the diagnosis of PBC after excluding bile duct obstruction on ultrasound. Although there has been a slight increase, PBC remains rare in India, with a hospital-based study over a period of 13.5 years diagnosing 1.5% of suspected autoimmune liver disease with AMA positivity. In India, PBC occurs in middle-aged women and appears to have an aggressive course, with 60% having cirrhosis at the time of presentation [12]. Patients with PBC who respond to treatment with ursodeoxycholic acid will usually have stable, non-progressive disease. Second-line treatments include fibrates and obeticholic acid.

Wilson's Disease

Wilson's disease is an autosomal recessive disorder of copper metabolism caused by an *ATP7B* gene mutation. In India, there are no community-based incidence and prevalence studies but the WHO estimates the global prevalence of Wilson's disease to be 1/10 000–1/30 000. In patients in whom Wilson's disease is suspected, serum ceruloplasmin levels less than 20 mg/dl, 24-hour urine copper greater than 40 μg, and the presence of Kayser–Fleischer rings confirms the diagnosis of Wilson's disease. The gold standard, dry liver copper estimation on liver biopsy is often difficult; it is not easily available and may be fraught with logistic and quality issues [13]. Genetic analysis of *ATP7B* gene mutation of siblings has also become routine. The age of presentation varies from 4 to 60 years, with most presenting before 30 years. The manifestations are more likely to be hepatic in early childhood and neurological in adolescents, with most patients with Wilson's disease demonstrating some degree of liver disease. Commonly, the disease, presents as chronic liver disease with chronic hepatitis, prolonged jaundice, hepatosplenomegaly, edema, ascites, and other signs of liver cell failure. It also presents as acute hepatitis like a typical attack of acute viral hepatitis, and sometimes rapidly deteriorating in to acute liver failure [13]. Early and lifelong chelation treatment of excessive copper with agents like D-penicillamine or trientine, together with zinc, prevents progression of the disease. Liver transplant is indicated in acute liver failure and chronic liver disease presenting as acute on chronic or in patients worsening despite treatment.

Drug-Induced Liver Injury

Although the exact prevalence of DILI in India is not known, the high prevalence of TB in the population and the use of traditional and complementary medicines suggests that it is likely to be significant [14]. DILI was implicated as a cause in 10.5% of Asian patients with acute on chronic liver failure with complementary and alternative medications (71.7%) being the most common insult, followed by anti-TB drugs (27.3%). Three patterns of DILI, categorized as hepatocellular, cholestatic, or mixed injury, are based on the baseline serum ALT and ALP ratio from the first available biochemical test. Early recognition and prompt withdrawal of the offending agent, together with future avoidance is sufficient in most cases, except those leading to liver failure. Although evidence is insufficient to recommend cholestyramine, carnitine, n-acetyl cysteine, and ursodeoxycholic acid in DILI, they may be helpful in specific situations [14].

Other Cholestatic Diseases

Diseases such as portal biliopathy and primary sclerosing cholangitis (PSC) causing cholestasis are reported in small numbers in India and are thus grouped in the category of other cholestatic diseases of hepatobiliary origin.

Portal biliopathy pertains to the abnormalities in the biliary tract occurring predominantly in patients with extrahepatic portal venous obstruction (EHPVO) with portal cavernoma. Over the years, the incidence of EHPVO has decreased and so has the burden of portal biliopathy. The largest reported series of patients with EHPVO as the cause of portal hypertension reported 20% of patients having symptomatic portal biliopathy [15]. Patients with EHPVO usually have a longstanding disease, lasting for 8–10 years before they present with symptoms. All patients with symptomatic biliopathy present with a history of jaundice with cholangitis present in around half to two thirds of patients. Patients with symptomatic biliopathy usually have jaundice, splenomegaly, and hepatomegaly, together with raised bilirubin and ALP. Treatment of symptomatic portal biliopathy is approached in a phased manner: first, biliary clearance endoscopically; second, portal decompression, either radiologically or surgically; and third, persistent biliary obstruction with biliary drainage surgery.

Primary Sclerosing Cholangitis (PSC) is a cholestatic disorder of autoimmune etiology that is rare in India. It affects young people with symptoms of jaundice, pruritus, clay-colored stools, abdominal pain, or symptoms of cholangitis with rapid progression to decompensation. The prevalence of inflammatory bowel disease in PSC is lower in India and the proportion of small-duct PSC is higher than that observed in the Western population [16].

Hemochromatosis

Genetic hemochromatosis is uncommon in India. Almost 10% of patients with non-alcoholic chronic liver disease in India have iron overload but have negative hemochromatosis genotyping. During population screening, Asians had the highest levels of serum ferritin and mean transferrin saturation but the lowest prevalence (0.000039%) of hemochromatosis with genotyping [17].

Gilbert's Syndrome

Gilbert's syndrome is an inherited condition identified in around 6% of healthy population but the exact prevalence in India is unknown. It is associated with reduced activity of uridine diphosphate-glucuronosyltransferase (UGT1A1), characterized by persistent, mild elevation of blood levels of unconjugated bilirubin with all other liver tests being normal. Although the syndrome is usually benign, bilirubin levels may increase during fasting or illnesses including systemic infections, or following certain drugs. Gilbert's syndrome in the Indian setting is important because incidental detection of raised bilirubin leads to complementary medicines use, which may cause enhanced toxicity via UGT1A1 polymorphisms [18] predisposing individuals to DILI.

Non-hepatic Causes of Liver Enzymes Elevation

After exclusion of hepatobiliary causes of elevated liver tests, non-hepatic causes include muscle disorders, cardiac (congestion/ischemia), thyroid disease (both hypo and hyper), celiac disease, sarcoidosis, and, rarely, adrenal insufficiency should be considered and investigated. In India, particular emphasis should be placed on TB, which can present in multiple ways, including liver injury, which poses difficulties in management, with anti-TB drugs affecting the liver tests.

Isolated Raised Alkaline Phosphatase

Isolated raised alkaline phosphatase poses a diagnostic challenge, but a clinical diagnosis can be arrived in around 80% of isolated ALP elevations based on history, physical examination and routine laboratory tests. Although there are no data on the most likely causes of an isolated raised ALP in an asymptomatic population, the most common cause is likely to be vitamin D deficiency or bone related [19]. Persistent elevation of isolated serum alkaline phosphatase can be attributed to either bone or renal disease given the high prevalence of vitamin D deficiency and chronic kidney diseases in India.

Conclusions

Viral hepatitis remains the most common reason for abnormal liver tests in India. The increasing prevalence of NAFLD and ARLD due to demographic and epidemiologic transition of liver disease burden in view of increase in per capita income, together with DILI due to complementary and alternative medications, contributes to the remaining major abnormal liver tests in India.

Far East Perspective

As chronic hepatitis B (CHB) virus infection remains endemic in the Far East, occult HBV infection [20] must be excluded in the patient with unexplained abnormal liver tests (i.e. HBsAg and anti-HCV both negative). Occult HBV infection is a status of undetectable serum HBsAg yet detectable serum and/or intrahepatic HBV DNA. It may result either from a self-limiting acute hepatitis; or in patients with CHB who achieved HBsAg sero-clearance, which refers to the loss of detectability of serum HBsAg with or without anti-HBs in patients with CHB. Anti-HBc is as prevalent as in 30% of patients being worked up for abnormal liver tests in East Asia [21]. In the absence of serum HBsAg, a low quantity of HBV DNA less than 200 iu/ml was often detected in the serum and liver tissue biopsy by real-time polymerase chain reaction [20]. However, a potentially life-threatening condition would be reactivation of an occult HBV infection in patients during immunosuppression therapy, especially in the setting of high-dose corticosteroid therapy [22], intensified immunosuppression including in onco-hematologic patients, those receiving hematopoietic stem cell transplantation and treated with the anti-CD20 monoclonal antibody (e.g. rituximab; Table 3.4) [23].

Lean NAFLD is a distinct phenotype of NAFLD which develops despite the patients being non-obese (body mass index $< 25\,kg/m^2$) [24]. Lean NAFLD occurs in up to one quarter of Asian patients with NAFLD; it usually represents the milder end of a continuous spectrum [25]. Severe liver disease did occur in some lean patients: advanced fibrosis was found in 26.1% of patients [25].

Table 3.4   Immunosuppressants and risk of reactivation of occult hepatitis B.

Agent	Risk of reactivation (%)
B cell-depleting agents (e.g. rituximab)	> 10
TNFα inhibitors (e.g. infliximab)	1
Tyrosine kinase inhibitors (e.g. imatinib)	1
Doxorubicin and epirubicin	1–10
Azathioprine, 6-mercaptopurine, methotrexate	≪ 1
Immunotherapy (e.g. pembrolizumab, nivolumab)	< 2
Systemic corticosteroids:	
Moderate to high dose > 4 weeks	1–10
Moderate to high dose < 1 week	≪ 1
Low dose > 4 weeks	< 1

TNFα, tumor necrosis factor alpha.
Source: Summarized from Perrillo et al. [30] and Wong et al. [31].

Another easily missed reason of unexplained abnormal liver tests is DILI, as use of some drugs and herbal and dietary supplements may be easily missed by the healthcare practitioners and even by the patients themselves. The proportion of herbal and dietary supplement-related liver injury can be as high as 60% in Asian patients [26]. Seeds of *Psoralea corylifolia* (Boh-Gol-Zhee), chaparral leaf, and Shou Wu Pian are some of the commonly used specific herbal remedies that have been linked to DILI [27]. Because of the lack of information on the hepatotoxic potential and signature of the majority of herbal compounds, establishing such diagnosis may be challenging. The Roussel–Uclaf causality assessment method score is a commonly used tool to establish the diagnosis of DILI. It has the issue of lack of sensitivity for herbal and dietary supplement-related liver injury. A high index of suspicion and exhaustive inquiry into the use of any medications and herbal and dietary supplements, be it prescribed or sold over the counter, would be the important first step of diagnostic process.

Recurrent pyogenic cholangitis is a distinct condition in Far East resulting from repeated infections of the biliary tree (cholangitis), which was first described in Hong Kong in 1930. It is also called Oriental cholangiohepatitis, Hong Kong disease, Oriental infestation cholangitis, or hepatolithiasis [28]. It is rarely seen in the West, with a prevalence less than 2%, and its incidence is highest in Far East has been decreasing at the same time over the past few decades, mainly from the improving sanitation of the region [29].

Africa Perspective

Liver diseases are increasing in Africa, probably due to an increased use of drugs, alcohol, and other chemicals, in addition to some highly prevalent infections. Most patients with raised liver enzymes are discovered incidentally, as it is not common for people with no medical complaints to seek care. Such incidental discoveries happen because liver function tests are increasingly becoming part of routinely requested investigations by clinicians. However, most patients with raised liver enzymes are not often identified since they are likely to be asymptomatic. Patients with symptoms are mainly identified in primary care and the next step is to investigate the cause of the raised liver enzymes.

Why Liver Disease in Primary Care?

Liver disease contributes significantly to mortality and morbidity in Africa. It should therefore be given serious attention in primary care, where most of the patients are seen and cared for. Liver enzymes are part of the first assessment tests for liver disease.

Liver Enzymes

The liver enzymes of clinical relevance are AST, ALT, ALP, and GGT. These enzyme tests are the ones commonly used in clinical laboratories in most parts of Africa. There are other liver enzymes such as 5′-nucleotidase that are raised in cases of cholestasis but these tests are not commonly done due to lack of resources.

It is important to remember that these liver enzymes are also found in other body tissues/ organs like the heart, skeletal muscles, kidneys, lungs, brain, pancreas, among others. Primary care clinicians therefore need to use a broader approach in dealing with a patient with unexplained raised liver enzymes.

Common Causes of Raised Enzymes

Liver enzymes are released into the blood circulatory system as a result of cell death or cell membrane damage. Common causes of raised serum liver enzymes are:

- Infections: including viral (common; hepatitis A, B, and C, HIV, and several others), parasitic (*Entamoeba histolytica*, *Echinococcus granulosus*, etc.).
- Drugs, including traditional medicines, which are commonly used in Africa.
- Chronic alcohol abuse: if you suspect alcohol-related liver disease, estimate AST : ALT ratio. If this ratio is more than 2 : 1, this greatly suggests alcohol related liver disease.
- Poisoning and use of other chemicals commonly chemicals related to agricultural use (e.g. pesticides).
- Malignancies (hepatocellular carcinoma and other secondary cancers involving the liver).

Non-hepatic causes of raised serum liver enzymes include:
- connective tissue diseases
- severe sepsis
- diabetes mellitus particularly type 2.

When evaluating a patient with abnormal serum liver enzymes, the clinician should be guided by these common causes of liver disease, as they will form the differential diagnoses.

What to Do When a Patient Has Unexplained Liver Enzymes

- Take a comprehensive history.
- Perform a focused physical examination to exclude some causes that can be demonstrated clinically. Most facilities in Africa do not have advanced diagnostic equipment.
- Request for clinically relevant laboratory and radiological investigations.

Clinical Features

Look for the following clinical features (which may indicate liver disease) in a patient with raised liver enzymes:

- yellowing of the eyes and other mucous membranes
- hair and skin texture
- swelling of the feet and abdomen
- presence of collateral vessels on the abdomen
- enlarged liver (hepatomegaly) on examination of the abdomen.

Relevant Investigations

When a patient is identified with raised serum liver enzymes, the following laboratory and radiological investigations should be performed to guide the next course of action:

- Urinalysis: check for appearance (may appear yellow in a jaundiced patient), shake to produce froth which will also appear yellow. Also check for protein.
- Stool analysis: stools will appear pale in a patient with biliary obstruction.
- Full blood count.
- Abdominal ultrasonography, abdominal computed tomography, and magnetic resonance imaging are becoming increasingly used in Africa.
- Bleeding and clotting time.

When to Refer

- Failure to identify the cause of persistently raised liver enzymes.
- Worsening in the patients' clinical condition.
- For specialized treatment, particularly common for HBV and HCV infections.

Infections

Africa suffers high prevalence of hepatitis viruses mainly A, B, and C, as well as HIV, all of which are associated with elevation of liver enzymes. In infectious cases, AST and ALT are the main liver enzymes affected. They may be moderately or severely raised depending on the severity of the condition. Bilirubin both direct and indirect may also be mildly raised.

In parasitic infections, including *E. histolytica*, which causes amoebic liver abscess, and *Echinococcus,* among others, the liver enzymes are usually within normal ranges.

Liver Cirrhosis

Chronic liver/hepatocellular injury commonly results into cirrhosis. In Africa, most diseases including those of the liver present late. Therefore, cirrhosis is one of the most common presentations of liver disease. In cirrhosis, the liver enzymes may be normal or elevated.

When cirrhosis is suspected, ultrasonography of the abdomen to visualize the liver appearance and texture should be done.

Drugs

In Africa, the use of traditional medicine is high. Africa is believed to be the cradle of mankind and use of traditional medicine may be as old, making African traditional medicine the oldest of such treatment modalities. African traditional medicine involves use of herbs, herbal materials, preparations, and products. Use of traditional medicine is common in Africa as there is limited access to modern medicines and trained providers. Traditional medicine providers are thus culturally acceptable and their methods are more patient-centered.

The use of pharmacological drugs is also on the increase but with lack or limited regulation. Therefore, most drugs including antibiotics and restricted drugs can easily be accessed across the counter in Africa without prescription. This practice allows an individual to use several drugs at the same time with possibilities of drugs interactions but also without consideration of hepatotoxicity. Clinically indicated and prescribed drugs can also cause liver damage.

Drugs cause transient raise in AST, ALT, and GGT, coupled with a slight raise in bilirubin. Sometimes, the bilirubin levels are normal. The clinician needs to identify the offending drug and make a decision whether to stop it or not. There is need to weigh the benefits against the risks of continuing with the drug. If a decision to continue with the drug is made, then there is need to reassure the patient and the patient should make a commitment to regularly report back for clinical and laboratory monitoring. If the serum levels of the enzymes continue raising, then the drug(s) must be stopped.

Issues to Note in Africa

- Lack of continuity of care coupled with limited resources makes it difficult to monitor the trends of liver enzymes. In the majority, serum enzyme estimations are done only once, with a possibility of making a clinical decision on transient abnormalities.
- Historically, most books about liver diseases are written in the context of high income/ countries with wider access to primary care, as well as specialist services as part of quality health system.
- There is poor health-seeking behavior among most African populations/communities, with most diseases presenting late/in advanced stages.
- Normative ranges used in interpretation of serum liver enzymes are not set in Africa. This should be considered by the clinicians.

Conclusion/Take Home Message

A clinician faced with a patient who has abnormal serum liver enzymes should take a history, perform a physical examination, and request clinically relevant investigations.

References

1. Tapper, E.B., Saini, S.D., and Sengupta, N. (2017). Extensive testing or focused testing of patients with elevated liver enzymes. *J. Hepatol.* 66 (2): 313–319.
2. Mokdad, A.A., Lopez, A.D., Shahraz, S. et al. (2014). Liver cirrhosis mortality in 187 countries between 1980 and 2010: a systematic analysis. *BMC Med.* 12: 145.
3. Mukherjee, P.S., Vishnubhatla, S., Amarapurkar, D.N. et al. (2017). Etiology and mode of presentation of chronic liver diseases in India: a multi centric study. *PLoS One* 12 (10): e0187033.
4. Kumar, T., Shrivastava, A., Kumar, A. et al. (2015). Viral hepatitis surveillance: India, 2011–2013. *Morb. Mortal. Wkly. Rep.* 64 (28): 758–762.
5. Shalimar, Acharya, S.K., Kumar, R. et al. (2020). Acute liver failure of non-A-E viral hepatitis etiology-profile, prognosis, and predictors of outcome. *J. Clin. Exp. Hepatol.* 10 (5): 453–461.

6. National Notifiable Diseases Surveillance System. *Surveillance Case Definitions for Current and Historical Conditions*. https://ndc.services.cdc.gov. Accessed 27 April 2022.

7. Acharya, S.K., Batra, Y., Bhatkal, B. et al. Seroepidemiology of hepatitis A virus infection among school children in Delhi and north Indian patients with chronic liver disease: implications for HAV vaccination. *J. Gastroenterol. Hepatol.* 2003 (18, 7): 822–827.

8. Sarin, S.K., Kumar, M., Eslam, M. et al. (2020). Liver diseases in the Asia-Pacific region: a Lancet Gastroenterology and Hepatology Commission. *Lancet Gastroenterol. Hepatol.* 5 (2): 167–228.

9. Duseja, A., Singh, S.P., Saraswat, V.A. et al. (2015). Non-alcoholic fatty liver disease and metabolic syndrome-position paper of the Indian National Association for the study of the liver, Endocrine Society of India, Indian College of Cardiology and Indian Society of Gastroenterology. *J. Clin. Exp. Hepatol.* 5 (1): 51–68.

10. Amarapurkar, D., Dharod, M., and Amarapurkar, A. (2015). Autoimmune hepatitis in India: single tertiary referral centre experience. *Trop. Gastroenterol.* 36 (1): 36–45.

11. Wang, G., Tanaka, A., Zhao, H. et al. (2021). The Asian Pacific Association for the Study of the Liver clinical practice guidance: the diagnosis and management of patients with autoimmune hepatitis. *Hepatol. Int.* 15: 223–257.

12. Minz, R.W., Kaur, N., Anand, S. et al. (2012). Complete spectrum of AMA-M2 positive liver disease in north India. *Hepatol. Int.* 6 (4): 790–795.

13. Nagral, A., Sarma, M.S., Matthai, J. et al. (2019). Wilson's disease: clinical practice guidelines of the Indian National Association for Study of the Liver, the Indian Society of Pediatric Gastroenterology, Hepatology and Nutrition, and the Movement Disorders Society of India. *J. Clin. Exp. Hepatol.* 9 (1): 74–98.

14. Devarbhavi, H., Aithal, G., Treeprasertsuk, S. et al. (2021). Drug-induced liver injury: Asia Pacific Association of Study of Liver consensus guidelines. *Hepatol. Int.* 15: 258–282.

15. Agarwal, A.K., Sharma, D., Singh, S. et al. (2011). Portal biliopathy: a study of 39 surgically treated patients. *HPB (Oxford)* 13 (1): 33–39.

16. Tibdewal, P., Bhatt, P., Jain, A. et al. (2019). Clinical profile and outcome of primary sclerosing cholangitis: a single-centre experience from western India. *Indian J. Gastroenterol.* 38 (4): 295–302.

17. Adams, P.C., Reboussin, D.M., Barton, J.C. et al. (2005). Hemochromatosis and iron-overload screening in a racially diverse population. *N. Engl. J. Med.* 352 (17): 1769–1778.

18. Farheen, S., Sengupta, S., Santra, A. et al. (2006). Gilbert's syndrome: high frequency of the (TA)7 TAA allele in India and its interaction with a novel CAT insertion in promoter of the gene for bilirubin UDP-glucuronosyltransferase 1 gene. *World J. Gastroenterol.* 12 (14): 2269–2275.

19. Newsome, P.N., Cramb, R., Davison, S.M. et al. (2018). Guidelines on the management of abnormal liver blood tests. *Gut* 67 (1): 6–19.

20. Yip, T.C. and Wong, G.L. (2019). Current knowledge of occult hepatitis B infection and clinical implications. *Semin. Liver Dis.* 39 (2): 249–260.

21. Chan, T.T., Chan, W.K., Wong, G.L. et al. (2020). Positive hepatitis B core antibody is associated with cirrhosis and hepatocellular carcinoma in nonalcoholic fatty liver disease. *Am. J. Gastroenterol.* 115 (6): 867–875.

22. Wong, G.L., Wong, V.W., Yuen, B.W. et al. (2020). Risk of hepatitis B surface antigen seroreversion after corticosteroid in patients with previous hepatitis B virus exposure. *J. Hepatol.* 72 (1): 57–66.

23. Phipps, C., Chen, Y., and Tan, D. (2016). Lymphoproliferative disease and hepatitis B reactivation: challenges in the era of rapidly evolving targeted therapy. *Clin. Lymphoma Myeloma Leuk.* 16: 5–11.

24. Francque, S. and Wong, V.W. (2022). NAFLD in lean individuals: not a benign disease. *Gut* 71: 234–236.

25. Leung, J.C., Loong, T.C., Wei, J.L. et al. (2017). Histological severity and clinical outcomes of nonalcoholic fatty liver disease in non-obese patients. *Hepatology* 65 (1): 54–64.

26. Weber, S., Wong, G.L.H., Wong, V.W.S. et al. (2020). Monocyte-derived hepatocyte-like cell test: a novel tool for *in vitro* identification of drug-induced liver injury in patients with herbal or dietary supplements. *Digestion* 20: 1–4.

27. Lin, N.H., Yang, H.W., Su, Y.J., and Chang, C.W. (2019). Herb induced liver injury after using herbal medicine: a systemic review and case-control study. *Medicine (Baltimore)* 98 (13): e14992.

28. Gupta, A. and Simo, K. (2022). Recurrent pyogenic cholangitis. In: *StatPearls*. Treasure Island, FL: StatPearls Publishing https://www.ncbi.nlm.nih.gov/books/NBK564308. Accessed 27 April 2022.

29. Lee, K.F., Cheung, Y.S., Chong, C.C. et al. (2016). Laparoscopic and robotic hepatectomy: experience from a single centre. *ANZ J. Surg.* 86 (3): 122–126.

30. Perrillo, R.P., Gish, R., and Falck-Ytter, Y.T. (2015). American Gastroenterological Association Institute technical review on prevention and treatment of hepatitis B virus reactivation during immunosuppressive drug therapy. *Gastroenterology* 148: 221–244.e3.

31. Wong, G.L., Wong, V.W., Hui, V.W. et al. (2021). Hepatitis flare during immunotherapy in patients with current or past hepatitis B virus infection. *Am. J. Gastroenterol.* 116: 1274–1283.

Section 3

Take-Home Primers

Managing Unexplained Abnormal Serum Liver Tests in Secondary Care

4

Intensive Care

William Bernal and Sheital Chand

Institute of I iver Studies, Kings College Hospital, London, UK

KEY POINTS

- Abnormalities of liver tests are common in patients in the intensive care setting and reflect the underlying condition.
- The degree of abnormality is often minor, and abnormal results resolve as the patient's condition improves.
- Common causes of severe liver damage in the intensive care setting include sepsis, hypoxic (ischemic) hepatitis, drug-induced liver injury; less common causes are acute viral hepatitis (especially hepatitis A, B, and E), acute Budd–Chiari syndrome, acute hepatic veno-occlusive disease, undetected pre-existing liver disease, and hepatic malignant infiltration. Enteral nutrition may also be associated with abnormal liver tests.
- High levels of serum bilirubin and liver should prompt appropriate serological and imaging tests to determine the cause of liver abnormalities.
- The onset of hepatic encephalopathy, high levels of blood lactate or ammonia in the context of liver abnormalities should prompt discussions with a liver specialist.

Classification and Prevalence

Liver injury may be identified on initial admission of a patient to an intensive care unit (ICU) or may develop during the course of their admission. It may reflect the severity of systemic illness precipitating ICU admission or, alternatively, can be acquired as a complication of medical treatment or intervention delivered in ICU. It may also be a first manifestation of previously unrecognized underlying chronic liver disease.

The severity of blood test abnormalities may vary widely. Most commonly, abnormalities are at the more minor end of the severity spectrum, with transient and minor elevations in liver biochemical tests, with liver enzyme elevations to two to three times

---

The Liver in Systemic Disease: A Clinician's Guide to Abnormal Liver Tests, First Edition.
Edited by Gideon M. Hirschfield, Paramjit Gill, and James Neuberger.
© 2023 John Wiley & Sons Ltd. Published 2023 by John Wiley & Sons Ltd.

the upper limit of normal [1]. These elevations are typically self-limiting without the need for intervention, and with little impact on the overall clinical course of the patient. At the other end of the spectrum, there may be rare major abnormalities in liver biochemical tests with enzyme elevations over 20 times the upper limit of normal, associated with loss of liver function and lactic acidosis, hyperammonemia, encephalopathy, and coagulopathy that require specific critical care support. Patients in ICU who develop abnormal liver biochemical tests can be assigned to three broad clinical groupings:

- *Acute liver injury*: where abnormal liver enzyme biochemical tests are identified but without evidence of significant hepatic functional compromise. Abnormal results of blood tests reflecting liver injury are seen commonly in patients in the ICU and may be present in more than half of all critically ill patients over the course of an ICU admission.
- *Acute hepatic dysfunction*: where abnormal liver enzyme biochemical tests are associated with laboratory evidence of synthetic and metabolic compromise, manifest either as the development of jaundice or coagulopathy. Liver dysfunction has prognostic implications: jaundice is seen approximately 10% of critically ill of patients early after ICU admission and is a specific and independent risk factor for death (Figure 4.1).
- *Acute liver failure*: where there is evidence of major hepatic functional compromise with the development of encephalopathy, in the absence of pre-existing chronic liver disease. This is often associated with other extrahepatic organ failure and is a rare medical emergency that often requires specialist management and, occasionally, liver transplantation.

Depending on the nature and severity of the insult responsible for liver injury and the presence or absence of pre-existing liver disease, some patients may remain within the liver injury category alone or may only show evidence of minor dysfunction. Others may

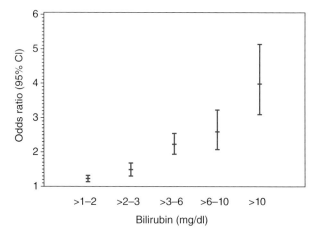

Figure 4.1 Adjusted risk of hospital mortality stratified by maximum bilirubin level within 48 hours of intensive care unit (ICU) admission; $n = 38\,036$ first ICU admissions. Exclusion of patients with acute or acute on chronic liver disease and with adjustment for age, sex, primary diagnosis, and non-hepatic organ dysfunction. DILI, drug-induced liver injury; NAFLD, non-alcoholic fatty liver disease. Source: Kramer et al. 2007 [1] / Wolters Kluwer Health, Inc.

rapidly progress from liver injury to dysfunction and then failure over the course of hours. The latter course is rare, but its early recognition and prompt and effective management may be lifesaving.

Some patients with pre-existing liver disease may present to the ICU and, in some cases, the presence of pre-existing liver damage may not be known. Common causes of hepatic decompensation requiring intensive care include sepsis, gastrointestinal bleeding (from varices, gastric erosions, or other causes), electrolyte disturbance, alcohol, or drug adverse effects. These causes require appropriate investigation and management, in conjunction with a hepatologist.

Patterns of Liver Test Abnormalities

Many factors may contribute to the development of liver injury and dysfunction in this setting, acting either in isolation or in concert. However, using clinical presentation and standard laboratory measures, patients with novel hepatic dysfunction in the setting of critical illness can be broadly classified into two categories of cholestatic or hepatocellular patterns of injury, with the former the more commonly observed. However, a "mixed" pattern may also be observed, and the pattern of abnormality may change over the course of illness.

Hepatocellular Pattern of Liver Injury

Hepatocellular abnormality is defined by predominant elevation of the serum aminotransferases alanine transaminase (ALT) and aspartate transaminase (AST). AST is released into the circulation as a result of hepatocyte damage and has a plasma half-life of 12–24 hours. AST is also released by cellar injury of skeletal and cardiac muscle and from erythrocytes, all of which may be injured in critical illness, so elevated AST levels do not always imply liver cell damage. ALT has a plasma half-life of 36–50 hours and its release is more specific for hepatic injury. Major hepatocellular biochemical abnormalities may develop very rapidly, over hours, particularly in hypoxic hepatitis or severe drug-induced hepatic necrosis, and may be detected well before the onset of clinically apparent jaundice. The decrease in serum aminotransferase levels is usually more gradual and the rate of resolution may reflect the effectiveness of the correction of the cause of liver injury. The major causes of severe hepatocellular liver injury are shown in Box 4.1.

Box 4.1 Principal Causes of Severe Hepatocellular Acute Hepatic Dysfunction
• Hypoxic hepatitis • Drug-induced liver injury • Acute viral hepatitis • Acute Budd–Chiari syndrome • Acute hepatic veno-occlusive disease • Hepatic malignant infiltration

Principal Causes of Hepatocellular Liver Injury

Hypoxic or Ischemic Hepatitis

The high metabolic activity of the liver and its complex vascular supply render it at risk of injury from hemodynamic insults, and "hypoxic" or "ischemic" hepatitis results from hepatocellular necrosis provoked by acute cellular hypoxia resulting from impaired hepatic oxygen delivery [2]. The prevalence of hypoxic hepatitis in hospital admissions is around 1/1000 but is probably at least an order of magnitude more common in ICU admissions. Diagnostic criteria vary but have included the triad of:

1) an appropriate clinical setting of cardiac, respiratory, or circulatory failure
2) an abrupt increase in serum transaminases reaching at least 20 times the upper limit of normal, and
3) exclusion other causes of acute liver cell necrosis, particularly severe viral or major drug-induced liver injury (Figure 4.2a).

Major elevation of transaminases is usually of short duration and may be followed by coagulopathy, reflecting transient hepatic synthetic compromise. Significant jaundice follows in about 30% of patients and, if present, is associated with increased risk of complications and death [4]. Liver biopsy is seldom required or performed, but typically shows extensive centrilobular necrosis, reflecting the sensitivity of "zone 3" hepatocytes to ischemic insults.

Heart failure, respiratory failure, and septic shock are responsible for more than 90% of cases of hypoxic hepatitis, with these factors acting alone or in combination in individual patients (Figure 4.3). Compromise of cardiac output resulting from acute cardiac events, such as myocardial infarction, dysrhythmia, or pericardial tamponade, may reduce blood flow and oxygen delivery to the liver, with an important role now also recognized from passive congestion of the liver from right-heart failure. The latter may occur in the setting of severe pulmonary disease, where concurrent hypoxemia may also contribute. Sepsis and the evoked inflammatory response play an important permissive role in the development of hypoxic hepatitis through the development of hepatic "dysoxia" and impairment of hepatic cellular respiratory function oxygen utilization and microcirculatory changes.

Effective management of hypoxic hepatitis depends on its early recognition and addressing the causative factors. In the ICU setting, this frequently involves assessment and monitoring of cardiac function through invasive or non-invasive means. Electrocardiography and echocardiography are mandatory early diagnostic investigations. Prognosis is variable, depending on the trigger(s) for the development of hypoxic hepatitis, although death seldom results from liver failure alone, but rather from multiple organ failure from the underlying conditions responsible. Recognition of hypoxic hepatitis may be challenging, as its presence may be confounded by the absence of a classical "shock state."

Drug-Induced Acute Hepatocyte Necrosis

Sudden and extensive hepatocyte death that causes massive release of hepatocellular enzymes into the circulation may also result from drug-induced liver injury. Although a number of drugs and toxins may be responsible (Figure 4.4), in the UK, United States, and Western Europe, paracetamol/acetaminophen-induced hepatocyte necrosis, usually after overdose, is by far the most common cause. The pattern and magnitude of abnormalities of

(a)   Hypoxic Hepatitis.

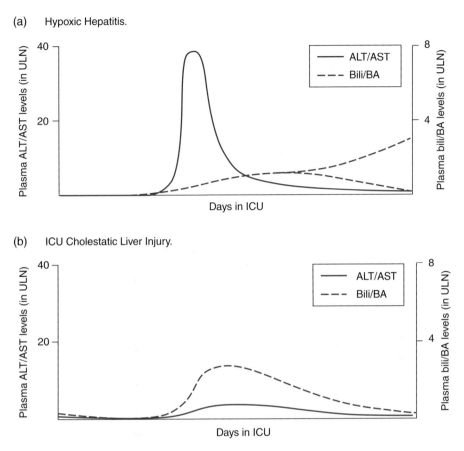

(b)   ICU Cholestatic Liver Injury.

Figure 4.2   Illustrative changes in liver biochemistry in hypoxic hepatitis and critical illness cholestatic liver injury. (a) Hypoxic hepatitis. In hypoxic hepatitis, oxygen supply to the liver is impaired, resulting in hepatocyte cellular necrosis. Alanine aminotransferase (ALT) and aspartate aminotransferase (AST), and to a lesser degree ALP and gGT, are released into the circulation. Excretory function as measured by means of bilirubin (Bili) and bile acids (BA) levels may be mildly impaired. In the recovery phase, oxygen supply to the liver is restored, and hepatocytes regenerate. In 30% of patients, clinical jaundice develops after hypoxic hepatitis. (b) Intensive care unit (ICU) cholestatic liver injury. During ICU cholestasis, intrahepatic alterations in the liver transport machinery result in higher circulating Bili and BA levels. Biliary stasis promotes release of ALP and gGT from cholangiocytes. Mild elevation of ALT and AST levels may also be present. Source: After Jenniskens et al. 2018 [3]. With permission of Elsevier.

liver tests, particularly elevation of AST, closely mimics that seen hypoxic hepatitis and may be difficult to distinguish from it. Circumstantial evidence of overdose and/or detectable paracetamol in the blood may aid diagnosis, and its identification is clinically urgent, as there is a narrow time window for the maximal efficacy of the antidote N-acetyl cysteine (NAC). However, the hepatic injury may not be apparent until paracetamol and its metabolites have become undetectable in blood and urine; thus, the absence of detectable levels of paracetamol or its metabolites do not preclude paracetamol toxicity. Some clinical risk factors may increase susceptibility to major paracetamol-induced liver injury (Box 4.2). Given

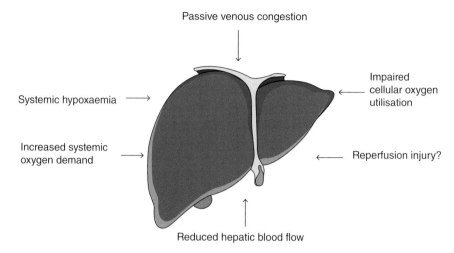

Passive venous congestion

Systemic hypoxaemia →

Increased systemic
oxygen demand →

Impaired
cellular oxygen
utilisation

← Reperfusion injury?

Reduced hepatic blood flow

Figure 4.3 Factors contributing to the development of hypoxic hepatitis.

the very limited adverse effect profile of NAC, if there is clinical suspicion of paracetamol-induced liver injury being responsible for or contributing to abnormal liver tests, there is little to be lost by its administration while confirmation is sought. If other drugs are suspected as being responsible for liver injury, their early withdrawal is key while alternative causes are excluded, and the severity of liver injury assessed (see Chapter 20).

Acute Viral Hepatitis

Globally, the most common case of gross hepatocellular blood test abnormalities in the critically ill is likely to be from severe acute viral hepatitis infections. Jaundice is often more prominent than in hypoxic hepatitis or acute drug-induced hepatic necrosis. As detailed elsewhere in this volume, these infections include those from hepatitis A (HAV), hepatitis B (HBV), and hepatitis E (HEV) viruses. Other viruses that less commonly cause hepatitis include cytomegalovirus (CMV), herpes simplex virus (HSV), and Epstein–Barr virus (EBV), with a very large number of other infective causes described. The majority of acute hepatitis infections are likely to go unrecognized. If they are clinically apparent, infections usually resolve with supportive management alone, although in some instances targeted antiviral therapy is required. Virus-specific serologic tests may be diagnostic and enable characterization of acute or more chronic infection, but assessment of liver injury severity uses more generic laboratory tests. as described below.

Hepatitis A and E are transmitted via the fecal–oral route and are common in developing countries or in travelers returned from endemic countries; symptomatic infection is uncommon and major liver injury is very rare. Acute hepatitis B infection is also usually asymptomatic and self-resolves, but on rare occasions it may also present with liver failure. Reactivation of hepatitis B in the context of chemotherapy or B-cell depleting immunosuppression is a potentially fatal event and may present many months after the precipitating treatment. Treatment is with immediate antiviral therapy.

CMV infection typically presents as reactivation in later life in an immunocompromised host, although acute hepatitis can also occur in immunocompetent individuals. Treatment

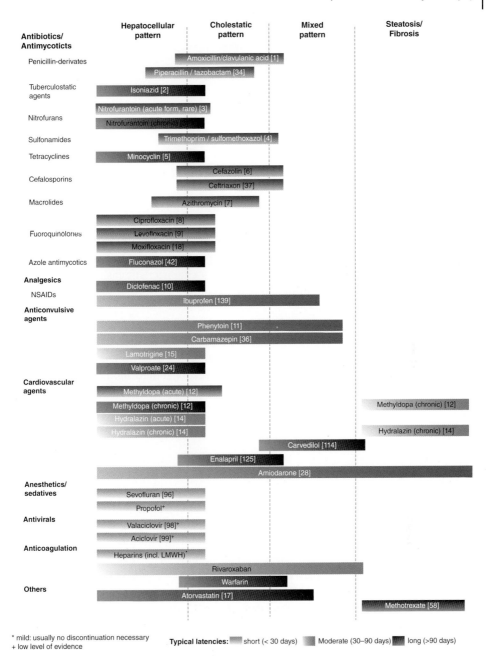

Figure 4.4 Medication most commonly responsible for drug-induced liver injury in intensive care and pattern of liver dysfunction. NSAIDs, non-steroidal anti-inflammatory drugs. Source: Based on Horvatits et al. (2019) [4]. For reference citations in this figure, please refer to Horvatits et al. (2019).

Box 4.2   Clinical Risk Factors for Enhanced Paracetamol-Induced Hepatotoxicity

- Anorexia and undernutrition
- Low body mass index
- Prolonged fasting
- Enzyme-inducing medication
- Chronic alcohol use
- Presentation over 24 hours after overdose
- Staggered overdose

---

with antiviral agents is indicated in many cases, with reduction in immunosuppression if relevant.

HSV infection rarely causes hepatitis, but when present is usually severe in nature and often fatal. Risk factors are the third trimester of pregnancy, immunosuppression, and advanced age. Symptoms maybe non-specific and a characteristic rash is not frequently evident. A high index of suspicion should be maintained for early diagnosis and immediate antiviral treatment is essential.

Other Causes

Other causes of severe hepatocellular liver dysfunction and failure are much rarer but will often become apparent on investigation with cross-sectional imaging. These include acute Budd–Chiari syndrome, hepatic veno-occlusive disease, and diffuse malignant infiltration. A "fulminant" first presentation of autoimmune liver disease can also present in this way and may have characteristic immunoglobulin and autoantibody changes.

Cholestatic Pattern of Liver Injury

Cholestatic liver injury is characterized by elevation in alkaline phosphatase (ALP) and gamma-glutamyl transferase (GGT), with or without the presence of elevated bilirubin. ALP has a plasma half-life of 72 hours and is released by the liver, but also by the kidney, bone, placenta, and ileum. GGT has a plasma half-life of 7–10 days, and is primarily secreted by cholangiocytes in the liver.

Cholestatic liver dysfunction typically has a more insidious onset than hypoxic hepatitis, usually manifest in a critically ill patient days after ICU admission, with progressive elevation of bilirubin, ALP, and GGT (Figure 4.2b). Investigation is hampered by a lack of universally accepted diagnostic criteria, but in clinical practice a bilirubin of over 2–3 mg/dl and ALP and GGT of two to three times normal may be accepted [4]. Overt mechanical obstruction of bile ducts is seldom the cause, although biliary "sludge" may be observed on hepatic imaging, cholestatic liver dysfunction is thought to result from critical illness-induced alteration of hepatobiliary transport mechanisms. Clinical risk factors for its development include sepsis, both through endotoxemia and the evoked inflammatory cytokine response, parenteral nutrition and hyperglycemia, and super-added drug-induced cholestasis (Box 4.3). A wide variety of drugs may be responsible (Figure 4.4).

Box 4.3   Principal Contributory Factors for Cholestatic Liver Injury in Critical Illness
• Drug-induced liver injury
• Parenteral nutrition
• Hyperglycemia
• Sepsis
• Systemic inflammation

A complex series of hepatobiliary transporter proteins exist to take up biliary components from the blood, traffic them through the hepatocyte and secrete them into the bile canaliculi. This tightly regulated process is markedly altered in critical illness where uptake transporters on the basolateral surface of the hepatocyte are downregulated and alternate export transport proteins upregulated, while transport proteins located on the apical canalicular surface are downregulated [3]. The net effect of these changes is reflected by increasing circulating levels of conjugated bile acids and bilirubin. Detrimental effects from cholestasis may include the modulation of intestinal flora and an increased release of endotoxin to the systemic circulation, and impairment of xenobiotic excretion with clinically important effects upon drug metabolism and handling.

Assessment of Severity of Liver Injury

Although the extent of elevation of hepatocellular and cholestatic enzymes and severity of jaundice may give indications of the nature and broad magnitude of liver injury, other laboratory markers may be better indicators of immediate hepatic synthetic and metabolic function and have greater prognostic utility.

International Normalized Ratio

With the exception of von Willebrand factor, all major proteins in the coagulation cascade are synthesized in the liver. The activity of the intrinsic coagulation pathway, including the actions of factors II, V, and X, can be assessed in the laboratory using the prothrombin time, standardized as the international normalized ratio (INR). As the half-lives of these factors are often only a few hours, reduction in their production resulting from impaired hepatic function can be reflected rapidly in changes in the INR. Its ready availability in most standard clinical laboratories and rapid determination make it a robust and practical measure to assess changes in liver synthetic function, and it is included in many systems for the assessment of prognosis in acute liver failure. Its interpretation is complicated by the administration of blood clotting products including fresh frozen plasma, and it may be prolonged by vitamin K deficiency or coumarin therapy. An increased INR does not necessarily reflect an increased bleeding tendency; when it results from liver injury as the balanced loss of hepatically synthesized pro- and anticoagulant factors may have a net neutral effect on functional coagulation status that is not evaluated by standard laboratory tests. Functional testing using viscoelastic methods such as thromboelastography are available as point-of-care tests in many critical care units, and may give a better reflection as to whether there is significant bleeding risk.

Lactate

Lactate concentration is usually tightly maintained at less than 2 mmol/l in arterial blood, although transient elevations may be seen after vigorous exercise. Persistent lactate elevation in critical illness is near universally associated with poor outcome. It may be rapidly measured using point-of-care testing (usually as part of a blood gas analysis) and, as such, is available in most critical care units. Its circulating concentration reflects the interaction of increased peripheral production from anaerobic metabolism resulting from tissue hypoperfusion, hypoxia or dysoxia from severe sepsis or systemic inflammation, with impaired clearance from the circulation. As the liver is the principal site of lactate metabolism, persistent hyperlactatemia after restoration of circulating volume and peripheral perfusion can be a sensitive marker of the magnitude of hepatic metabolic compromise and is an excellent indicator of illness severity and prognosis.

Ammonia

The liver is the principal site of ammonia clearance from the circulation, and ammonia is now recognized as having toxic effects on multiple tissues, including brain, muscle, and immune function. In acute liver failure, ammonia is the principal neurotoxin responsible for the development of encephalopathy and cerebral edema, and its circulating levels are closely related to the risks of encephalopathy and fatal intracranial hypertension. As such, it may serve a useful role in assessing the severity and likely consequences of acute hepatic injury and liver dysfunction. Its blood concentration may be measured both in standard biochemical laboratories, and in some critical care units using specialized point-of-care testing. The normal arterial blood concentration is less than 32 mmol/l. In the setting of acute liver dysfunction, any elevation should raise concern, with sustained levels greater than 150 mmol/l closely associated with the development of severe hepatic encephalopathy, and those greater than 200 mmol/l with a risk of symptomatic cerebral edema.

Albumin

Albumin is synthesized in the liver and is secreted solely by hepatocytes, with up to 25 g of albumin produced daily by the adult liver. In healthy individuals, its serum half-life is about 21 days. Albumin is part of the acute phase response, and concentrations often decrease with the onset of a major stress. In critical illness, low circulating levels may develop rapidly but are not necessarily an indicator of impaired hepatic synthetic function as they may also reflect altered vascular permeability, malnutrition, or hemodilution from intravenous fluid therapy, rather than hepatic dysfunction. It should not be relied upon as a measure of acute hepatic functional compromise.

Sequential Clinical Assessment

Liver functional compromise may change rapidly, and in some cases of severe acute hepatocellular necrosis this can be over the course of a few hours. When liver injury is first identified, a baseline assessment of severity of liver injury is required, using INR, blood lactate and glucose, and ammonia, if available. If there are concerns raised by these initial results, these tests should be repeated at four- to six-hourly intervals to assess the trajectory of liver functional compromise and response to supportive care. Clinical assessment is also key, and the presence of encephalopathy is of major importance, reflecting major functional impairment, and may require both specific clinical interventions and discussion with a liver unit.

Approach to Supportive Care

The basic approaches to the care of patients in intensive care in whom new liver dysfunction is identified are straightforward (Box 4.4).

1) Establish severity of hepatic functional compromise.
   Using both clinical assessment and the laboratory measures outlined above the magnitude of liver functional impairment and its trajectory are assessed. In this way, the urgency of interventions and/or need for referral to a specialist liver center can be determined.
2) Identify and treat cause of liver injury.
   Understanding the cause of liver injury is key, as in some etiologies specific therapies may limit or interrupt its development. A basic panel of investigations will include a paracetamol level and urgent screen for acute and chronic viral infection, imaging thorough ultrasound and/or cross-sectional imaging to exclude mechanical biliary obstruction, assess liver structure for possible underlying chronic liver disease and confirm hepatic vascular patency. Given the prevalence and importance of hypoxic hepatitis as a cause of hepatocellular injury in a critical care setting, the assessment of cardiac structure and function through echocardiography is mandatory for these patients. All medication is reviewed, and any potentially contributory agents discontinued. In patients with a hepatocellular pattern of liver injury and any suspicion of a contributory role of paracetamol-induced hepatotoxicity, intravenous NAC should be immediately commenced.
3) Establish physiologic stability.
   Steps are taken to achieve metabolic and hemodynamic stability: restoring adequate blood pressure and flows to improve systemic perfusion, and the correction of hypoxia,

---

Box 4.4 Approach to Supportive Care of Liver Injury in Intensive Care

- Establish severity of hepatic functional compromise
- Identify and treat cause of liver injury
- Establish physiologic stability
- Seek and treat sepsis.
- Minimize other secondary insults
- Discuss serious cases with a specialist liver unit

acid–base disturbance and electrolyte abnormalities. In doing so, the conditions for hepatic regeneration will be optimized.

4) Seek and treat sepsis.

Infection is common in patients with significant liver injury, and may act as a co-factor for injury and impair hepatic regeneration. Sepsis should be sought, and a low threshold for antimicrobial therapy should be maintained, with the proviso that any agent should not contribute to an increased risk of liver injury.

5) Minimize other secondary insults.

The steps above address factors identified as directly contributing to liver injury, but others may also be potential cofactors. General steps may include withdrawal of all non-essential medication and where possible parenteral nutrition should be discontinued. If possible, nutritional support should be delivered through the enteral route. Liver injury from parenteral nutrition is likely to be more common when the prescription results in overprovision of calories, lipids, or carbohydrates, and may be limited when its administration is cyclical and/or combined with enteral feeding.

Discussion with a Specialist Liver Unit

The great majority of patients who develop abnormal liver biochemical tests during ICU admission will have only minor abnormalities that will correct with minimal intervention and reflect the overall severity of critical illness. In general, discussion with a specialist liver unit will be required only for those where there are significant or unexplained abnormalities, most often associated with liver dysfunction and functional compromise. However, a low threshold should be maintained for contact with a liver center, especially where there is diagnostic uncertainty, as guidance can be offered on the interpretation of test results and further investigation and management. Transfer is required of only a very small minority of cases. The presence of significant liver dysfunction or associated extrahepatic organ failure are features of concern; the development of encephalopathy and the syndrome of acute liver failure mandates discussion as it within this category that liver transplantation may become a possible therapeutic option.

References

1. Kramer, L., Jordan, B., Druml, W. et al. (2007). Austrian epidemiologic study on intensive care ASG. Incidence and prognosis of early hepatic dysfunction in critically ill patients: a prospective multicenter study. *Crit. Care Med.* 35 (4): 1099–1104.
2. Bernal, W. and Quaglia, A. (2016). Normal physiology of the hepatic system. In: *Oxford Textbook of Critical Care*, 2e (ed. A. Webb, D.C. Angus, S. Finfer, et al.), 815–818. Oxford: Oxford University Press.
3. Jenniskens, M., Langouche, L., and Van den Berghe, G. (2018). Cholestatic alterations in the critically ill: some new light on an old problem. *Chest* 153 (3): 733–743.
4. Horvatits, T., Drolz, A., Trauner, M., and Fuhrmann, V. (2019). Liver injury and failure in critical illness. *Hepatology* 70 (6): 2204–2215.

5

Infections Affecting the Liver in the Immunosuppressed

Dinesh Jothimani, Radhika Venugopal, Srividya Manjunath, and Mohamed Rela

Dr. Rela Institute and Medical Centre, Chromepet, Chennai, India

---

KEY POINTS

- Many bacteria, viruses and other infectious agents may affect the liver.
- Clinical presentation of liver infections may vary from the standard mode depending on the host immunity.
- Clinicians should have a high index of suspicion of the inciting agent; a detailed history, including a travel, may guide diagnosis.
- Patients may require follow up despite complete resolution of infection to watch for occasional delayed complications and consideration of treatment if needed.
- Specialist guidance may be required in the clinical management of liver infections.

Introduction

The liver is constantly exposed to a wide variety of bacterial products, environmental and food toxins. Microorganisms escaping host immune control can directly or indirectly affect the liver, causing a wide variety of clinical manifestations ranging from asymptomatic enzyme elevations to acute liver failure or progressive liver fibrosis leading to cirrhosis.

The liver can be targeted by viruses, bacteria, fungi, and parasites (Table 5.1). Viruses that exclusively survive in the liver are called "hepatotropic." Hepatitis A (HAV) and E (HEV) cause acute hepatitis, whereas hepatitis B (HBV) and C (HCV) are associated with chronic hepatitis leading to long-term damage.

Systemic and non-hepatotropic viruses may cause abnormal elevation in liver function tests (LFTs). Understanding of the pathophysiology and pattern of injury by these organisms is essential in the management of such conditions. Hepatic injury may occur as a

The Liver in Systemic Disease: A Clinician's Guide to Abnormal Liver Tests, First Edition.
Edited by Gideon M. Hirschfield, Paramjit Gill, and James Neuberger.
© 2023 John Wiley & Sons Ltd. Published 2023 by John Wiley & Sons Ltd.

Table 5.1 Some infections affecting the liver in immunocompetent and immunocompromised patients.

Pattern of liver abnormality	Patients	
	Immunocompetent	Immunocompromised
Hyperbilirubinemia	Malaria, *Mycoplasma*	
Hepatitis		
Bacterial	*Salmonella*, *Leptospira*, *Brucella*, scrub typhus, Rocky Mountain spotted fever, Q fever, lyme disease	
Viral:		
Hepatotropic	HAV, HEV, HBV, HDV, HCV	HAV, HEV, HBV, HDV, HCV
Non-hepatotropic	HSV1, HSV2, EBV, CMV, VZV, HHV 6, dengue	HSV1, HSV2, EBV, CMV, VZV,HIV
Parasitic:		
Helminthic	Malaria	
Cholestatic	Tuberculosis	Atypical mycobacteria
	Fasciola hepatica, *Clonorchis sinensis*, biliary ascariasis	AIDS cholangiopathy: CMV, *Cryptospora*, *Isospora*
Granulomatous:		
Bacterial	Tuberculosis, *Yersinia*, melioidosis, nocardosis, brucellosis, *Bartonella*, chlamydia	Tuberculosis, *Mycobacterium avium* complex
Fungal		Histoplasmosis, coccidiomycosis, Blastomycosis, Candidiasis, aspergillosis, mucormycosis
Parasitic	Visceral leishmaniasis, schistosomiasis, visceral larva migrans, strongyloidiasis, giardiasis	
Portal hypertension	Schistosomiasis, *Fasciola hepatica*	
Liver abscess	*Entamoeba histolytica*, *Echinococcus granulomatosis*, hepatosplenic candidiasis	

result of direct invasion, mediated by toxins, or may be immunologically induced. An immunocompromised patient may react to an infection severely in comparison with an immunocompetent host. Various non-hepatotropic organisms implicated in liver injury are enumerated in Figure 5.1. There is a considerable geographical heterogeneity in these organisms across the world. Clinicians should be familiar with infectious agents in their

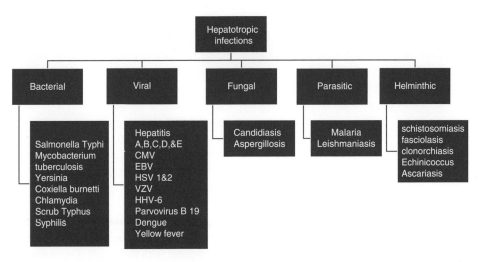

Figure 5.1 Non-hepatotropic organisms implicated in liver injury.

locality and should also be aware of infections in other parts of the world related to travel. Adequate clinical knowledge regarding this geographic variations is required to guide patient management.

Viral Infections

Hepatitis A

HAV is a single-stranded RNA virus belonging to the family Picornaviridae. It has six genotypes, of which genotypes 1–3 cause human infection. About 1.5 million people are infected with hepatitis A virus annually. Viral transmission occurs from person to person through oral–fecal route, usually through contaminated food and water. HAV causes acute necroinflammation in the liver, which usually resolves completely. However, between 3% and 20% of patients may encounter viral relapse in first few weeks following recovery. This relapse is marked by elevation in alanine amino transferase (ALT) and viremia and may last up to 24 weeks before complete resolution, particularly in the immunocompromised host. About 50% of patients with acute HAV infection are asymptomatic, others may present with cholestatic jaundice. HAV infection does not lead to chronic liver disease, but rarely cause life threatening fulminant liver failure characterised by jaundice, coagulopathy and hepatic encephalopathy. Detection of anti-HAV immunoglobulin (Ig) M is diagnostic of acute infection, and the occurrence of this antibody correlate with maximum rise in liver enzymes. The rise in aminotransferase levels precedes bilirubin increase and reduces prior to the resolution of jaundice.

Hepatitis E

HEV is a single-stranded RNA virus belonging to the family Hepeviridae, more common in India and surrounding countries. It has five major genotypes, of which genotypes 1 and 2 are human pathogens, and 3 and 4 are of swine origin causing zoonotic infections in humans. Similar to HAV, HEV is also transmitted through oral–fecal route, mostly through contaminated water (genotype 1 and 2); HEV related hepatitis is usually a self-limiting illness, but increasingly reported to cause chronic infection (persistent of HEV viremia beyond three months) in immunocompromised hosts. Chronic hepatitis E infection has been shown to cause allograft injury in solid-organ transplant recipients. The incubation period can vary from 15–60 days and patients become symptomatic about 3–4 weeks following infection. Aminotransferase elevations greater than 10–15 times the upper limit of normal (ULN) have been observed in patients with acute HEV infection; detection of anti-HEV IgM in the serum or the presence of HEV RNA is diagnostic, but the latter is not widely available. Aminotransferase elevation may persist for up to three months. The incidence of HEV is high in pregnant women and are associated with acute liver failure particularly in the third trimester leading to maternal and fatal mortality. ALF has been reported in 0.5-4% of patients with a case fatality rate of up to 4%. Acute HEV infection may precipitate acute on chronic liver failure (ACLF) in patients with pre-existing liver disease. Because of the self-limiting nature of the disease treatment of acute HEV infection is usually supportive. Ribavirin is widely used in the management of HEV infection in the immunocompromised patient Sofosbuvir has been shown to be effective in chronic HEV infection in patients where Ribavirin is ineffective, but no large data. Reduction in immunosuppression drug levels is recommended in solid organ transplant recipients.

Hepatitis B

HBV is a double-stranded incomplete DNA virus belonging to the family Hepadnaviridae. Its transmission is through blood or body fluids of infected individuals in the West, and by perinatal transmission in the East. HBV infection is mostly asymptomatic, and persistence of hepatitis B surface antigen (HBsAg) for longer than six months is considered chronic. The Presence of hepatitis B envelope antigen (HBeAg) or HBV DNA indicates active viral replication. The majority of acute hepatitis B infection acquired in the adulthood resolves unlike those acquired during childhood. It is important to monitor those with acute HBV infection to ensure complete HBsAg clearance followed by development of protective anti-has antibody titres Failure of viral clearance may lead to chronic infection and may cause cirrhosis and liver cell cancer. Those who remain HBsAg positive for six months or longer should be referred to an appropriate virologist or hepatologist, as effective antiviral therapy using drugs such as entecavir or tenofovir may be required. It is important that contacts and family members are screened and vaccinated if HBsAg negative. Those who have cleared HBV infection are still at risk of viral reactivation in the presence of suppressed immunity such as following organ transplantation, those or if receiving chemotherapeutic drugs because of the presence of covalently closed circular HBV DNA remains within the hepatocytes.

Hepatitis C

HCV is a single-stranded RNA virus belonging to the family Flaviviridae. It comprises six genotypes. HCV accounts for about 15–20% of all acute hepatitis. Primary HCV infection is usually asymptomatic, and is characterized by non-specific symptoms such as nausea, fatigue, and low-grade fever, with no clinically evident jaundice. HCV viremia can occur even without elevations in liver enzymes. Acute HCV infection is diagnosed when HCV RNA is detectable in the absence of HCV antibody in a person with recent high-risk exposure. Approximately 20% of those who present with acute HCV infections have spontaneous clearance within six months. ALT levels fluctuate during the acute phase, but other causes should be considered, such as alcohol toxicity, HBV co-infection, and drug-induced liver injury. Persistence of HCV RNA beyond six months is considered to be a chronic HCV infection. Around 50–80% of patients with acute hepatitis develop chronic HCV infection, and 15–40% clear the infection spontaneously. Chronic HCV is an indolent infection, leading on to cirrhosis of the liver in 20% of patients and hepatocellular carcinoma, at a rate of 4–5% a year in those with cirrhosis. Around 10–40% of patients with chronic HCV will have normal ALT levels. Patients with chronic HCV infection should be treated with direct acting anti-viral therapy if RNA positive. With the current generation antiviral therapy, the viral clearance or sustained virological response rate has improved to 99%. Patients with advanced liver disease due to chronic hepatitis C infection should be managed in a specialist liver centre.

Yellow Fever

Yellow fever is a zoonotic disease caused by a flavivirus spread by *Aedes aegypti*, the yellow fever mosquito. It causes viral hemorrhagic fever and may present with jaundice. Over 90% of cases are reported from Africa and the remainder from South American countries. Clinical manifestations range from asymptomatic infections (5–50%) to multisystem involvement (20%). The disease process occurs in three phases.

The first phase lasts for three to six days, with peaking of the viral load manifesting as fever, chills, nausea, and vomiting. Elevated transaminases with leucopenia is often the laboratory finding. The majority of patients recover completely over the next 48 hours with long-term immunity.

About 15–20% of patients may develop an "intoxication" phase characterized by abdominal pain, jaundice, bleeding tendencies due to coagulopathy, and renal failure. These patients have elevated transaminase levels in proportion to the disease severity. Aspartate amino transferase (AST) levels are higher than ALT because of cardiac and skeletal muscle involvement. Non-survivors were found to have much higher AST and ALT levels compared with survivors. There is a mortality of 20–50%. A direct viral cytopathic effect on hepatocytes and ischemia contribute to liver injury, together with host cytokine dysregulation. Histopathology of the liver shows hepatic necrosis in mid-zones sparing the portal and central veins. The infected hepatocytes undergo apoptosis, which is characterized by eosinophilic condensed chromatin, called councilman bodies. The diagnosis is by IgG and IgM enzyme-linked immunosorbent assay (ELISA). There are no specific treatments available.

Dengue

Dengue is a vector-borne disease prevalent in tropical and subtropical regions of world. It is one of the major public health concerns, as it results in multisystem involvement leading to multiorgan dysfunction. Although the liver is not the main target organ, widespread hepatic injury has been reported in dengue infection, particularly in severe cases. Fever, abdominal pain, anorexia, and nausea, together with hepatomegaly, are common clinical features. LFTs may show modest elevation in up to 80% of patients, with AST or ALT two or more times ULN, usually around day 5–7, which normalizes in three weeks. Elevated bilirubin may occur in up to 20% of patients. Rarely, dengue fever can present as acute liver failure with ALT greater than 1000 iu/l, hyperbilirubinemia, coagulopathy, and encephalopathy, particularly noted in children.Patients with solid organ transplants may develop a lower frequency of fever and two thirds may have allograft dysfunction. Immunocompromised host may develop severe disease with more thrombocytopenia and higher mortality (37.5% vs 5%) in comparison to immunocompetent host. Most cases of liver injury recover with supportive care.

Epstein–Barr Virus

Epstein–Barr virus (EBV) is gamma herpes virus replicates, primarily in nasopharyngeal epithelial cells and B lymphocytes. More than 95% of population worldwide is infected with EBV and about 50% acquire the infection before the age of five years. Most EBV infections are asymptomatic or mildly symptomatic. Around 75% of adolescents and young adults develop clinical manifestations of infectious mononucleosis, characterized by fever, sore throat, and lymphadenopathy. Liver involvement ranges from a mild hepatitis to clinically evident jaundice with hepatosplenomegaly, and rarely acute liver failure. EBV hepatitis can occur without clinical features of infectious mononucleosis in the immunocompromised patient, where it is characterized by a febrile illness. Only 5% have clinically evident jaundice. Up to 60% have mild elevation in alkaline phosphatase and 45% have elevated bilirubin. In EBV hepatitis, ALT levels rarely exceed 1000 iu/l and, characteristically, patients have a lymphocytosis greater than 5×10^9/l, which helps to differentiate EBV infections from other causes of viral hepatitis.

Liver histology shows sinusoidal infiltration of mononuclear cells and ballooning of hepatocytes with vacuolization. Chronic active EBV infection may lead to lymphoproliferative disorders, especially in patients who are immunocompromised post-transplant. Up to 30% of patients develop post-transplant lymphoproliferative disease; the risk depends on age, type of graft, and the degree and type of immunosuppression.

Cytomegalovirus

Human cytomegalovirus (CMV) is a beta-herpes virus. It usually causes asymptomatic or subclinical infection in adults who are immunocompetent. Primary CMV is acquired in early childhood and the virus may remain latent in myeloid cell lineage. The virus may reactivate with reduced immunity as in patients post-transplant or those with acquired immunodeficiency syndrome. The mononucleosis-like illness in immunocompetent hosts is associated with elevations in AST level in 90% of patients. However, only 2.8% had bilirubin levels above 2.0 g/dl. The incidence of CMV hepatitis varies from 2% to 34% in post-transplant patients, depending on the donor recipient serostatus, use of antiviral prophylaxis, and immunosuppressive regimen.

Herpes Simplex Virus

Hepatic involvement of herpes simplex virus (HSV) is rare, except in the immunocompromised hosts, where HSV infection is disseminated disease and occasionally acute liver failure. Clinical presentation includes fever, abdominal pain, hepatomegaly (reported in up to 50% of patients), and abnormal LFTs in about 70% of patients. Aminotransferase can be greater than 100 times ULN with no or minimal rise in bilirubin. The presence of fever, leukopenia, thrombocytopenia, and markedly elevated liver enzymes, with normal bilirubin in an immunocompromised host should raise a suspicion of HSV hepatitis, where early initiation of treatment with antiviral therapy is associated with improved survival.

Other Viral Infections

Many other viruses can infect the live,r and abnormalities of liver function are seen with agents such as influenza virus. Recently, there has been an interest in liver abnormalities associated with COVID-19 (SARS-Cov-19). Up to 60% of patients develop various degrees of liver damage. Hepatic involvement in COVID-19 could be related to the direct cytopathic effect of the virus, an uncontrolled immune reaction, sepsis or drug-induced liver injury. The postulated mechanism of viral entry is through the host angiotensin-converting enzyme 2 (ACE2) receptors that are abundantly present in type 2 alveolar cells. ACE2 receptors are also expressed in the gastrointestinal tract, vascular endothelium, and cholangiocytes of the liver. The effects of COVID-19 are uncertain. The degree of liver test disturbance correlates with mortality.

Bacterial and Parasitic Infections

Enteric Fever

Enteric fever caused by *Salmonella typhi* is a common systemic infection seen mainly in tropical and subtropical regions. Symptoms commence one to two weeks after acquiring the infection, and have non-specific clinical manifestations such headache, leukopenia, and hepatosplenomegaly. Hepatic involvement in enteric fever may occur either though hematogenous seedling during bacteremic phase, or through infection of the reticuloendothelial system. Jaundice is seen in up to 18% of patients with enteric fever. However, there may be liver abnormalities even in the absence of jaundice in up to two thirds. Serum AST is usually higher than the ALT.

Hepatic involvement may develop in the second or third week of the illness, presenting as an acute hepatitis. An ALT/LDH ratio less than 4.0 favors enteric fever, whereas a ratio greater than 5.0 in acute viral hepatitis.

Diagnosis is established by positive blood cultures. Bone-marrow cultures remain positive for longer duration. Treatment includes fluroquinolones or third-generation cephalosporins for 7–10 days. Liver involvement does not require specific treatment and warrants only supportive therapy.

Brucellosis

Brucellosis is commonly caused by *Brucella melitensis*, a Gram-negative diplococcus, which spreads by either aerosols or direct contact with infected animals. Fever, chills, and constitutional symptoms are the common presenting symptoms. Hepatomegaly with elevated aminotransferases occurs in about 20–40% of patients. Jaundice is a rare occurrence. *Brucella* hepatitis has a mild clinical course and no cases of acute liver failure have been reported. *Brucella suis* infection can cause hepatic abscesses. Diagnosis is made by serum agglutination assays with a titer greater than1/160. Blood culture has a sensitivity of 15–70%, but bone-marrow cultures have higher sensitivity. *Brucella* hepatitis does not require specific therapy and is usually self-limiting. Brucellosis is treated with doxycycline for six weeks, with or without rifampicin for six weeks, or streptomycin for two weeks.

Leptospirosis

Leptospirosis is a zoonotic disease caused by spirochetes of the genus *Leptospira*. Disease transmission occurs by contact with urine of infected animals, such as rodents. Leptospirosis runs a biphasic course, where the first phase is characterized by non-specific symptoms such as fever, headache, and myalgia. In the second phase of illness over 90% of cases are anicteric. About 5–10% have a severe icteric form known as Weil's disease or icterohemorrhagic fever with multiorgan involvement. Liver involvement is characterized by elevation of transaminases of about two to three times ULN, AST greater than ALT. There is mild increase in alkaline phosphatase, and serum bilirubin may rise up to 30–40 mg/dl. An AST/ALT ratio greater than three indicates a poor prognosis, also associated with severe coagulopathy as a result of immune complex mediated endothelial injury and thrombocytopenia. Liver histology shows non-specific changes with mild periportal hepatitis, hepatocanalicular cholestasis, and an increase in mitotic activity suggesting regenerative changes and no necrosis. Diagnosis is by ELISA for IgG and IgM antibodies, positive agglutination tests and polymerase chain reaction (PCR). Mild cases are treated with oral doxycycline or amoxicillin, severe cases require parenteral penicillin or third-generation cephalosporins.

Syphilis

Syphilis is a rare sexually transmitted disease caused by *Treponema pallidum*. The disease progresses through primary secondary and tertiary stages. Liver involvement occurs commonly in early syphilis, where over one third with early syphilis and up to half with secondary syphilis have abnormal aminotransferase levels. A few may develop syphilitic hepatitis, which is characterized by mild elevation of aminotransferases and marked rise in alkaline phosphatase and gamma-glutamyl transferase (GGT). However hepatic involvement during different stages of syphilis is very rare in the antibiotic era. Treatment with penicillin may sometimes trigger a Jarisch–Herxheimer reaction, resulting in jaundice, fever, chills, and rash. The incidence of syphilis is higher in patients with HIV infection should be borne in mind when treating patients infected with HIV with elevated liver enzymes. Liver histology is characterized by bile duct inflammatory infiltration and hepatic granuloma.

Lyme Disease, Q Fever, Rocky Mountain Spotted Fever

Lyme disease is caused by *Borrelia burgdorferi* and is the most common vector-borne disease in North America and Europe. Hepatic involvement occurs in 20% of patients, and is characterized by elevated AST, ALT, and GGT. Borrelia hepatitis is usually detected as an incidental asymptomatic enzyme elevation. Histopathology shows granulomatous hepatitis.

Q fever is a zoonotic disease caused by *Coxiella burnetti*. Infection occurs after inhaling infectious particles. Q fever hepatitis is seen commonly in younger patients in high-risk areas. About 50% show involvement of the liver and clinically manifest as anicteric hepatitis with elevated liver enzymes of up to two to three times ULN. The diagnosis of hepatic involvement is often made retrospectively, by immunofluorescent assays, and treatment is with doxycycline for 10–14 days. The disease may be asymptomatic in pregnant women and may be associated with a poor fetal outcome. Early treatment will help to prevent cardiac damage, such as endocarditis and valvular damage.

Rocky mountain spotted fever is caused by *Rickettsia rickettsii* and liver involvement is clinically manifested as jaundice.

Tuberculosis

Hepatic tuberculosis (TB) occurs as a consequence of hematogenous dissemination of the bacillus or by local spread from the gastrointestinal. The miliary form accounts for 79% cases, and the hepatic form 21%; however, biliary TB is rare. Hepatic TB was more frequently observed in patients with HIV/AIDS compared with immunocompetent individuals. Miliary hepatic TB is characterized by diffuse seeding of the liver with tubercles 0.6–2.0 mm in diameter in the hepatic lobules. Dissemination is via the hepatic artery from a lung focus. Interestingly, tubercles greater than 2 mm disseminate to the liver via the portal vein, usually from a gastrointestinal focus. Patients may present with fever, pain abdomen, weight loss, cough, and ascites. Jaundice is more common in hepatic TB compared with military TB. LFTs show an infiltrative pattern, with elevated alkaline phosphatase and GGT, and occasional elevation of transaminases, with mild elevation of bilirubin. These patients also have albumin–globulin reversal.

In miliary hepatic TB, computed tomography (CT) may reveal hepatomegaly without nodular intrahepatic lesions, abdominal lymphadenopathy with peripheral lymph node enhancement and/or calcifications. On the other hand, hepatic TB appears on CT as one large solitary nodule or two to three low-density nodules. Liver biopsy with mycobacterial culture is the most specific test for establishment of diagnosis. Treatment is with antitubercular therapy for one year. Treatment requires specialist advice and management.

Schistosomiasis

Schistosomiasis is a parasitic infection caused by blood fluke trematodes known as schistosomes. There are 200 million people worldwide with schistosomiasis, of whom 60% have symptomatic disease and 20 million suffer from severe disease [1]. All four species except *Schistosoma haematobium* cause hepatic involvement. Clinical presentation of schistosomiasis may vary from asymptomatic infection, self-limited dermatitis, acute, and chronic schistosomiasis. Acute infection manifests as Katayama fever, and some have hepatomegaly in this phase. Chronic disease is characterized by granulomas and hepatosplenomegaly due to egg deposition in portal venules, which subsequently manifest as pipestem fibrosis with preserved hepatocyte functions.

Malaria

Malaria is a protozoal infection caused by one of the four species of the genus *Plasmodium*. It is a vector-borne disease common in tropical countries where anopheles mosquitoes flourish. The disease classically has two phases: the hepatic phase, at the end of which the hepatocytes rupture to release mature merozoites, and erythrocytic phase for erythrocytic schizogony. Some 60% of patients with falciparum or vivax malaria have hepatosplenomegaly. Clinically evident jaundice is more common in falciparum malaria and is seen in up to half of patients. Both unconjugated and conjugated hyperbilirubinemia may occur, as jaundice may be a result of hepatocellular dysfunction, intravascular hemolysis, septicemia, disseminated intravascular coagulation, or antimalarial drug induced. Diagnosis is by thick and thin peripheral smears or immunological assays. Treatment depends on the species of infection and the prevalence of drug resistance in that geographical area. Chloroquine is the usual drug of choice for treatment, and primaquine for eradication of hepatic hypnozoites.

Fungal Infections

Fungal infections can involve the liver, either as a part of opportunistic infection in an immunocompromised host, or as an endemic infection in a normal host. The liver maybe involved as a part of disseminated infection, together with renal, pulmonary, cardiac, and neurological involvement.

Candida

Candida species are the most common cause of invasive fungal infections, especially in oncohematologic and immunosuppressed patients. *Candida albicans* is the leading cause of invasive fungal infections, followed by *Candida glabrata*, *Candida Parapsilosis*, *Candida krusei,* and *Candida tropicalis*. Hepatosplenic candidiasis is a type of chronic disseminated candidiasis, occurring in those with prolonged neutropenia (> 10 days) during the recovery phase. Clinical features include persistent fever, nausea, abdominal pain, tenderness, and jaundice. LFTs may show higher elevation of alkaline phosphatase compared with transaminases and GGT. The organism is less frequently isolated from blood cultures. Abdominal imaging with a CT or magnetic resonance imaging in the arterial phase may show hyperattenuating rim surrounding a hypoattenuating center, giving a "bullseye" appearance, and formation of microabscesses. Echinocandins are the drugs of choice in the treatment of invasive candidiasis (caspofungin, micafungin, anidulafungin).

Other infections caused by *Candida* in the setting of liver disease include the complication of hepatic abscess in patients with chronic granulomatous disease, spontaneous fungal peritonitis in liver cirrhosis and in hepatic abscess post-liver transplant (non-albicans).

Candida can also colonize the biliary tract, especially in patients with primary sclerosing cholangitis. *C. albicans* and *C. glabrata* have been reported to complicate cholecystitis in diabetic and immunosuppressed patients.

Aspergillosis

Invasive aspergillosis is caused most commonly by *Aspergillus fumigatus*, and carries a high risk of death (50–70%). The disease may affect those with hematologic malignancies, stem-cell transplant recipients, solid-organ transplant recipients, patients treated with prolonged corticosteroid therapy, tumor necrosis factor alpha antagonists and long-term patients in intensive care units. Although pulmonary infections are most common, extrapulmonary sites such as gastrointestinal tract and liver may also be involved. Hepatic pathologic findings include abscess formation, infarction, intrahepatic hemorrhage, and infiltration of hyphae in the liver parenchyma. Diagnosis is established by a positive beta galactomannan assay in the serum or bronchoalveolar lavage PCR assay. Early initiation of antifungal treatment is key for amelioration. The drug of choice is voriconazole or amphotericin B.

Histoplasmosis

Histoplasmosis is caused by *Histoplasma capsulatum*, an endemic mycosis seen in North and South America, Latin America, and China. However, it can also present as an opportunistic infection in those with immunosuppressed states, like HIV. Primarily a pulmonary disease, the liver is often involved as a part of disseminated disease, especially in an immune compromised patient. Clinical presentation includes fever, anorexia, weight loss, hepatosplenomegaly, pallor, lymphadenopathy, and skin rash. Laboratory investigations may show pancytopenia, elevated erythrocyte sedimentation rate, and lung nodules. LFTs may reveal elevated alkaline phosphatase. Diagnosis is established by antigen detection, culture or biopsy. Drug of choice is either amphotericin B and itraconazole.

Blastomycosis

Blastomycosis is an infection caused by the dimorphic fungi *Blastomycosis dermatitidis* and *Blastomycosis gilchristii*. Infection is acquired by inhalation and can cause primary pneumonia central nervous system, cutaneous or disseminated disease affecting the liver. As with *Histoplasma*, the organism can affect healthy and immunocompromised patients (HIV, steroid, anti-tumor necrosis factore therapy, etc.).

Cryptococcosis

Cryptococcosis is an encapsulated yeast, of which *Cryptococcus neoformans* and *Cryptococcus gatti* produce disease in humans. There is higher risk of infection in those with malignancy, solid-organ transplantation and HIV/AIDS (CD4 < 100/µl). *Cryptococcus* predominantly causes central nervous system and pulmonary infections; however, other organs may be involved as a part of disseminated disease. Hepatic cryptococcosis is usually seen in immunocompromised host. Liver biopsy shows granuloma with yeast like organisms.

Conclusion

The liver is constantly exposed to gut-derived and bloodborne pathogens and functions as an immunological barrier to a variety of viruses, bacteria, and other microorganisms. It is not uncommon to develop hepatic derangement following these infections. It is important to distinguish deranged liver function secondary to hepatotropic from the systemic infection, because the treatment may vary in these scenarios. In addition, a detailed history including travel, drug intake, and high exposure is mandatory as a guide to identifying the infective cause. Infections attributable to the local geographic location should be borne in mind by the treating clinician. A prompt identification will enable initiation of appropriate treatment to curtail disease severity.

Reference

1. Chitsulo, L., Loverde, P., and Engels, D. (2004). Schistosomiasis. *Nat. Rev. Microbiol.* 2 (1): 12–13.

Further Reading

Aslan, A.T. and Balaban, H.Y. (2020). Hepatitis E virus: epidemiology, diagnosis, clinical manifestations, and treatment. *World J. Gastroenterol.* 26 (37): 5543–5560.

Djokic, V., Rocha, S.C., and Parveen, N. (2021). Lessons learned for pathogenesis, immunology, and disease of erythrocytic parasites: plasmodium and babesia. *Front. Cell. Infect. Microbiol.* 11: 685239.

Jothimani, D., Venugopal, R., Abedin, M.F. et al. (2020). COVID-19 and the liver. *J. Hepatol.* 73 (5): 1231–1240.

Manns, M.P., Buti, M., Gane, E. et al. (2017). Hepatitis C virus infection. *Nat. Rev. Dis Primers* 3: 17006.

Nguyen, M.H., Wong, G., Gane, E. et al. (2020). Hepatitis B virus: advances in prevention, diagnosis, and therapy. *Clin. Microbiol. Rev.* 33 (2): e00046-19.

Seto, W.K., Lo, Y.R., Pawlotsky, J.M., and Yuen, M.F. (2018). Chronic hepatitis B virus infection. *Lancet* 392 (10161): 2313–2324.

6

The Postoperative Patient

Louise China and Douglas Thorburn

Royal Free London NHS Foundation Trust, London, UK

KEY POINTS

- Abnormalities of liver tests are common after surgery and, in most cases, do not require changes in management.
- Clinical, serological investigations, and imaging will usually enable a cause of deranged liver tests to be identified.
- Common causes of deranged liver tests include drug-induced liver injury (DILI), ischemic insults, infections, and sepsis.
- Occasionally, abnormalities of liver tests post-surgery may be the first manifestation of pre-existing liver disease.

Introduction

Abnormality in liver function tests (LFTs) is a common situation encountered in patients who have recently undergone surgery. Many of these patients do not have primary liver disease, as most of the commonly performed markers labeled "LFTs" are not specific for the liver and are affected by many factors unrelated to the liver. Also, many of these tests (like liver enzyme levels) do not measure the function of the liver, but are markers of liver injury, which is broadly of two types: hepatocellular and cholestatic. A combination of a careful history and clinical examination, together with interpretation of pattern of liver test abnormalities, can often identify the type of liver injury or etiology of liver disease, allowing for focused investigation (Figure 6.1).

Most postoperative patients with abnormal LFTs will have no symptoms in relation to their liver. Most commonly the test abnormalities will be iatrogenic and caused by the surgery, its complications or the supportive care before or after surgery. Sometimes, patients manifest an underlying pre-existing liver disease in the postoperative period. For example, a patient with compensated liver cirrhosis and previously normal blood tests may

The Liver in Systemic Disease: A Clinician's Guide to Abnormal Liver Tests, First Edition.
Edited by Gideon M. Hirschfield, Paramjit Gill, and James Neuberger.

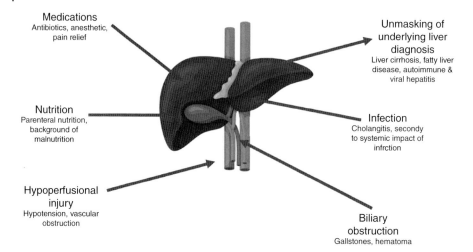

Figure 6.1 Common hepatic causes of abnormal liver function tests after surgery.

decompensate with ascites or hepatic encephalopathy in the postoperative period. Taking a careful history from the patient, their general practitioner, and reviewing preoperative blood tests may allow distinction between these problems.

There should be a low threshold for discussing abnormal LFTs with the local gastroenterology or hepatology team after an initial history has been sought, with differentials considered.

Common Liver Problems Associated with the Postoperative Patient

Common Postoperative Causes of a Predominant Hepatocellular Injury

Common postoperative causes of a predominant hepatocellular injury will usually present with a predominant rise in alanine amino transferase (ALT) and aspartate amino transferase (AST). Depending on the severity of the injury the bilirubin and international normalized ratio (INR)/prothrombin time (PT) can also be deranged [1].

Drug-Induced Liver Injury
DILI can be classified according to the pattern of liver tests observed (hepatocellular, cholestatic, or mixed) [2]. Amoxicillin–clavulanate is the most common drug implicated in DILI and is commonly used in the postoperative setting. Other drugs commonly responsible for DILI that are used in postoperative patients are listed in Table 6.1. Timing of onset of LFT abnormality varies and can occur within days or sometimes weeks post-medication introduction.

Vascular Liver Injury
Ischemic hepatitis, caused by liver hypoperfusion, is most commonly caused by a systemic hypotensive episode with rapid onset of liver enzyme abnormalities after the event. There is usually a large rise in serum ALT and AST, which peaks at 25–250 times the upper limit

Table 6.1 Common postoperative medications causing drug induced liver injury.

Type of drug	Common example
Antibiotics	Co-amoxiclav, flucloxacillin
Halogenated anesthetic agents	Halothane (pediatrics)
Pain relief	Paracetamol, non-steroidal anti-inflammatory drugs
Cardiac	Amiodarone

of normal (ULN) within one to three days of the hypotensive event. Less frequently, raised serum bilirubin and alkaline phosphatase (ALP) are observed and to a much lesser extent (two to four time the ULN). In the absence of continuing hypotension, liver enzymes usually return to normal within 7–10 days, with AST falling first due to its shorter half-life. Rarely, hepatic synthetic function is impaired.

Rarer forms of perfusional liver injury, which may be seen in the postoperative setting, are:

- *Hepatic infarction* represents a focal ischemic injury to the liver and typically results from an occlusion of a single branch of the hepatic artery. Inadvertent ligation of the hepatic artery (usually right) has been described after laparoscopic cholecystectomy.
- *Prothrombotic vascular occlusion* usually happens in patients who have a hypercoagulable state or in patients undergoing hepatic surgery.
- *Congestion due to cardiac failure*: any cause of right-sided heart failure can result in hepatic congestion and should be considered in patients with pre-existing heart conditions that could deteriorate postoperatively or in those who are undergoing cardiac surgery.

Blood-Transmitted Viral Infection

This is rare but it is possible for hepatitis viruses (A/B/C/E), cytomegalovirus, Epstein–Barr virus, and herpes viruses to cause a hepatocellular injury, and should be considered during discussions with the gastroenterology and virology team in unexplained cases.

Common Postoperative Causes of a Predominantly Cholestatic Injury

This category of liver problems will usually present with a predominant rise in ALP (with or without bilirubin). Depending on the severity of the injury, the bilirubin and INR/PT may also be elevated.

Intrahepatic Cholestatic Injury

- *Drugs.*
- *Parenteral nutrition*: the use of excessive amounts of calories is the largest risk factor for liver dysfunction [3].
- *Infiltrative disease*: most commonly lymphoma.
- *Sepsis*: the etiology of sepsis-induced cholestatic liver injury is likely to be multifactorial, resulting from hypoperfusion, drugs, and systemic inflammation.

Extrahepatic Cholestasis
- *Choledocholithiasis*: common bile duct obstruction can occur with retained stones post-cholecystectomy. Mirizzi syndrome occurs when an acutely inflamed gallbladder containing stones compresses the common hepatic duct.
- *External compression*: postoperatively, this could be with hematoma or a focal collection. Other possible causes in a surgical patient are malignancy and pancreatitis (usually in the setting of a pseudocyst).
- *Biliary strictures* would not usually present themselves in the initial postoperative period apart from in the setting of liver transplantation. Distal bile duct stricture may present in the setting of chronic pancreatitis.
- *Biliary injury* is a rare cause if LFTs alone are abnormal; it usually presents with focal peritonitis.
- *Following gallbladder surgery*: retained stones can cause jaundice post-cholecystectomy.

Unmasking Underlying Chronic Liver Conditions

Liver Cirrhosis

Patients with well-compensated liver cirrhosis (no ascites, jaundice, or hepatic encephalopathy) can have normal blood tests and not be aware of their underlying condition [4]. The stress of a general anesthetic, surgical procedure, new medications, and postoperative infection can precipitate the first episode of decompensation. This may begin with blood test abnormalities (usually a high bilirubin, low albumin, and prolonged INR/PT) and can manifest clinically as:

- *New ascites with or without peripheral edema*: in patients with abdominal drains postoperatively, liver cirrhosis may go unnoticed for some days, with unexplained high serous drain output. Drain fluid analysis (protein, white cell count, bilirubin) can help to differentiate (Table 6.2) [5].

Table 6.2 Drain fluid analysis in postoperative patients with deranged liver function tests.

	Cirrhosis/portal HTN	Cirrhosis/portal HTN (+SBP)	Heart failure	Malignancy	Pancreatitis	Bile leak
WCC $(n)^a$	Low (<100)	> 250 neutrophils	Low (<100)	Low or ↑ lymphocyte	Low or ↑ lymphocyte	↑ (all)
Protein (g/dl)	<3	Low (<2)	Usually >2 but <3	>3	>3	>3
SAAG $(g/dl)^{a,b}$	>11	>11	>11	<11	<11	<11
Bilirubin	<serum bilirubin	<serum bilirubin	<serum bilirubin	<serum bilirubin	<serum bilirubin	>serum bilirubin
Amylase (u/l)	<100	<100	<100	<100	>100	>100

SAAG, serum albumin ascites gradient; WCC, white cell count.
[a] A reactive lymphocytosis is common in any abdominal drain fluid.
[b] Serum albumin minus ascites albumin.

- *Hepatic encephalopathy*: in its milder forms, the mild disorientation may be difficult to distinguish from other causes of postoperative obtundation. Hepatic encephalopathy can be exacerbated by opiate drugs and constipation in the postoperative period. The diagnosis is usually made by excluding other factors and making a diagnosis of underlying liver disease with portal hypertension. Occasionally, blood ammonia can contribute to supporting a diagnosis, but it is not diagnostic and levels are often raised with other medical problems in an unwell postoperative patient. Sometimes, electroencephalography will show characteristic features but it is rarely performed in this context.
- *Portal hypertensive bleeding* usually manifests as overt hematemesis or melena rather than a gradual hemoglobin drop.

Non-Alcoholic Fatty Liver Disease

Non-alcoholic fatty liver disease (NAFLD) is a very common disorder that occurs secondary to fat accumulation in the liver in the absence of alcohol misuse [6]. Overweight individuals with the metabolic syndrome are most commonly affected, but it may be seen in other conditions such as diabetes mellitus. The disorder covers a wide spectrum and can range from simple fat infiltration with or without mild LFT abnormalities in patients with advanced fibrosis or decompensated cirrhosis.

In the postoperative period, patients who may have previously undiagnosed mild NAFLD are more susceptible to liver injury from postoperative insults, such as drugs and hypoperfusion.

Autoimmune and Metabolic Liver Disease

Autoimmune and metabolic liver disease may be present, previously undiagnosed, in younger patients, but it would be very rare for the diagnosis to be made in the postoperative period.

Approach to Abnormal Liver Function Tests in the Postoperative Patient

The following approach to abnormal LFTs in the postoperative patient can be taken (Figure 6.2):

- What were the LFTs preoperatively (or preadmission)? Is this a new problem?
- Is the pattern an isolated abnormality with one test? (Is it a liver problem at all?)
- Is the picture more hepatic (ALT/AST rise) or cholestatic (ALP/bilirubin)?
- What are the risk factors for liver problems:
  - prehospital (e.g. alcohol, obesity)?
  - hospital: underlying pathology being treated, type of surgery, new drugs, episodes of hypotension, thrombosis?
- What is the trend in the deterioration of the blood tests:
  - days/weeks?
  - rate of rise?
  - fluctuation in association with risk factors (e.g. drugs or infection)?
  - how abnormal are the tests (compared with ULN)?

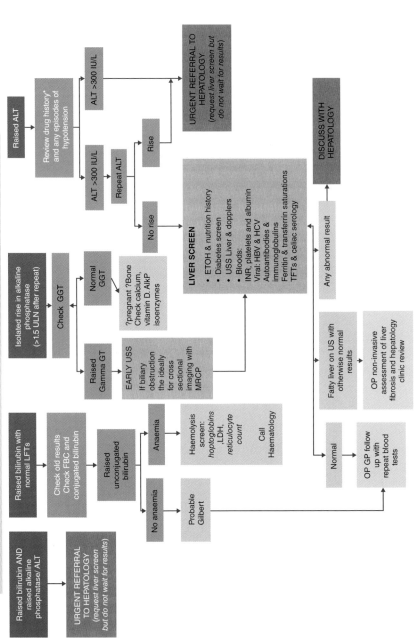

Figure 6.2 Approach to diagnostic evaluation of abnormal liver function tests after surgery. AlkP, alkaline phosphatase; ALT, alanine amino transferase; ETOH, ethanol; FBC, full blood count; GGT, gamma-glutamyl transferase; GP, general practitioner; HBV, hepatitis B virus; HCV, hepatitis C virus; INR, international normalized ratio; LFTs, liver function tests; OP, outpatient; TFTs, thyroid function tests; USS, ultrasound scan

- What are the markers of severity:
  - synthetic dysfunction: albumin, clotting?
  - acute liver injury: glucose, pH, lactate?
- Are there any physical manifestations of advanced chronic liver disease:
  - clinical jaundice?
  - ascites?
  - liver flap or confusion that may be hepatic encephalopathy?

Imaging the Liver When Liver Function Tests are Deranged Postoperatively

Ultrasound
In a stable patient with deranged LFTs, ultrasound is nearly always the first-line imaging modality. It should be conducted urgently if biliary obstruction is a possibility (cholestatic tests). Doppler flow assessment of the portal and hepatic veins is essential if there is concern about vascular obstruction.

Computed Tomography
In a deteriorating patient, computed tomography with contrast (arterial and venous phase) will provide more detailed information about extrahepatic organs, possible bleeding, and perfusion of the liver. Renal function needs to be considered and should be discussed with radiology and renal teams if there is concern.

Magnetic Resonance Cholangiopancreatography
Magnetic resonance cholangiopancreatography is the modality of choice (usually after ultrasound) if a more detailed delineation of the biliary system is required; for example, in suspected retained gallbladder stones or biliary strictures.

Technetium^{99m} Hepatobiliary Iminodiacetic Acid
Technetium^{99m} hepatobiliary iminodiacetic acid radionuclide imaging, or HIDA, involves tracers taken up by hepatocytes and excreted into biliary system. This modality is rarely used in the acute setting. It can be useful in bile leaks and biliary strictures in certain settings.

When Postoperative Abnormal Liver Function Tests are Unrelated to a Primary Liver Pathology

Alkaline Phosphatase
ALP can be produced by hepatocytes but is also released in bony injury and from the placenta. Gamma-glutamyl transferase (GGT) is usually raised when an ALP rise is from a liver source. If GGT is normal, a bony source should be sought by checking calcium levels, and vitamin D, and reviewing any history of bone injury. In women with child-bearing potential, a pregnancy test should be completed. If the cause remains obscure, abdominal imaging to exclude biliary obstruction is warranted. Where isolated elevation of ALP is present and unexplained, laboratories may be able to check isoenzymes, which will help establish whether the ALP elevation is of hepatic origin.

Liver Enzymes

The liver enzymes ALT and AST are also released from muscle. A patient who has had a muscular injury or rhabdomyolysis in the context of a disorder such as compartment syndrome will often have raised ALT and AST. AST will be predominantly elevated and should correlate with a high creatine kinase. This, alongside the clinical history, normal bilirubin, and liver synthetic function, will confirm a muscular source.

Coagulation

The liver produces proteins required for coagulation therefore prolonged coagulation time (INR) is often reflective of poor synthetic liver function and decreased production of clotting factors, particularly in the setting of acute liver injury. Other acquired (non-immune-mediated) factor deficiencies may results in isolated abnormal coagulation postoperatively. Examples can be divided into the following categories:

- *Increased destruction*: as seen in disseminated intravascular coagulation.
- *Abnormal production*: for example, in warfarin therapy (interferes with vitamin K-dependent gamma carboxylation or certain clotting factors), nutritional deficiency (e.g. vitamin K).
- *Loss and sequestration*: as seen in plasmapheresis or massive blood loss when product replacement has not been balanced, or in conditions such as nephrotic syndrome.
- *Inactivation*: usually pharmacological (e.g. direct thrombin inhibitors such as argatroban).

Albumin

Albumin is produced by the liver; a low albumin can therefore be a marker of poor liver function. However, in catabolic states, such as with infection in the postoperative period, albumin is broken down at a faster rate than it can be produced, so this is more commonly the reason for a low albumin in the postoperative period. Albumin loss through the kidneys or bowel may also contribute to low albumin levels.

Bilirubin

If a raised isolated bilirubin is unconjugated then the source is usually from bilirubin released during red cell breakdown, or it can sometimes be a patient who has previously undiagnosed Gilbert syndrome. Checking the hemoglobin, past medical history, and previous blood test results will direct to either of these diagnoses. In the postoperative setting, a transfusion reaction (fever around the time of transfusion) is the most common cause of hemolysis.

References

1. Horvatits, T., Drolz, A., Trauner, M., and Fuhrmann, V. (2019). Liver injury and failure in critical illness. *Hepatology* 70: 2204–2215.
2. European Association for the Study of the Liver (2019). EASL clinical practice guidelines: drug-induced liver injury. *J. Hepatol.* 70: 1222–1261.
3. Grau, T., Bonet, A., Rubio, M. et al. (2007). Liver dysfunction associated with artificial nutrition in critically ill patients. *Crit. Care* 11: R10.

4. (2018). EASL Clinical Practice Guidelines for the management of patients with decompensated cirrhosis. *J. Hepatol.* 69: 406–460.

5. Aithal, G.P., Palaniyappan, N., China, L. et al. (2021). Guidelines on the management of ascites in cirrhosis. *Gut* 70: 9–29.

6. European Association for the Study of the Liver, European Association for the Study of Diabetes, European Association for the Study of Obesity (2016). EASL-EASD-EASO clinical practice guidelines for the management of non-alcoholic fatty liver disease. *J. Hepatol.* 64: 1388–1402.

7

Pregnancy

Francesca E.M. Neuberger

North Bristol NHS Trust, Bristol, UK

KEY POINTS

- The normal range of liver tests differs in the pregnant woman.
- Abnormalities of liver tests need prompt investigation and intervention when indicated.
- Liver diseases seen in the pregnant woman may be considered as:
  - liver diseases of pregnancy (especially hyperemesis gravidarum, acute fatty liver, HELLP syndrome, and intrahepatic cholestasis of pregnancy)
  - liver disease occurring during pregnancy
  - liver disease pre-existing the pregnancy.

Introduction

Abnormal liver tests are relatively common, occurring in approximately 3–5% of pregnancies. Due to physiological changes of pregnancy, the reference ranges for liver tests are different in this group. Abnormal liver tests in pregnancy can broadly be divided into three categories; results that can be attributed to pregnancy-associated disease, and results that are due to non-pregnancy-related disease, which may be pre-existing underlying disease, sometimes unmasked by the pregnancy, or newly acquired.

A knowledge of normal pregnancy physiology and pregnancy-specific conditions enables the clinician to avoid over- or under-investigating pregnant women, so giving the best chance of an optimum pregnancy outcome. Interpretation of liver tests in pregnant women starts with a careful history and examination.

The Liver in Systemic Disease: A Clinician's Guide to Abnormal Liver Tests, First Edition.
Edited by Gideon M. Hirschfield, Paramjit Gill, and James Neuberger.
© 2023 John Wiley & Sons Ltd. Published 2023 by John Wiley & Sons Ltd.

Normal Pregnancy

History

Many women will experience some of the symptoms of normal pregnancy, which overlap with those of liver disease (Box 7.1). It is very common to have a degree of lethargy, particularly in the first trimester. It is prudent to exclude anemia as a contributor. The abdominal distension associated with a gravid uterus is usually easily distinguishable from that of ascites or hepatomegaly, but a pregnancy test should be carried out in any women of childbearing age, presenting with this symptom, or any other acute medical presentation. A degree of ankle swelling is also very common, but it needs to be further investigated with a blood pressure check and urine dip to look for the presence of proteinuria, which may indicate pre-eclampsia, or more rarely an underlying renal disorder (Box 7.2).

Pruritus in pregnancy affects approximately one in five women. It warrants further investigation toward the end of pregnancy, with a blood test to measure total bile acids (TBAs), to diagnose/exclude intrahepatic cholestasis of pregnancy (ICP). This condition is most commonly diagnosed in the third trimester, but it can occur as early as eight weeks of gestation. Occasionally, as discussed below, some chronic cholestatic diseases present during pregnancy with pruritus (such as primary sclerosing cholangitis, PSC, and primary biliary cholangitis, PBC).

Investigations

Reference ranges for pregnancy differ from those used for non-pregnant women. The most common changes in normal pregnancy are an isolated raised alkaline phosphatase (ALP), and a low albumin (Table 7.1). There is a hemodilution effect, resulting in lower normal values for hemoglobin and creatinine. Table 7.2 details suggested initial investigations for pregnant women with unexplained abnormal liver tests.

Box 7.1 Overlapping Symptoms of Normal Pregnancy and Liver Disease

- Common and usually normal:
  - Lethargy, particularly in first trimester
  - Abdominal distension
  - Mild ankle swelling
  - Nausea and vomiting, particularly in first trimester
- Requires further investigation:
  - Pruritus
  - Jaundice
  - Dark urine
  - Pale stools
  - Weight loss
  - Easy bruising
  - Upper abdominal pain

Box 7.2   Overlapping Signs of Normal Pregnancy and Liver Disease

- Common and usually normal
  - Spider naevi in third trimester
  - Abdominal distension
  - Palmar erythema
- Requires further investigation
  - Jaundice
  - Flap
  - Encephalopathy

Table 7.1   Reference ranges in pregnancy.

	Non-pregnant	Pregnant	1st	2nd	3rd
			Trimester		
Hb (g/l)	120–150	105–140			
WBC×10⁹/l	4–11	6–16			
Plts×10⁹/l	150–400	150–400			
MCV (fl)	80–100	80–100			
Urea (mmol/l)	2.5–7.5		2.8–4.2	2.5–4.1	2.4–3.8
Creatinine (μmol/l)	65–101		52–76	44–72	55–77
K (mmol/l)	3.5–5	3.3–4.1			
Na (mmol/l)	135–145	130–140			
Protein creatinine ratio (mg/mmol)		<30			
Bilirubin (μmol/l)	0–17		4–16	3–13	3–14
Total protein (g/l)	64–86	48–64			
Albumin (g/l)	35–46	28–37			
AST (iu/l)	7–40		10–28	11–29	11–30
ALT (iu/l)	0–40	6–32			
GGT (iu/l)	11–50		5–37	5–43	3–41
ALP (iu/l)	30–130		32–100	43–135	133–418
Bile acids (μmol/l)	0–14	0–14			
FT4 (pmol/l)	9–26		10–16	9–15.5	8–14.5
FT3 (pmol/l)	2.6–5.7		3–7	3–5.5	2.2–5.5
TSH (mu/l)	0.3–4.2		0–4.5	0.5–3.5	0.5–4

Source: Adapted from Nelson-Piercy [1].

Table 7.2 Investigations in pregnancy.

Investigation	Consideration in pregnancy
Liver ultrasound	Safe at any gestation
Chest x-ray	Safe at any gestation
Liver biopsy	Not contraindicated at any gestation if benefit > risk
	Ideally undertaken in second trimester
FibroScan	Not validated in pregnancy
Magnetic resonance imaging	Not contraindicated at any gestation
Computed tomography	Can be performed at any gestation if benefit > risk
	The patient must be counseled about radiation exposure to herself and the fetus
Gastroscopy	Safe during pregnancy
	Ideally undertaken in second trimester, but can be done at any gestation if indicated
	Low-dose sedation is recommended, and fetal monitoring should be offered pre- and post-procedure
	Left lateral position in the second half of pregnancy

Alkaline Phosphatase in Normal Pregnancy

ALP increases over the course of the pregnancy. If it is raised in isolation, a useful test is ALP isoenzymes, which can differentiate placental ALP from other causes of raised ALP (Figure 7.1). Occasionally ALP levels greater than 1000 iu/l are seen in normal pregnancy. If it is not possible to check ALP isoenzymes, it is prudent to perform a basic liver screen (Box 7.3). A normal gamma-glutamyl transferase would also support an elevated ALP being from a placental source.

Albumin drops in normal pregnancy due to hemodilution. If albumin is lower than the reference range, consider proteinuria (which can be excluded with a urine dip), protein losing enteropathy, or liver disease as possible causes.

Abnormal Liver Tests Attributable to Pregnancy-Related Disease

In diagnosing pregnancy-related liver disease, it is helpful to be mindful of the woman's gestation, medical history, and obstetric history when considering the differentials. The majority of pregnancy-related causes of liver disease occur in the third trimester (Table 7.3). It is important to establish the correct diagnosis, not only to guide immediate management, including whether it is prudent to deliver the fetus to aid maternal recovery, but to be able to counsel the woman about potentials risks in future pregnancies.

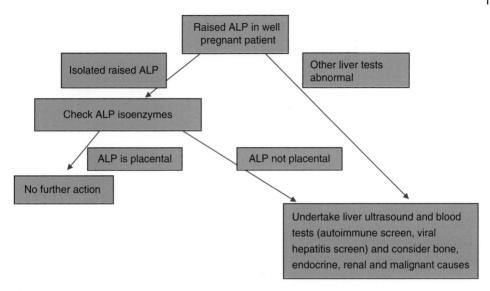

Figure 7.1 Approach to investigating raised alkaline phosphatase (ALP) in pregnancy.

Box 7.3   Initial Tests to Consider to Investigate Abnormal Liver Tests in Pregnancy

- Clotting screen
- Full blood count
- Renal function
- Liver tests to include gamma-glutamyl transferase and AST
- Glucose
- Lactate
- C-reactive protein
- Viral hepatitis serology (A/B/C/E)
- CMV and EBV serology
- Anti-nuclear antibody
- Anti-mitochondrial antibodies
- Anti-smooth muscle antibodies
- Immunoglobulins
- Liver ultrasound ± Dopplers

Hyperemesis Gravidarum

Up to 80% of women experience nausea and vomiting of pregnancy, which usually subsides by 16–20 weeks' gestation. Hyperemesis gravidarum (HG) is much less common and is more severe. It is associated with persistent vomiting, loss of at least 5% of body weight, dehydration, electrolyte abnormalities, and ketosis.

Table 7.3 Pregnancy-related causes of abnormal liver function tests.

	Trimester			
Condition	First	Second	Third	Postpartum
Hyperemesis gravidarum	Most common	Unusual	Unusual	Does not present postpartum
Acute fatty liver of pregnancy	Does not occur	Occurs rarely	Most common	Occurs rarely
HELLP syndrome	Does not occur	Occurs rarely	Most common	Can occur
Intrahepatic cholestasis of pregnancy	Does not occur	Occurs rarely	Most common	Does not occur

Source: Adapted from Acute Care Toolkit 15 [2].

Women with HG are treated with antiemetics, intravenous fluid, and electrolyte supplementation. Cases of Wernicke's encephalopathy have been reported, so it is prudent to replace B vitamins.

Approximately half of women who require hospital admission for HG will have abnormal liver tests. The most common liver test abnormality observed is a mild transaminitis (up to approximately 200 iu/l. Other abnormalities observed include ALP elevation to twice the upper limit of normal, and bilirubin up to 40 μmol/l [3]. The liver tests normalize within a few days of the cessation of symptoms, and no further investigations are necessary. A transient biochemical hyperthyroidism is also observed in some cases, with the woman being clinically euthyroid.

Fulminant liver disease secondary to HG has not been described. The pathophysiology of liver involvement in HG is poorly understood. No further liver investigations are needed in straightforward cases where the diagnosis is secure. An abdominal ultrasound should be undertaken in women with abdominal pain, and consideration of alternative diagnoses in refractory or atypical cases.

Acute Fatty Liver of Pregnancy

Acute fatty liver of pregnancy (AFLP) is a rare disorder, which typically presents in the third trimester, or in the early postpartum period. It is more common in primiparous women, and is associated with male fetuses and multiple pregnancies. It can lead to multiorgan failure and maternal and fetal death. Early diagnosis can be challenging, in part because it can be difficult to distinguish from related conditions such as severe preeclampsia or hemolysis, elevated liver enzymes, low platelets (HELLP).

The main symptoms are vomiting, abdominal pain, and polyuria. Any woman presenting with abdominal pain and vomiting in the third trimester should have blood tests to look for liver dysfunction. On examination, there may be evidence of encephalopathy and abdominal tenderness.

> **Box 7.4 Swansea Criteria (Six or More with No Other Explanation)**
>
> - Vomiting
> - Abdominal pain
> - Polydipsia/polyuria
> - Encephalopathy
> - Elevated bilirubin (>14 μmol/l)
> - Hypoglycemia (<4 mmol/l)
> - Elevated urate (>340 μmol/l)
> - Leucocytosis (>11 × 109/l)
> - Ascites or bright liver on ultrasound
> - Elevated transaminases (ALT/AST > 42 IU/l)
> - Elevated ammonia (>47 μmol/l)
> - Renal impairment (creatinine >150 μmol/l)
> - Coagulopathy (PT > 14 s or APTT > 34 s)
> - Microvascular steatosis on liver biopsy
>
> Source: Adapted from Ch'ng et al. [4].

Key findings in AFLP are coagulopathy, elevated transaminases (3–10-fold) and an elevated ALP. There may be hypoglycemia, elevated ammonia, and there is often an associated acute kidney injury. Diabetes insipidus may also coexist. Typically, a fatty liver is seen on ultrasound, and liver biopsy shows microvascular steatosis, although this is rarely needed to make the diagnosis.

The Swansea criteria can be an aid to diagnosis. The Swansea criteria are met if six or more features are present, in the absence of another explanation (Box 7.4).

Early liaison with a liver unit is recommended, and women with AFLP should be managed in an intensive care setting. Management involves prompt delivery of the fetus, and supportive care of the woman. Hypoglycemia should be treated, and coagulopathy corrected, and there should be a low threshold for antibiotic therapy if infection is suspected. N-acetylcysteine can be considered. Features of pre-eclampsia, such as hypertension, can coexist and should be managed with antihypertensives. Women with fulminant liver failure may require transplantation.

Recurrence rate is low (data are limited), but in cases where it is associated with fetal homozygosity for disorders of β-fatty acid oxidation, such as long-chain 3-hydroxyacyl-coenzyme A dehydrogenase deficiency, recurrence rate is around 25%.

Hypertensive Disorders of Pregnancy

Pre-eclampsia, eclampsia, and HELLP are closely related. Pre-eclampsia is diagnosed after 20 weeks of gestation when there is:

- Hypertension (blood pressure higher than 140/90 mmHg) *and* one or more of:
  - proteinuria ≥300 mg/day or protein creatinine ratio >30 mg/mmol
  - maternal organ dysfunction (renal or hepatic)
  - uteroplacental dysfunction (fetal growth restriction).

Abnormal liver tests are commonly seen in pre-eclampsia, usually a transaminitis and/or a raised bilirubin. These abnormalities should normalize in four to eight weeks following delivery.

HELLP Syndrome

HELLP is regarded as a severe form of pre-eclampsia. It usually presents in the third trimester, but can present in the early postpartum period. Two thirds of women with HELLP will experience right upper-quadrant pain, and approximately one third will have nausea and vomiting. The features of pre-eclampsia (hypertension and proteinuria) may be mild.

Women may not have all three features to make the diagnosis, and it can be diagnosed in the absence of hemolysis, with elevated liver enzymes and low platelets only. There is a risk of liver hematoma and rupture, placental abruption, acute kidney injury, and disseminated intravascular coagulation.

Management of HELLP is by treating hypertension, correcting coagulopathy, and delivery of the fetus. Platelet transfusion is not usually required.

Women with HELLP have a much higher risk of pre-eclamptic toxemia in future pregnancies, but the risk of HELLP reoccurring is comparatively low.

Distinguishing HELLP from Acute Fatty Liver of Pregnancy

HELLP syndrome shares features in common with AFLP, and they can be difficult to distinguish. AFLP is more commonly associated with hypoglycemia, hyperuricemia, a bright liver on ultrasound, and an early coagulopathy (Table 7.4).

Table 7.4 Differential diagnosis of HELLP Syndrome from AFLP.

Symptom/result	HELLP	AFLP
Epigastric pain	++	+
Vomiting	+/−	++
Hypertension	++	+
Proteinuria	++	+
Elevated liver enzymes	+	++
Hypoglycemia	+/−	++
Hyperuricemia	+	++
DIC	+	++
Thrombocytopenia	++	+/−
Elevated WBC	+	++
Imaging	Normal/hepatic hematoma	Bright liver on ultrasound
Multiple pregnancy		+
Primiparous	++	+
Male fetus	50%	70%

Source: Adapted from Nelson-Piercy [1].

Intrahepatic Cholestasis of Pregnancy

ICP, sometimes known as obstetric cholestasis, affects 0.7% of pregnancies in the UK, with a higher incidence among Asian ethnic groups. It is characterized by pruritus in the absence of a skin rash, with abnormal liver tests, typically with raised TBAs.

The pruritus associated with ICP typically has a preponderance for the palms and the soles of the feet. Pruritus is a common symptom during pregnancy, and the vast majority of women with pruritus do not have ICP, but any woman who presents with this symptom, particularly in the second half of pregnancy, should have their liver function tested and TBAs measured. This diagnosis can be made once alternative causes of pruritus and liver dysfunction have been excluded.

Management of ICP involves giving ursodeoxycholic acid (UDCA), which may improve liver function, but does not affect pregnancy outcomes. Aqueous cream with menthol may provide symptomatic relief. Rifampicin is occasionally used as an additional therapy if UDCA is ineffective, and clotting should be corrected with vitamin K. There is evidence of adverse fetal outcomes if TBAs are greater than 100 μmol/l, and early delivery may be offered, to reduce this risk. It should be noted that while UDCA is recognized as treatment for ICP, its use in this condition is off license.

Ischemic Hepatitis

Major obstetric hemorrhage can cause a transient ischemic hepatitis, often associated with an acute kidney injury. This usually resolves over days, once circulating volume is restored.

Pre-existing Liver Disease

Non-alcoholic Fatty Liver Disease

Non-alcoholic fatty liver disease (NAFLD) is extremely common, and affects up to 25% of the general population. Individuals with NAFLD may go on to develop non-alcoholic steatohepatitis, which can progress to liver fibrosis and cirrhosis. It is associated with type 2 diabetes, obesity, hyperlipidemia, and older age. NAFLD is often diagnosed in asymptomatic individuals with abnormal liver tests (typically raised transaminases), where no other cause has been identified. However, NAFLD can be present in people with normal liver tests.

Outside pregnancy, transient elastography (FibroScan®, Echosens) can be used to assess the level of fibrosis, but this increases in pregnancy, so it is less helpful in this group. Ultrasound of the liver can show characteristic changes. A liver biopsy is occasionally used to aid diagnosis, but this is very rarely required in pregnancy.

There are few data to guide management of NAFLD in pregnancy, but the principles of management involve healthy eating, exercise, and alcohol avoidance. During pregnancy, any coexisting conditions such as diabetes need to be managed proactively, in the usual way.

Cirrhosis

Fertility is often reduced in women with cirrhosis, but pregnancy can still occur. Liver tests may appear to be normal and there may be minimal symptoms, but all women with cirrhosis are at risk of deteriorating in pregnancy, and should be managed by a team of experts, regardless of the liver tests.

The women at highest risk of adverse maternal and perinatal outcomes are those with a high model for end-stage liver disease/UK model for end-stage liver disease score.

For women with varices, bleeding is a particular risk in the second and third trimesters, and screening with an endoscopy with or without treatment should be performed in the second trimester. Women with portal hypertension who take regular beta-blockers should continue to take these during pregnancy. In women with portal hypertension, it is prudent to screen for splenic artery aneurysm with an ultrasound scan, prior to conceiving.

Liver Transplant

Women who have undergone a liver transplant are advised to delay pregnancy until they have been stable for at least one year. Pregnancy should be managed by a multidisciplinary team of experts, regardless of their liver tests. Immunosuppression should be continued, with the exception of mycophenolate, sirolimus, and everolimus, as these are highly teratogenic. Any change in the immunosuppressive regimen should be discussed with the transplant team. Registry data suggest that there is a slightly greater risk of prematurity in transplant recipients.

Gall Bladder Disease

Gall stones are common in women of childbearing age, and rarely causes complications in pregnancy. Women with right upper-quadrant pain and/or cholestatic liver tests should have investigations including abdominal ultrasound. Biliary colic and acute cholecystitis are both managed in the same way as for a non-pregnant woman. Often, conservative measures are sufficient, but laparoscopic cholecystectomy can safely be performed if needed, preferably in the second trimester. Endoscopic retrograde cholangiopancreatography (ERCP) can be performed if needed.

Primary Biliary Cholangitis

PBC may present with features of cholestasis (dark urine and pale stools), and pruritus, and is associated with cholestatic liver tests, and positive anti-mitochondrial antibodies in 95% of cases. Most women with PBC who have stable liver function prior to pregnancy have uneventful pregnancies, and UDCA can be started/continued if needed.

Primary Sclerosing Cholangitis

PSC is a rare disorder associated with inflammatory bowel disease (usually ulcerative colitis) in over 70% of cases. It causes progressive inflammation and fibrosis of the intra- and extrahepatic ducts. It is associated with symptoms of cholestasis, as well as weight loss and right upper-quadrant pain. The diagnosis is confirmed with characteristic findings at magnetic resonance cholangiopancreatography and ERCP. It is associated with a 15% lifetime risk of developing cholangiocarcinoma.

PBC and PSC are both associated with an increased risk of preterm birth, related to maternal TBAs.

Hereditary Hemochromatosis

Hereditary hemochromatosis is an autosomal recessive condition resulting in iron deposition in tissues, which can cause cardiomyopathy, diabetes, and cirrhosis. It is unusual in pregnancy, and the pregnancy risk depends on the end-organ damage of the individual. Treatments such as therapeutic phlebotomy can continue in pregnancy, if needed.

Wilson's Disease

Wilson's is a rare disease, leading to copper accumulation in organs such as the liver and the brain. It can be treated with chelating agents, which can be continued in pregnancy.

Acquired Non-Pregnancy-Related Disease

Budd–Chiari Syndrome

Most pregnant women with Budd–Chiari syndrome (hepatic venous outflow obstruction) have the diagnosis prior to pregnancy, although the incidence is greater in pregnancy than otherwise. The diagnosis should be considered in patients presenting with right upper-quadrant pain, ascites, and jaundice. Ultrasound of the liver with Doppler to assess flow in the portal and hepatic veins is the initial investigation of choice in a patient with abnormal liver tests where Budd–Chiari syndrome is one of the differentials.

Drug-Induced Liver Injury

Worldwide, pregnant women frequently take medication, including herbal treatments. Drugs associated with liver injury are alpha-methyldopa, propylthiouracil, and nevirapine.

Autoimmune Hepatitis

Autoimmune hepatitis (AIH) can be pre-existing or can be acquired during pregnancy. It is three to four times more common in women more than men, including women of childbearing age. AIH may be asymptomatic, and abnormal liver tests may be the only feature, or they may be symptomatic, with lethargy, pruritus, joint pain, and abdominal discomfort.

Transaminases can be very high, and ALP may also be elevated. Autoantibodies are found in the majority of cases, typically antinuclear antibodies and anti-smooth-muscle antibodies. Liver biopsy can help to confirm the diagnosis. Management is with immunosuppression, often with steroids/azathioprine. There is a risk of flare in the postpartum period.

Table 7.5 Viral hepatitis in pregnancy.

Virus	Considerations in pregnancy
Hepatitis A	Transmitted via fecal–oral route
	Usually self-limiting
	Mother-to-child transmission (MTCT) is rare
	Neonate should be given immunoglobulin at birth in cases of MTCT
Hepatitis B	Bloodborne virus
	Course of hepatitis B is unchanged in pregnancy
	MTCT is common in women who are e-antigen positive
	Neonates whose mothers have hepatitis B should be vaccinated within 24 hours of delivery, and may need immunoglobulin
Hepatitis C	Bloodborne virus
	MTCT rates are low in the absence of coexisting HIV infection, in which case antiviral drugs should be considered
Hepatitis E	Transmitted via fecal–oral route
	Pregnant women are at greater risk of contracting hepatitis E
	Usually a mild, self-limiting illness outside of pregnancy, but can cause fulminant hepatic failure in up to 20% of pregnant women
Epstein–Barr virus	Primary infection in pregnancy does not pose any particular risk to the fetus
	Course of infection unchanged in pregnancy
Cytomegalovirus	Primary maternal infection in pregnancy poses a risk of congenital defects in the fetus
	Course of infection unchanged in pregnancy
Herpes simplex virus	Rare cause of fulminant hepatitis in pregnancy, but high mortality due to immunosuppression caused by pregnancy

Viral Hepatitis

Globally, viral hepatitis is the most common cause of liver dysfunction in pregnancy (Table 7.5). Women should be tested for viral hepatitis in cases of jaundice, new unexplained liver dysfunction, or if the clinical history supports the diagnosis (typically nausea/vomiting, fever, and malaise).

References

1. Nelson-Piercy, C. (2020). *Handbook of Obstetric Medicine*, 6e. Boca Raton, FL: CRC Press.
2. Royal College of Physicians (2019). *Managing Acute Medical Problems in Pregnancy*. Acute Care Toolkit 15. London: RCP.
3. Gaba, N. and Gaba, S. Study of liver dysfunction in hyperemesis gravidarum. *Cureus* 2020;12 (6): e8709.
4. Ch'ng, C.L., Morgan, M., Hainsworth, I., and Kingham, J.G. (2002). Prospective study of liver dysfunction in pregnancy in Southwest Wales. *Gut* 51: 876–880.

Further Reading

Frise, C. and Collins, S. (2020). *Obstetric Medicine*. Oxford: Oxford University Press.

Mackillop, L. and Neuberger, F. (2018). Maternal medicine. In: *Davidson's Principles and Practice of Medicine*, 23e (ed. S.R. Ralston, I. Penman, S. MWJ and R. Hobson), 1269–1286. Edinburgh: Elsevier.

Royal College of Obstetrics and Gynaecology. *The Management of Nausea and Vomiting of Pregnancy and Hyperemesis Gravidarum*. Green-top Guideline No. 69. London: RCOG; 2016.

8

Endocrinology and Metabolic Diseases (Including Diabetes)

Laura Cristoferi[1,2], Stefano Ciardullo[1,3], Pietro Invernizzi[1,2], Gianluca Perseghin[1,3], and Marco Carbone[1,2]

[1] University of Milano-Bicocca, Monza, Italy
[2] European Reference Network on Hepatological Diseases, San Gerardo Hospital, Monza, Italy
[3] Policlinico di Monza, Monza, Italy

KEY POINTS

- Abnormal liver tests are not uncommon in patients with endocrine diseases.
- Liver diseases may be associated with endocrine disturbance and, conversely, endocrine diseases may be associated with liver diseases; some patients may have unrelated liver and endocrine disorders.
- Autoimmune liver diseases (especially autoimmune hepatitis and primary biliary cholangitis) are associated with autoimmune diseases, especially thyroid disorders.
- Non-alcohol fatty liver disease and hepatitis C viral infection are associated with diabetes; genetic hemochromatosis should be considered in those with diabetes and liver disease.
- Some untreated endocrine diseases, such as thyroid disease, may be associated with abnormal liver tests which settle after treatment of the endocrine disorder.
- Drug-induced liver injury should always be considered in the differential diagnosis of abnormal liver tests.

Introduction

The liver plays a central role in the regulation of the metabolic homeostasis and is therefore a potential target of several metabolic and endocrine disorders. Often, endocrinologists find abnormal liver function tests (LFTs) in the context of common diseases such as thyroid disease and type 2 diabetes mellitus (T2DM), and these are frequent indications for referral to the liver specialist.

Physicians should be aware of the potential impact of endocrine disorders on liver function and the development of chronic liver diseases, and of the effects of liver function on the endocrine system. For instance, obesity/visceral obesity, uncontrolled T2DM, hypothyroidism, growth hormone deficiency, and polycystic ovary syndrome might all lead to

The Liver in Systemic Disease: A Clinician's Guide to Abnormal Liver Tests, First Edition.
Edited by Gideon M. Hirschfield, Paramjit Gill, and James Neuberger.
© 2023 John Wiley & Sons Ltd. Published 2023 by John Wiley & Sons Ltd.

non-alcoholic fatty liver disease (NAFLD). On the other hand, adrenal failure is increasingly reported in patients with end-stage liver disease and in patients who have received a liver transplant, which suggests a bidirectional relationship between liver and endocrine functions.

In this chapter, we review the most common causes of abnormal LFTs that endocrinologists face in their daily practice and provide advice on how to perform the first assessment, how to interpret those tests, and when to refer the patient to the liver specialist.

The Liver: Crossroads of Nutrient Homeostasis

The liver is the site of many metabolic pathways. It is the site of storage and release of carbohydrate, lipoproteins, vitamins, minerals, and metals, which are made available when required. In turn, the metabolic function of the liver is regulated by hormones secreted by the alpha (glucagon) and beta-cells (insulin) within the endocrine component of the pancreas, the thyroid, and the adrenal glands.

The liver maintains carbohydrates stores by synthesizing glycogen and generating glucose from lactate, pyruvate and amino acids (gluconeogenesis). In chronic liver diseases, it is common to observe altered fasting glucose, altered glucose tolerance, and insulin resistance, likely secondary to a decreased glucose uptake by muscle and reduced glycogen storage in the liver and muscle.

In the lipid metabolism, the liver releases cholesterol and phospholipids, many of which are re-esterified and packaged within lipoproteins. Bile acids are synthetized in the liver from cholesterol and they are both secreted into the bile, which represents the major route for cholesterol excretion.

When Will the Endocrinologist See Unexplained Abnormal Liver Function Tests?

LFTs are commonly used in clinical practice to screen for liver diseases, to monitor the progression of a known chronic disease, and to monitor the effects of potentially hepatotoxic drugs. The last represents a common setting when abnormal LFTs are detected by endocrinologists. In addition, LFTs are routinely checked in patients with T2DM and obesity to stage multiorgan damage and explore the presence of NAFLD.

- *Endocrinologic conditions associated with chronic liver disease*: The most common cause of elevated LFTs faced by endocrinologists is NAFLD in obesity/visceral obesity and T2DM. Cholestasis is common in hypothyroid myxedema, while thyrotoxicosis is associated with raised transaminases. Particular attention should be paid in patients with autoimmune diseases (i.e. Graves' disease, Hashimoto thyroiditis, and type 1 diabetes mellitus); in these patients, abnormal LFTs, particularly elevated transaminases, and/or raised markers of cholestasis should trigger the suspicion of a concomitant autoimmune disease of the liver (i.e. autoimmune hepatitis) or of the biliary three (primary biliary cholangitis and primary sclerosing cholangitis), respectively. This topic is developed below.

- *Drug-induced liver injury* (DILI; Table 8.1) may be common in patients using statins, propylthiouracil, sulfonamides, anabolic androgenic steroids, and estrogens/progestins, where idiosyncratic DILI can develop. Liver damage can present with a hepatocellular pattern; that is, if alanine aminotransferase (ALT) alone is elevated five-fold or higher above the upper limit of normal (ULN); a cholestatic pattern, if alkaline phosphatase (ALP) alone is elevated two-fold or higher above ULN, or a mixed pattern. Chronic DILI is described when DILI with acute presentation has evidence of persistent liver injury at over one year after its onset. To avoid severe acute liver damage with the potential for organ failure, early recognition (possibly by checking LFTs after introducing a potentially hepatotoxic drug) and prompt withdrawal of the medication with regular monitoring of LFTs until normalization are of key importance.

Workup for Excluding Alternative Causes

Irrespective of the suspicion and of the level and duration of abnormality, all patients with abnormal LFTs should undergo liver etiology screen. It represents standard practice to retrieve previous blood test records before requesting additional investigations and referrals (Figure 8.1).

The diagnosis of NAFLD and DILI largely relies on the exclusion of alternative causes of liver damage. These include a hepatitis B panel (HBsAg, HBsAb, HBcAb), hepatitis C antibody (with follow-on polymerase chain reaction if positive), autoimmune panel, including anti-mitochondrial antibody, anti-nuclear antibody, anti-smooth muscle antibody, serum immunoglobulins, serum ferritin (generally elevated in case of acute hepatitis as an acute-phase protein), and transferrin saturation and ceruloplasmin. Anti-liver kidney microsome antibody and anti-transglutaminase antibodies should be requested, particularly in children and adolescents. An abdominal ultrasound is necessary to rule out bile duct and vessel obstruction, and chronic damage, with or without indirect signs of portal hypertension. The tests of liver function – bilirubin, albumin, international normalized ratio (INR) – and platelet count should be requested. Liver disease is generally silent and symptoms should not be awaited before LFTs are requested.

Collecting a thorough medical history is relevant. The amount of alcohol drunk weekly should be estimated using units (or grams), bearing in mind the World Health Organization's recommended maximum of ≤14 units/week in woman and ≤18 units/week in men. One unit of alcohol is equal to a small glass of wine (125 ml), half a can or 440 ml of lager/beer/cider 5.5% alcohol by volume (ABV), a small shot of spirits (25 ml, ABV 40%). However, when body mass index is greater than 35 kg/m^2 and when chronic liver disease is already established, the risk of liver disease exponentially increases. The type of alcohol, drinking patterns, duration of exposure, and (generally unknown) individual/genetic susceptibility should be taken into account.

Hepatic viral diseases are more common in injecting drug users, migrants, and people with multiple sexual partners; autoimmune liver disease is more common in patients with, or with a family history of, concomitant autoimmune diseases such as primary sclerosing cholangitis (PSC) in patients with inflammatory bowel disease, primary biliary cholangitis

Table 8.1 Liver injury type and frequencies in most routinely used drugs in endocrinology.

Drug	Type	Frequency
Allopurinol	Hepatocellular, cholestatic or mixed	Minor liver test alterations in 2–6% of patients; rare acute liver injury
Dipeptidyl peptidase 4 inhibitors	Cholestatic or mixed liver injury that generally arises 1–4 weeks and resolves without residual injury within 1–3 months	Rare
Metformin	Cholestatic, hepatocellular, and mixed liver injury. Liver injury usually appears after 1–8 weeks, typically with symptoms of weakness and fatigue followed by jaundice; recovery is usually rapid after metformin is stopped	1% minor liver test alterations; acute hepatitis is rare
Repaglinide	Cholestatic, hepatocellular and mixed liver injury. Onset from 2–8 weeks; recovery after withdrawal	Rare
Second-generation sulfonylurea	Cholestatic, hepatocellular and mixed liver injury. Onset within 3–12 weeks; rare instances of hepatic injury arising after many months or years of therapy have been reported, particularly soon after an increase in dosage	Rare
Troglitazone	Latency to onset of injury typically 1–6 months; hepatitis can be severe and even fatal and may become chronic	ALT $> 3 \times$ ULN in 1.9%. ALT $> 10 \times$ ULN occurred in 0.5% of patients. Clinically significant injury was occurring in 1 : 1000 to 1 : 10,000 recipients
Fibrates	All fibrates are associated with mild-to-moderate serum aminotransferase elevations during therapy; typically transient, asymptomatic and may resolve even without discontinuation. All agents have been linked to cases of clinically apparent acute liver injury, fenofibrate most frequently and convincingly	Mild, transient serum aminotransferase elevations develop in up to 20% of patients receiving fenofibrate, but values above 3 times normal in only 3–5%
Statins	Majority of cases are hepatocellular but cholestatic hepatitis is also well described for most statins. Liver injury ranges from mild to moderate LFT elevation to clinically apparent acute liver injury. Latency to onset varies considerably and can be more than 6 months or even several years after starting	1–3% mild elevation, 1% $> 3 \times$ ULN
Ezetimibe	Cholestatic and hepatocellular. Most elevations were self-limited and not associated with jaundice or symptoms	Low rate of serum enzyme elevations (0.5–1.5%)
Antithyroid agents (propylthiouracil and methimazole)	Propylthiouracil is associated with hepatocellular injury and an acute hepatitis syndrome arising 2–12 weeks after starting medication. Injury can be severe; many fatal cases have been described. Methimazole typically causes cholestatic injury arising 1–8 weeks after starting	Liver injury from methimazole appears to be less frequent than with propylthiouracil (~1 : 10,000 vs ~1 : 1,000 people exposed)

ALT, alanine amino transferase; LFT, liver function test; ULN, upper limit of normal.

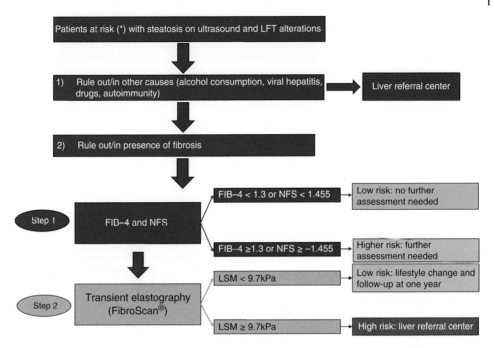

Figure 8.1 Flowchart for the management of patients with non-alcoholic fatty liver disease (NAFLD) and elevated liver function tests. (*) Patients with type 2 diabetes, metabolic syndrome, and obesity. FIB-4: fibrosis score 4; LFTs: liver function tests; NFS: NAFLD fibrosis score; LSM: liver stiffness measurement.

(PBC) in patients with autoimmune thyroid disease, Sjögren syndrome or scleroderma; iron storage can be suspected in patients with diabetes and/or brown skin.

Alcoholism and NAFLDs can coexist in the same patient with metabolic risk and drinking habits above the safe limit. Likewise, other chronic liver conditions can coexist in patients with NAFLD. A full history should be taken of current medications, including herbal preparations and dietary supplements, particularly those recently introduced.

Abnormal Liver Function Tests in Patients with Known Endocrinology Disease

Type 2 Diabetes Mellitus

T2DM is strongly associated with NAFLD and it is estimated that 60–70% of patients with T2DM have NAFLD. NAFLD has been under-recognized in the recent past and was often labeled as cryptogenic liver disease. Today, it represents the most common cause of chronic liver disease in the Western countries, together with alcoholic liver disease. Its prevalence parallels that of obesity, metabolic syndrome and its components.

NAFLD is a clinical–pathological condition represented by a spectrum ranging from steatosis without inflammation, to non-alcoholic steatohepatitis (NASH), with liver steatosis and inflammation that may or may not include fibrosis. NAFLD is defined by the absence of or minimal alcohol consumption.

Steatosis is characterized by the deposition of triglycerides within greater than 5% of hepatocytes, with or without necroinflammatory activity and fibrosis, associated with insulin resistance. Histological lesions defining NASH are macrovesicular steatosis, ballooning degeneration, scattered lobular inflammation, and apoptotic bodies, Mallory–Denk bodies, and fibrosis. The oxidant stress, adenosine triphosphate depletion, and mitochondrial dysfunction might all contribute to hepatocyte injury.

While steatosis was initially considered benign, we are today aware that its inflammatory variant (i.e. NASH) can lead to cirrhosis, which represents one of the causes of death of patients with metabolic syndrome, together with cardiovascular accidents, and for the complication of end-stage liver disease, including hepatocellular carcinoma.

Natural History and Prognosis

NAFLD is a common condition and only a minority of patients eventually develop NASH and its complications. The rate of progression depends on the resolution of the underlying metabolic syndrome with lifestyle changes or medications, but is generally estimated to be equal to one stage of fibrosis every seven years in patients with NASH; this can speed up in the presence of additional components of metabolic syndrome, particularly arterial hypertension.

Epidemiological studies highlight that the risk of developing hepatocellular carcinoma (HCC) is raised in patients with NALFD, T2DM, and obesity, which may develop even in the pre-cirrhotic stage. NAFLD-related HCC may, however, be diagnosed at an advanced stage, owing to the lack of systematic surveillance and curative treatment for the disease. Unfortunately, the high prevalence of NAFLD makes a surveillance program for HCC with six-monthly ultrasound impracticable, and should only be undertaken in the subgroup of patients with NAFLD-related cirrhosis.

NAFLD can be present even in patients of normal weight, the so called "lean NAFLD" or "non-obese NAFLD." This condition has a stronger genetic susceptibility (e.g. *PNPLA3* gene). It is more common in Asian populations and is often associated with bodyweight gain, even within normal weight limits, and high fructose and cholesterol intake. The principle of management through lifestyle changes and caloric restrictions in lean steatosis are the same as for those who are obese. Many clinical trials exclude lean patients and this may limit the application of novel, potential therapies in NASH.

Investigations

Metabolic workup should include a careful assessment of all components of metabolic syndrome. As regards as liver investigations, a common pattern of liver damage in insulin resistance is raised gamma-glutamyl transferase (GGT) and ALT. When GGT is raised along with ALP, it represents a marker of cholestasis, while isolated elevated GGT has a positive association with insulin resistance, alcohol intake, and drug toxicity. Indeed, elevated GGT is very common in T2DM, overweight and obesity. When diabetes is well controlled, LFTs are generally normal.

Systematic screening for NAFLD in patients with T2DM is recommended by the EASL-EASD-EASO guidelines [1]. Steatosis should be sought by ultrasound examination, which is widely available and inexpensive, and shows the characteristic "bright" liver. On the other hand, American Association for the Study of Liver Diseases does not recommend systematic screening in this population, but calls for a high index of suspicion. The detailed quantification of liver fat content is not relevant, although the comparison with kidney echogenicity informs the severity of the steatosis, allowing the clinician to distinguish mild, moderate and severe steatosis. Ultrasound has poor sensitivity for detecting steatosis, particularly when steatosis is less then 20% or in patients who are obese, so FibroScan® (Echosens) should be considered (as discussed below).

Simple, isolated LFTs are not a reliable indicator of the amount of fibrosis, which is the strongest predictor of liver-related events in patients with NAFLD. However, non-invasive scores are available that support the identification of those with worse prognosis (e.g. severe NASH), monitor disease progression, and predict response to therapeutic interventions.

Risk Stratification

Patients with NAFLD should undergo risk stratification to assess their risk of developing long-term complications. This is based mainly on exploring the presence or absence of fibrosis. First-line testing should use either Fibrosis-4 Index for Liver Fibrosis (FIB-4, which includes age, AST, ALT, and platelet count) or NAFLD Fibrosis Score (NFS, which includes, in addition to the FIB-4, body mass index, the presence of impaired fasting glucose, or diabetes and serum albumin), with the latest overestimating the risk in patients with diabetes. Second-line testing requires a quantitative assessment of fibrosis with tests such as the serum Enhanced Liver Fibrosis (ELF; a proprietary test, which is not widely available) or FibroScan/acoustic radiation force impulse elastography, simple devices generally available in every liver service.

If advanced fibrosis is ruled out by low values of FIB-4 (<1.3 for those aged <65 years or <2.0 for those >65 years [2], or low values of NFS (<-1.455 for those aged <65 years or <0.12 for those >65 years) [3], patients do not need escalation of the liver assessment in the medium term. Patients with high values of FIB-4 or NFS, suggesting fibrosis, or in the gray area of prediction, should undergo liver stiffness assessment by transient elastography (FibroScan). In those with NAFLD, FibroScan can discriminate fibrosis (METAVIR stage $\geq F3$) with a cut-off of 9.7 kPa (area under the curve 0.80, 95% confidence interval 0.75–0.84). If fibrosis cannot be ruled out, or if it is confirmed by non-invasive tests, patients should be referred to the liver service. Liver biopsy is necessary for the diagnosis of NASH and is the only procedure able to differentiate steatosis from NASH, despite its limitations due to sampling variability.

Action

No drug has currently been approved for NASH by regulatory agencies. Thus, any therapeutic treatment would be off-label. Monitoring aims at reducing the risk of disease progression by controlling the underlying factors, and to perform HCC surveillance. Patients with NASH and/or fibrosis should be monitored annually, those with NASH cirrhosis at six-month intervals.

Metabolic syndrome and NAFLD share common causes. Patient counseling on unhealthy lifestyles and sedentary behaviors and appropriate diet, with reduced intake of overall calories, excess saturated fats, refined carbohydrates, sugar-sweetened beverages, a high fructose intake should be provided. Dietary recommendations should include energy restriction, reduction of processed food, and high in added fructose. Glycemic control is the mainstay of the prevention of NAFLD progression in T2DM. Elevation of ALT within three times the ULN is not a contraindication for starting any oral antidiabetic or lipid-modifying therapy. On the contrary, antidiabetic agents have generally been shown to decrease ALT levels as tighter blood glucose levels are achieved. Rarely, antidiabetic agents or lipid-modifying therapy can themselves be a cause of liver injury.

Successful treatment of NASH should improve outcomes (i.e. decrease of NASH-related mortality and reduced progression to cirrhosis or HCC). The resolution of the histological lesions defining NASH is now accepted as a surrogate endpoint, particularly in clinical trials.

Thyroid Diseases

The function of the thyroid and the liver are closely intertwined. Thyroxine and tri-iodothyronine are necessary for normal hepatic function and hepatobiliary metabolism. Conversely, the liver is the site for thyroid hormone metabolism and plays a role in regulating their systemic effects. Thus, the dysfunction of one organ can impact on the metabolism of the other. In addition, both thyroid and liver are target for autoimmune and infiltrative disorders. Indeed, thyroid function tests should be requested in all patients with deranged LFTs.

Hypothyroidism

LFTs are (generally mildly) deranged in case of hypofunction of the thyroid, in particular markers of cholestasis (ALP and GGT), and they generally improve after thyroxin therapy. This happens as a consequence of reduced hepatic oxygen consumption and gluconeogenesis. However, no major histological lesions have been described. Generally, a prompt replacement therapy restores the liver impairment.

Hypothyroidism increases the risk of bile duct stones through the reduction of gallbladder motility, reduced bilirubin excretion, and hypercholesterolemia. Introduction of ursodeoxycholic acid might be evaluated if there are residual gallstones or biliary sludge amenable to be dissolute.

Thyroid hormones play an essential role in lipid mobilization, lipid degradation, and fatty acid oxidation. Indeed, hypothyroidism is common in patients with NAFLD compared with other liver conditions, with hepatocyte accumulation of lipids. Following replacement therapy with L-thyroxine, an improvement of the lipid profile is followed by improvement in LFTs.

Autoimmune thyroid disease with hypothyroidism, when associated with chronic cholestasis (elevated ALP and GGT), should prompt the search for anti-mitochondrial antibodies and/or specific anti-nuclear antibodies (anti gp210 or antisp100), which are hallmarks of primary biliary cholangitis, an autoimmune cholestatic disease commonly associated with autoimmune thyroid disease. Primary sclerosing cholangitis is also associated with autoimmune thyroid disease, and is characterized by stricturing and dilations of the large bile ducts. Investigation is by magnetic resonance imaging.

Finally, a long-term history of hypothyroidism (> 10 years) has been shown to confer an increased risk of HCC, even after adjusting for demographic factors, diabetes, hepatitis, alcohol consumption, cigarette smoking, and family history of cancer. This was not shown for hyperthyroidism.

Hyperthyroidism

Abnormal LFTs are common in thyrotoxicosis secondary to hypoxia of the hepatocytes. This can be seen in Grave's disease or other thyroid disorders, with no specific pattern of transaminases. ALP is more commonly raised (up to two third of patients) and may have a hepatic or bone origin. These abnormalities return to normal with the treatment of the thyroid disease; however, fulminant hepatitis has been described, precipitated by congestive cardiac failure and arrhythmia.

Importantly, among the drugs used to treat thyrotoxicosis, propylthiouracil is a common cause of DILI in up to 30% of patients, although severe cases are rare ($<0.1\%$). It is therefore advisable to check LFTs at baseline, and periodically thereafter whenever propylthiouracil is used. Owing to the toxicity profile of propylthiouracil, other drugs like carbimazole and methimazole are more commonly used nowadays.

Drugs to Treat Liver Disease Affecting Thyroid Function

Pegylated interferon-based regimen, commonly used to eradicate hepatitis C and associated with the development of autoimmune thyroiditis or subacute thyroiditis, has been recently replaced by direct antiviral agents, with no effect on thyroid disease.

Hypothyroidism may develop in patients treated with sorafenib, a biaryl urea with tyrosine protein kinase inhibitor properties employed orally in HCC therapy. Routine monitoring of thyroid function should be considered during sorafenib treatment in patients with advanced HCC.

Diseases that Concomitantly Affect the Thyroid and the Liver

Chronic alcohol abuse, a common cause of chronic liver disease, has been associated with abnormal level of thyroid hormones, including elevation of thyroxine and thyroxine-binding globulin with normal free thyroxine and thyroid-stimulating hormone. Several other conditions can involve both the liver and the thyroid, particularly infiltrating malignancies such as non-Hodgkin's lymphoma, or systemic diseases such as amyloidosis and hemochromatosis.

Dyslipidemia

NAFLD is also characterized by atherogenic dyslipidemia, postprandial lipemia, and high-density lipoprotein dysfunction. Patients with dyslipidemia have an increased risk of cardiovascular events, as long as there is a risk of developing fibrotic liver diseases. Statins are effective in improving LFTs and ultrasound findings, but also in reducing cardiovascular risk. Most importantly, statins are safe in patients with NAFLD (and in general with chronic liver disease), even with high baseline transaminases levels (less than three times ULN). Fibrates, used to treat hypertriglyceridemia, are also considered safe in patients with NAFLD.

Statin, Fibrates, and the Liver

Historically, there have been concerns about the potential hepatotoxicity of statins (and also fibrates), and various statin guidelines continue to warn of this risk. This concern is confused by the fact that many patients are ideal candidates for statin therapy (e.g. patients with cardiovascular risk factors, such as diabetes, high blood pressure, coronary artery disease, and dyslipidemia) have fatty liver and/or NASH, which raise LFTs.

However, the rate of DILI due to statins, which is an idiosyncratic drug reaction, is very low. Moreover, multiple retrospective studies have shown that statins are not only safe for use in patients with cirrhosis (and cardiovascular risk), but are also likely beneficial in reducing the risk of liver decompensation, HCC, infections, and death, and are currently under investigation for this purpose. Atorvastatin might be safer than simvastatin. Monitoring liver-associated enzymes in the first month of statin use and then perhaps every three to six months thereafter is suggested.

Caution must be exercised in the use of statins and fibrates in patients with decompensated cirrhosis (Child–Pugh score B-C), who may experience more harm than benefit associated with initiating or continuing these therapies.

In patients with PBC or chronic cholestasis in general, it is common to see elevation of cholesterol. However, there is no robust evidence to suggest that ischemic heart disease or other forms of atherosclerotic disease are seen at increased frequency in the condition. This is likely due to the fact that cholesterol elevation is typically high-density lipoprotein and lipoprotein-X. Liver guidelines suggest that patients with PBC with elevated cholesterol and increased overall cardiovascular risk should be offered statin therapy. Of note, fibrates are currently used as off-label second-line therapy in patients with an unsatisfactory response to ursodeoxycholic acid (first line therapy in PBC) for their choleretic effect.

Adrenal Diseases and the Liver

The relationship between the adrenal gland and the liver is complex, and the dysfunction of one of these organs tends to cause functional abnormalities in the other organ as well.

Adrenal Insufficiency and the Liver

Addison's disease is associated with mildly elevated aminotransferases, which can exceed two to three times ULN. This may be related to changes in body weight; notably, transaminase values generally return to normal after appropriate glucocorticoid replacement therapy.

Adrenal Excess and the Liver

Cushing's syndrome is associated with features of metabolic syndrome, including liver steatosis and insulin resistance. Hypertension caused by the upregulation of the renin–angiotensin system contributes to the development of NAFLD.

When to Refer to a Liver Specialist

In patients with evidence of advanced liver disease, for example with clinical or ultrasound features of cirrhosis, or portal hypertension, or from blood tests (low platelet counts, high FIB-4) and/or FibroScan reading suggesting fibrotic disease, it is recommended to refer the patient to the liver service. In addition, in cases of abnormal liver blood tests with no clear endocrinological explanation, even with a negative extended liver etiology screen and no risk factors for NAFLD, referral to or discussion with the liver specialist for further evaluation is recommended.

References

1. European Association for the Study of the Liver, European Association for the Study of Diabetes, European Association for the Study of Obesity (2016). EASL–EASD–EASO Clinical Practice Guidelines for the management of non-alcoholic fatty liver disease. *J. Hepatol* 64 (6): P1388–P1402.
2. Sterling, R. (2022). Fibrosis-4 (FIB-4) Index for Liver Fibrosis. *MDCalc* https://www.mdcalc.com/fibrosis-4-fib-4-index-liver-fibrosis. Accessed 29 April 2022.
3. Sterling, R. (2022). NAFLD (Non-Alcoholic Fatty Liver Disease) Fibrosis Score. *MDCalc* https://www.mdcalc.com/nafld-non-alcoholic-fatty-liver-disease-fibrosis-score. Accessed 29 April 2022.

Further Reading

Bellentani, S., Dalle Grave, R., Suppini, A., and Marchesini, G. (2008). Fatty Liver Italian Network. Behavior therapy for nonalcoholic fatty liver disease: the need for a multidisciplinary approach. *Hepatology* 47 (2): 746–754.

Chalasani, N., Younossi, Z., Lavine, J.E. et al. (2018). The diagnosis and management of nonalcoholic fatty liver disease: practice guidance from the American Association for the Study of Liver Diseases. *Hepatology* 67 (1): 328–357.

Ciardullo, S., Monti, T., and Perseghin, G. (2021). High prevalence of advanced liver fibrosis assessed by transient elastography among U.S. adults with type 2 diabetes. *Diabetes Care* 44 (2): 519–525.

9

Abnormal Serum Liver Tests in Cardiac Disease

James Neuberger

Queen Elizabeth Hospital, Birmingham, UK

KEY POINTS

- Abnormalities in serum liver tests are not uncommon in patients with heart disease.
- Abnormal liver tests may arise as a consequence of heart disease, when heart disease is a consequence of liver disease, when there is a common cause for both heart and liver disease, or when the patient has unrelated heart and liver diseases.
- Abnormalities of liver tests secondary to cardiac disease:
  - Derangements in serum liver tests seen in atrial fibrillation and left- and right-sided heart failure, and usually improve as the underlying cause is treated.
  - Severe heart failure may result in ischemic hepatitis, which can be manifest as liver failure. Prolonged right-sided heart failure can result in long-term consequences with the development of "cardiac" cirrhosis. Standard tests for estimating the severity of the liver disease, including elastography, in this situation are unreliable.
  - Cardiac abnormalities secondary to liver disease: cirrhosis may be associated with abnormalities of conduction and in cardiac function (hepatic cardiomyopathy).
- There are many causes for both cardiac and liver damage, which include infectious, metabolic, and toxic disorders.
- Drug-induced liver disease should also be included in the differential diagnosis.
- Patients with cardiac disease are also susceptible to liver disease unrelated to cardiac disease.

Introduction

Abnormal serum liver tests may be seen in many patients with cardiac disease. The abnormalities may reflect (Table 9.1):

- liver disease causing heart disease
- heart disease causing liver disease
- heart and liver disease caused by one condition
- liver disease unrelated to the heart disease
- drug-induced liver disease.

The Liver in Systemic Disease: A Clinician's Guide to Abnormal Liver Tests, First Edition.
Edited by Gideon M. Hirschfield, Paramjit Gill, and James Neuberger.

Table 9.1 Some causes of abnormal serum liver tests in patients with cardiac disease.

Classification	Examples
Liver diseases causing heart disorders	Hepatic cardiopathy
Heart disorders causing liver damage	Right-sided heart failure
	Ischemic hepatitis
	Fontan surgery
Diseases causing both heart and liver disorders	Diabetes mellitus
	Metabolic syndrome
	Hyperlipidemia
	Amyloid
	Hemochromatosis
	Alcohol-related disease
Drug-induced liver disease	Statins
	Amiodarone

When a patient with heart disease has abnormal liver tests, it is important to establish the cause of the liver abnormalities and to determine whether these abnormalities can be attributed to the cardiac problems or require additional treatment or alteration of the management of the patient. In practice, most patients under the cardiologist will have straightforward explanations for the liver abnormalities, which require little further investigation or change in management, but clinicians must be alert so as not to miss treatable disease.

Liver tests, especially transaminases in the upper end of the reference range, may be associated with reduced survival, especially in patients with cardiac disease. Furthermore, other studies have shown that increased levels of gamma-glutamyl transferase (GGT) are associated with an increase in all-cause mortality, as well as chronic heart disease events such as congestive heart failure and components of the metabolic syndrome (such as increased body mass index, diabetes, hyperlipidemia, and hypertension). GGT may be considered a biomarker for oxidative stress and a proatherogenic state, and so a marker for cardiovascular risk (hence one reason for its common use in life-insurance medical evaluations). With rising rates of metabolic syndrome, associated non-alcohol-related fatty liver disease (NAFLD) will become commonly seen in a cardiology practice. Patients with cardiac disease who have coexistent NAFLD have higher risks for poor cardiac outcomes.

Liver Disease Causing Heart Disease

Abnormalities of cardiac function are becoming increasingly recognized in those with cirrhosis. In most cases, there is a common cause for both cardiac and hepatic disorder (see below) but some abnormalities do seem dependent on the presence of cirrhosis. On the electrocardiography, prolongation of the QT interval is related to an increased mortality rate in chronic liver disease and may revert after liver transplantation. Other interactions between the liver and thoracic organs include hepatopulmonary syndrome and emphysema are discussed elsewhere (Chapter 10).

Cirrhotic Cardiomyopathy

In recent years, there has been increasing recognition of a cardiomyopathy seen in patients with end-stage liver disease; usually termed cirrhotic cardiomyopathy (CCM). This syndrome includes a combination of reduced cardiac contractility with systolic and diastolic dysfunction and electrophysiological abnormalities. CCM is characterized by an impaired contractile response to stress, so has become increasingly relevant to those being considered for liver transplantation. CCM is associated with the development of hepatic nephropathy and impaired survival. Liver tests are consistent with cirrhosis and, while the optimal approach to diagnosis is not yet fully established, imaging under circulatory stress testing, physiologically or pharmacologically induced, has been used to assess systolic dysfunction. Echocardiography with Doppler is probably the most preferred method to detect diastolic dysfunction, but increased use of magnetic resonance imaging is becoming established when additional investigations are needed.

Heart Disease Causing Liver Disease

The blood flow to and from the liver is affected by many factors. The blood supply to the liver is from the hepatic artery and the portal vein: since, in the normal situation, 70% of blood oxygen is supplied by the portal vein, reduced blood flow in the portal vein, as well as reduced hepatic artery flow, may result in ischemic changes in the liver. Conversely, reduced outflow (whether due to thrombosis or partial occlusion, raised pressure in the inferior vena cava) will have an impact on the liver which may in time lead to fibrosis and cirrhosis.

Liver tests may respond differently to raised right-sided filling pressure and low cardiac output (Table 9.2).

Table 9.2 Liver tests in cardiac disease.

	Raised right-side pressure	Low cardiac output
Transaminases	−/+	++
Alkaline phosphatase	+/++	−/+
Gamma-glutamyl transferase	++	−/+
Bilirubin	−/+	+/++
Lactate dehydrogenase	+/++	+/++

Right-Sided Heart Failure and Hepatic Congestion

Hepatic Congestion

In patients with right-sided heart failure, elevated right-sided right atrial or ventricular pressures or pericarditis, hepatic congestion may occur. The majority of patients with right-sided failure have few or no signs of symptoms related to hepatic congestion, but some may complain of right upper abdominal pain or discomfort. This is usually associated with hepatomegaly. Early series describe jaundice, ascites, cirrhosis, splenomegaly, and even liver failure in patients with right-sided heart failure, but with modern diagnosis and management of heart failure and other causes of raised pressures in the inferior vena cava, these are becoming less frequent manifestations. Jaundice is now rarely seen, and other features such as ascites or splenomegaly are very uncommon in adults. Before the advent of better diagnostic and therapeutic interventions, prolonged right-heart failure did lead to the development of cirrhosis ("cardiac cirrhosis") but, again, this is now uncommon in adults in most therapeutic settings, although the situation in those children with underlying cardiac disease is different (see below).

Clinically, the liver is enlarged and maybe tender and jugular venous pressure is elevated. Liver tests show a non-specific pattern of elevation, although a pattern of acute hepatitis is seen more with acute heart failure, and chronic disease more with a cholestatic pattern, but there is great overlap. The suspected diagnosis may be confirmed by liver ultrasound, which typically shows dilated hepatic veins. Liver histology may help to confirm the diagnosis but is rarely required. Histologically, acute cardiac insufficiency is characterized by centrilobular hepatocellular necrosis, whereas chronic disease is associated with centrilobular hepatocyte atrophy, dilated sinusoids, and perisinusoidal fibrosis, which, if untreated, may progress to bridging fibrosis and ultimately cirrhosis. Treatment is of the underlying condition.

Ischemic Hepatitis

Liver abnormalities are commonly seen in cases of ventricular failure. In the most severe form, there is a very marked hepatitis pattern of liver tests, with serum transaminases exceeding 10 000 iu/l. This may be associated with a significant rise on lactate dehydrogenase. The liver damage is usually apparent within 24–48 hours of a clinically obvious event associated with shock or hypotension. Common causes include:

- severe shock (major blood loss, cardiac arrhythmia, heat stroke, trauma)
- post-surgery
- acute myocardial infarction
- pulmonary embolism
- acute dysrhythmia
- cardiac tamponade.

The hepatitis may be severe enough to cause acute hepatic failure. The insult is usually relatively short lived and liver tests start to settle within a few days. Where there is doubt as to the diagnosis, liver histology may be helpful, and shows typical features of sinusoidal dilatation and congestion of the central veins, with extravasation of blood cells and centrilobular necrosis. Treatment is aimed at correcting the underlying cause and supportive treatment for the liver.

Acute Heart Failure

Abnormalities of liver tests are not uncommon in those with acute heart failure. This has been termed the cardiohepatic syndrome but the term has yet to receive widespread use. Analysis from the PROTECT study [1] found that the prevalence of abnormal liver tests at baseline was aspartate amino transferase (AST) 20%, alanine amino transferase (ALT) 12%, albumin 40%; and at day 14, 15%, 9%, and 26%, respectively. Elevations in serum alkaline phosphatase (ALP) values and serum bilirubin occur later. Abnormal tests were associated with an increased risk of death (which may well be a reflection of the underlying cardiac disease). In general, the severity of the heart failure parallels the degree of abnormalities of the liver tests.

Atrial Fibrillation

Mild derangements of liver tests are commonly seen in those with atrial fibrillation [2] but the cause is not clear.

Left-Ventricular Assist Devices and Cardiac Support Devices

Left-ventricular assist devices (LVADs) improve liver function in patients with mildly abnormal liver tests prior to implantation, and this improvement is maintained. Abnormal liver tests can also develop or worsen after LVAD implantation. This is due primarily to right ventricular failure. Liver tests usually show a predominantly cholestatic pattern. Abnormal liver tests persisting after LVAD implantation carries a poor prognosis.

Beyond LVAD devices, inevitably patients on critical care with cardiac failure requiring invasive support (including extracorporeal membrane oxygenation) very frequently have serum liver test abnormalities, proportionate to their degree of organ failure. Rarely, patients develop ischemic cholangiopathy in the context of critical illness and its treatments.

Liver Disease in Congenital Heart Disease

Abnormalities of liver function are seen in babies, children, and adults with congenital heart disease. Congenital abnormalities associated with liver damage and hepatocyte necrosis are most often associated with hypoplastic left-heart syndrome, coarctation of the aorta, anomalous pulmonary venous return, and transposition of the great vessels. Liver damage is rarely seen in other conditions such as Ebstein's anomaly, Fallot's tetralogy, or hypoplastic right heart. The liver abnormalities are similar to those in adults with right-heart failure; treatment is aimed at the underlying cause. The liver abnormalities will usually return to normal if and when the cause is treated.

Fontan's Physiology

In contrast to adults, significant liver damage is becoming increasingly recognized in those pediatric patients with Fontan's physiology, although it is thought that the liver abnormalities develop before surgical intervention. In these patients, abnormalities of liver function are common and significant liver disease often develops, with the development of cirrhosis and even liver cell cancer. As survival has improved into adulthood, it is not infrequently a clinical challenge to manage a patient with a failing Fontan, alongside significant Fontan-related liver cirrhosis.

Assessment of the degree of liver damage is difficult, as both liver tests and imaging (including the use of thromboelastography) are unreliable; liver histology is often required to assess fully the degree of liver damage. It is outside the scope of this chapter to discuss the optimal investigation and management of the liver aspect of those with Fontan's physiology, but it should be stressed that standard investigations of liver abnormalities are complex and should be carried out in collaboration with an experienced hepatologist [3].

Heart and Liver Disease Caused by a Common Disorder

There are many diseases that affect both the heart and the liver (Table 9.3).

Table 9.3 Some conditions which affect both the heart and the liver.

Type		Agent
Infection	Viral	Adenovirus
		Coxsackie
		Epstein–Barr
		Hepatitis C
		Influenza
		SARS-CoV-2 (COVID-19)
	Protozoan	*Trypanosoma cruzi*
		Toxoplasma gondii
	Bacterial	Brucella
		Leptospirosis
	Parasitic	Echinococcus
		Schistosoma
Toxins	Drugs	
	Alcohol	
	Iron	(as in hemochromatosis)
	Copper	(as in Wilson's disease)
	Immunologic	
Immune	Systemic lupus erythematosus	
	Sarcoidosis	
	Some systemic vasculitides	
Other	Hyperpyrexia	Amyloid
		Hyperlipidemia
		Thyroid disease
		Obesity
		Diabetes mellitus

Infections

Infections include viruses that may result in myocarditis as well as liver disease; for example, HIV, which may cause myocarditis or cardiomyopathy and may affect the liver with hepatitis and granulomas. Dengue fever may lead to hepatic necrosis as well as myocarditis. Sepsis, too, may lead to heart disease and liver damage (often manifested as cholestasis even in the absence of direct hepatic involvement). Malaria may be associated with massive hepatic involvement and cardiac failure.

Inflammatory Diseases

Sarcoidosis may involve the liver with non-caseating granulomas or merely non-specific inflammation and the heart with infiltration. Systemic lupus erythematosus may involve the liver with minor derangement of liver tests and sometimes hepatomegaly is found, and the heart involvement may manifest as endocarditis, non-septic pericarditis, myocarditis, and coronary angiopathy.

Metabolic Diseases

The most common diseases that affect both the heart and the liver are diabetes and obesity. Both conditions may result in fatty liver disease, which may be manifest simply as fatty infiltration (non-alcoholic fatty liver disease) or the more aggressive non-alcoholic steatohepatitis, which may progress to cirrhosis and liver cell cancer. Fatty liver disease may be a benign condition for many, but some will progress and therefore full evaluation of the liver is required (as outlined in Chapter 11). As treatments for fatty liver disease become more effective, appropriate management is needed by a hepatologist.

Iron Overload and Hemochromatosis

Iron overload may result from either genetic hemochromatosis or other causes, such as repeat blood transfusion. The cardiac effects include ventricular hypertrophy and increased end-diastolic and systolic volumes, even though frank heart failure is uncommon. In the liver, hemochromatosis may present as hepatomegaly, cirrhosis, and liver cell cancer. With iron overload, it is essential to exclude genetic hemochromatosis.

Amyloid

Amyloidosis is a rare cause of liver and heart dysfunction. Hepatic amyloid deposition leads to elevation of liver enzymes in early stages and, later, increased serum bilirubin and jaundice. Cardiac amyloidosis may lead to a restrictive cardiomyopathy. It should be recognized that there are many variants of amyloid, some have systemic involvement, such as AL (light-chain precursor), ATTR (transthyretin precursor), and AA (aposerum AA precursor), although amyloid light-chain (AL) amyloidosis primarily infiltrates the liver and transthyretin amyloidosis (TTR) mainly affects the heart.

Alcohol-Related Disease

Excessive alcohol consumption may lead both to liver disease (ranging from fatty liver disease to alcoholic hepatitis, cirrhosis, and liver cell cancer). In the heart, cardiomyopathy is the most common manifestation. While the two may develop independently, there is overall a correlation between the severity of the cardiomyopathy and the severity of liver damage.

Liver Abnormalities in Heart Transplant Recipients

In heart transplant recipients, abnormalities of liver tests may occur, and the differential diagnosis is large. Viral hepatitis, which may be present before transplant or acquired at transplant from the donor heart or associated blood or blood products. There are well described cases of hepatitis C (HCV) and hepatitis B (HBV) virus transmission by heart transplantation. Some blood donors, whose blood test negative by conventional testing (including individual nucleic acid testing) may still have circulating HBV DNA (occult blood infection) and this may lead to HBV infection in the recipient.

Immunosuppression may mask some of the signs or symptoms of infections and may lead to chronic infection (e.g. hepatitis E infection, most commonly resulting from blood or dietary intake of pork), may lead to chronic infection in the immunosuppressed, resulting in fibrosis and cirrhosis. Both HBV and HCV are more likely to run a chronic course in the immunosuppressed.

Drug Treatment

Finally, drug treatment should also be considered and calcineurin inhibitors are sometimes the cause of drug-induced liver injury (DILI; Table 9.4). Thus, unexplained and sustained abnormalities of liver tests in the heart allograft recipient should be investigated so that appropriate treatment may be instigated.

Table 9.4 Some drugs used in cardiac disease which may be associated with drug-induced liver injury.

Type	Drug
Hepatocellular	Amiodarone
	Diltiazem
	Lisinopril
	Losartan
	Non-steroidal anti-inflammatory drugs
	Omeprazole
	Statins
Cholestatic	Calcineurin inhibitors
	Clopidogrel
	Irbesartan
Mixed cholestatic/hepatitis	Angiotensin-converting enzyme inhibitors
	Azathioprine
	Bosentan
	Fibrates
	Orlistat
	Verapamil

Liver Disease Unrelated to Heart Disease

The patient with heart disease is not immune from liver disease, unrelated to the cause, consequences, or treatment of the heart disease. Therefore, the clinician should consider all liver diseases as appropriate to the individual patient and refer to a gastroenterologist or hepatologist if there is no clear explanation for the abnormal liver tests.

Drug-Induced Liver Injury

The diagnosis and management of DILI or disease is discussed in detail in Chapter 20. The clinician should remember that:

- Almost all medications (including over the counter, herbal remedies, and "natural" remedies) can cause liver damage.
- The pattern of liver damage seen in DILI covers the spectrum of liver disease and there are few (if any) diagnostic markers.
- The diagnosis of DILI is primarily one of exclusion.
- If a DILI is suspected, consideration should be given to discontinuing the drug where possible.

A frequent clinical dilemma concerns those who have abnormal liver tests and require statins for management of their cardiac disease. Guidelines [4] have confirmed that in those with mild pre-existing abnormalities of serum liver tests statins can be safely prescribed, although regular follow-up is indicated.

References

1. Biegus, J., Hillege, H.L., Postmus, D. et al. (2016). Abnormal liver function tests in acute heart failure: relationship with clinical characteristics and outcome in the PROTECT study. *Eur. J. Heart Fail.* 18: 830–839.
2. Makar, G.A., Weiner, M.G., Kimmel, S.E. et al. (2008). Incidence and prevalence of abnormal liver associated enzymes in patients with atrial fibrillation in a routine clinical care population. *Pharmacoepidemiol. Drug Saf.* 17: 43–51.
3. Emamaullee, J., Zaidi, A.N., Schiano, T. et al. (2020). Fontan-associated liver disease: screening, management, and transplant considerations. *Circulation.* 142: 591–604.
4. Newman, C.B., Preiss, D., Tobert, J.A. et al. (2019). Statin safety and associated adverse events: a scientific statement from the American Heart Association. *Arterioscler. Thromb. Vasc. Biol* 39 (2): e38, e81. Erratum in: *Arterioscler. Thromb. Vasc. Biol.* 2019;39(5):e158.

Further Reading

Correale, M., Tricarico, L., Leopizzi, A. et al. (2020). Liver disease and heart failure. *Panminerva Med.* 62: 26–37.

10

Respiratory Disease

Michael J. Krowka and Michael D. Leise

Mayo Clinic, Rochester, MN, USA

KEY POINTS

- Significant lung problems can develop due to unexpected liver issues.
  - Arterial hypoxemia, pulmonary hypertension, and pleural effusion prime examples.
- Liver–lung problems exist as part of systemic disorders.
  - Many liver–lung disorders have significant genetic links.
- Major clinical considerations exist when liver transplantation is to be considered in the setting of lung abnormalities.

Lung Problems Due to Unexpected Liver Issues

Two relatively common lung abnormalities – arterial hypoxemia and pulmonary artery hypertension (PAH) – may have a pathophysiologic origin in the diseased liver. Of course, the more common clinical presentation is that a liver disease manifests first and as part of that evaluation, a lung condition is uncovered. But the reverse is not uncommon (lung issue first), especially as seen in pulmonary subspecialty clinics. The clinical liver issues can be relatively asymptomatic or have such minimal expression as to not attract as much attention as the ongoing lung presentation. These two disorders have special clinical importance in that both have significant implications for potential liver transplant candidates, despite the severity of their lung presentation [1].

Arterial Hypoxemia

Arterial hypoxemia that occurs in the setting of occult of or covert liver dysfunction has been called "hepatopulmonary syndrome" (HPS) [2]. It is characterized by the triad of arterial hypoxemia, evidence for intrapulmonary vascular dilation and liver dysfunction. Clues of a possible liver aspect to the finding arterial hypoxemia (by pulse oximetry or arterial

The Liver in Systemic Disease: A Clinician's Guide to Abnormal Liver Tests, First Edition.
Edited by Gideon M. Hirschfield, Paramjit Gill, and James Neuberger.
© 2023 John Wiley & Sons Ltd. Published 2023 by John Wiley & Sons Ltd.

blood gas) start with the severity hypoxemia. Moderate to severe arterial hypoxemia (oxygen saturation by oximetry < 90% or partial pressure of oxygen, PaO_2 < 70 mmHg by arterial blood gas) and a normal chest radiograph can be challenging. Obtaining a careful liver history (heavy alcohol use, previous hepatitis C infection, longstanding obesity) may be a productive start. Laboratory-wise, the concomitant findings of thrombocytopenia and anemia may be present. Importantly, it is not unusual to note normal or minimally elevated serum bilirubin, aspartate amino transferase (AST), or alanine amino transferase (ALT) levels in the setting of HPS. The finding of modest elevations of alkaline phosphatase (ALP) can also suggest the possibility of nodular regenerative hyperplasia, which does not cause cirrhosis but can cause portal hypertension and is sometimes associated with HPS.

The possibility of liver disease as the culprit is significantly increased with physical examination findings of digital clubbing and spider angiomas over the upper thorax and extremities in the setting of arterial hypoxemia. The finding of ascites would also strongly suggest the possibility of liver disease.

From the liver perspective, we would advise a liver ultrasound with Doppler as the first imaging of choice, followed by consultation with a liver specialist. Cirrhosis can be diagnosed with non-invasive modalities such as magnetic resonance imaging or transient elastography. For non-cirrhotic portal hypertension entities (of which nodular regenerative hyperplasia would be most common in the context of HPS), a consultation with a hepatologist is imperative.

From the lung perspective, it is necessary to document the existence of intrapulmonary vascular dilation (IPVD) as the cause of the hypoxemia. This is easily done non-invasively using lung–brain perfusion scanning (Figure 10.1) or contrast-enhanced transthoracic echocardiography. A "positive" contrast echocardiogram demonstrates the passage of

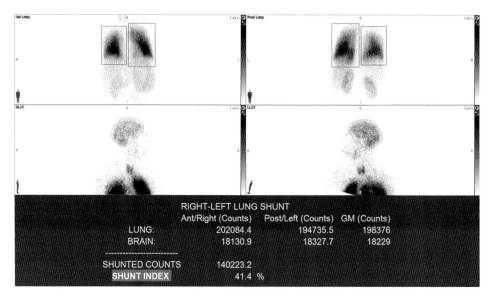

Figure 10.1 Lung–brain perfusion scan evaluation for severe arterial hypoxemia associated with cirrhosis. Patient had hepatopulmonary syndrome with PaO_2 50 mmHg and normal chest x-ray. Intrapulmonary shunt of 41% (normal < 5%).

agitated saline-induced microbubbles through dilated pulmonary capillary blood vessels, which, because of the dilation, interferes with the normal of oxygen from the alveoli into the capillary blood stream, thus causing hypoxemia.

It is unclear as that the factors that are either not metabolized or not produced by a diseased liver that cause the IPVD. However, a leading theory suggests that BMP9 (a bone morphogenetic protein made in the liver) is deficient in the those with HPS. This protein is needed to support a normal pulmonary vascular bed. Its deficiency leads to pulmonary vascular dilatations which cause the hypoxemia.

Importantly, the degree of hypoxemia is not necessarily related to the severity of liver dysfunction, measured either by the Child–Pugh score or the MELD (Model for End-stage Liver Disease) score or the type of liver disease. Usually, cirrhosis is liver issue that has been present, but HPS may occur only in the setting of portal hypertension without cirrhosis.

Severe arterial hypoxemia due to HPS (PaO$_2$ < 60 mmHg) is important to document as it warrants an expedited priority for liver transplantation. Finally, the importance of documenting this etiology for arterial hypoxemia rests on the well-documented experiences that HPS is expected to totally resolve weeks to months following a successful liver transplant.

Pulmonary Hypertension

Pulmonary hypertension can have grave consequences including right-heart failure and death. Importantly and often not appreciated, is that pulmonary hypertension should be categorized as either PAH or pulmonary venous hypertension (PVH) [3]. The distinction and diagnostic criteria for each type of pulmonary hypertension are established by right-heart catheterization measurements (pulmonary artery pressures and cardiac output) and subsequent calculations (pulmonary vascular resistance). The therapeutic implications for PAH compared with PVH can be dramatic and harmful if this distinction is not appreciated.

The third leading cause or association of PAH noted in French and US registries (roughly 10–15% of all PAH) is portal hypertension. PAH diagnosed in the setting of portal hypertension is known as "portopulmonary hypertension" (POPH; Figure 10.2). The cause of POPH in the setting of portal hypertension is unknown, but failure to metabolize substances emanating from the gut, which leads to pulmonary endothelial/smooth muscle proliferation and subsequent vascular obstruction, is the current conjecture.

During the diagnostic evaluation for pulmonary hypertension (which includes screening echocardiography to assess right ventricular size and function for evaluation of exertional dyspnea), the main clue as to the possibility of POPH is the presence of thrombocytopenia due to splenic enlargement/platelet sequestration due to portal hypertension. Serum AST and ALT may be normal or mildly elevated; total bilirubin may be increased. The international normalized ratio may be elevated. Clinical manifestations of portal hypertension (ascites, splenomegaly, history of gastrointestinal bleeding) may be subtle or absent.

Consultation with a liver specialist is advised to further explore the reasons for these laboratory abnormalities, possible portal hypertension and its clinical management. A variety of PAH medications are now available that improve pulmonary hemodynamics and right-heart function in the setting of POPH. POPH associated with autoimmune liver

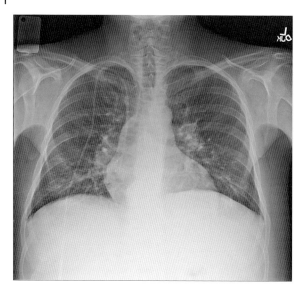

Figure 10.2 Chest x-ray showing pulmonary hypertension, enlarged pulmonary arteries, and portal hypertension. Patient had portopulmonary hypertension due to primary biliary cholangitis, which was treated with intravenous prostacyclin.

disease, primary biliary cholangitis (PBC), or primary sclerosing cholangitis may be more difficult to treat than other causes of liver disease.

Confirmation of POPH requires a documentation of portal hypertension (clinically or by portal pressure measurements) and PAH by right-heart catheterization (mean pulmonary artery pressure mPAP, > 21 mmHg and calculated pulmonary vascular resistance > 3 Wood units).

Importantly, severe POPH (mPAP > 45 mmHg) is considered an absolute contraindication to liver transplant consideration. Successful treatment with pulmonary vasomodulators may alter that consideration. Although pulmonary vasomodulating drugs are now available to treat POPH, the risk of intraoperative/immediate postoperative death is increased in transplant attempts with moderate POPH pressures (mPAP > 35 mmHg). Unlike HPS, resolution of lesser degrees of POPH following liver transplant is possible, but unpredictable.

Although both HPS and POPH are most commonly seen in centers that evaluate patients for liver transplantation, the surprise finding of these patients in the non-transplant settings, subspecialty clinics (pulmonary hypertension, chronic obstructive pulmonary disease) can be expected due to their subtle and not infrequent presentations.

Pleural Effusions

The accumulation of fluid around the lungs can be quite symptomatic and a diagnostic challenge (Figure 10.3) [4]. A key diagnostic step is to discern whether the fluid is transudative or exudative. This distinction made is primarily upon protein levels associated within the pleural fluid sample obtained from a diagnostic thoracentesis. Transudative effusions usually have low protein levels (< 2.5 mg/dl); exudative effusions are associated with high levels (> 3.5 mg/dl). Congestive heart failure, constrictive pericarditis, nephrotic syndrome, lung atelectasis, and liver disease are the main reasons for transudative effusions.

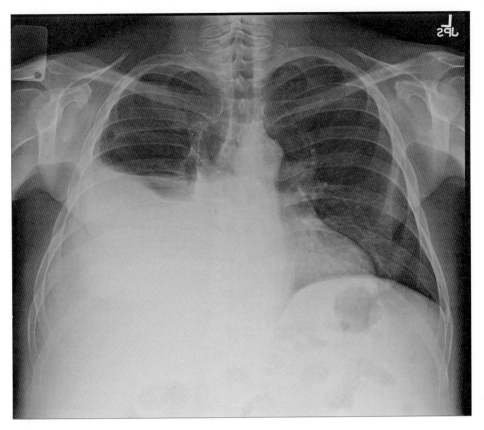

Figure 10.3 Chest x-ray showing pleural fluid and minimal ascites. Patient had portal hypertension due to portal vein thrombosis.

With respect to the liver, the accumulation of pleural fluid in the setting of a disease liver is referred to as "hepatic hydrothorax" and it usually occurs on the right side. Uncommonly, it can be bilateral or left sided only.

Clinically, the main clue implicating the liver as the source of pleural fluid is the presence of abdominal ascites. That finding should signal consultation with a liver specialist. Owing to the pressure of the abdominal fluid, leaks through the diaphragm and the negative pleural pressure generated with inspiration result in hepatic hydrothorax. It is not uncommon to document minimal ascitic fluid clinically yet to note the presence of pleural fluid. This is because of the strong negative pleural pressure that draws the fluid from the peritoneal cavity into the pleural space. Other stigmata of advanced liver disease may coexist in such cases, such as spider angiomata, muscle wasting, hypoalbuminemia, thrombocytopenia, and other typical findings.

A correct diagnosis of hepatic hydrothorax is desired since a spectrum of therapeutic options, ideally directed by liver specialist, exists in managing pleural fluid, which includes medical management (careful diuretic therapy) to minimize ascitic fluid and paracentesis/ thoracenteses as needed. For refractory hepatic hydrothorax, an indwelling pleural catheter, transjugular intrahepatic portosystemic shunt, and liver transplant would be considered.

Liver–Lung Problems as Part of a "Systemic" Presentation

Coexisting liver–lung abnormalities can present as part of a spectrum of systemic disorders. These disorders an effect both organs simultaneously, yet may be recognized at the same or different times, depending on the severity of the organ affected. Often the respiratory problem presents or is identified first, and a further liver evaluation is warranted based upon clinical or laboratory findings. These clinical situations do not represent specific lung consequences or complications of liver disease. For purposes of this review, we characterize these disorders as either genetic or inflammatory.

Genetic Lung Abnormalities with Associated Abnormal Liver Tests

Alpha-1 Antitrypsin Deficiency

Evaluation of any patient for chronic obstructive pulmonary disease, especially emphysema, should include testing for alpha1 antitrypsin deficiency. This includes obtaining a serum alpha-1 level and genetic phenotype. The normal alpha-1 allele is "M" [5]. The concerning alleles that cause lung abnormalities are "S" and "Z." A serum level less than 57 mg/dl (reference range 100–190 mg/dl) is thought to be associated with destructive lung disease, most commonly in the form of panacinar emphysema and bronchiectasis in relatively young patients. In such patients, liver tests may or may not be normal, but liver biopsies are always abnormal. The spectrum of lung abnormalities in a patient with the ZZ homozygous condition (the most concerning genetic scenario in terms of lung or liver problems) may range from no symptoms and normal pulmonary function tests to significant dyspnea and severe expiratory airflow obstruction due to emphysema, as well as bronchiectasis (Figure 10.4). Not all patients with the ZZ condition will have chest imaging (x-ray and computed tomography, CT) suggestive of emphysema or abnormal pulmonary function testing. For patients with serious alpha-1 protein deficiency and abnormal pulmonary function tests, replacement therapy with human-derived pooled alpha-1 protein is available to prevent further lung damage.

The spectrum of liver abnormalities in that same ZZ patient ranges from being asymptomatic to those with cirrhosis. Referral to a liver specialist for patients with abnormal transaminases or clinical evidence of cirrhosis is necessary. All ZZ patients will have abnormal livers with liver histology showing engorged hepatocytes with the mutant alpha-1 protein cannot be secreted into the circulation, thus the circulating alpha-1 deficiency. Liver function tests may be normal. Replacement therapy has no impact on alpha-1 liver abnormalities. Liver transplantation can be considered in those with end-stage liver disease due to alpha-1 deficiency, usually with ZZ or SZ phenotypes. The MZ phenotype is a synergistic co-factor with other liver disease, such as alcohol-related and non-alcoholic liver disease, which leads to a more progressive form of end-stage liver disease.

Interesting, most alpha-1 ZZ patients present with either pulmonary (emphysema) or hepatic (cirrhosis) issues, but it is uncommon to have both clinical manifestations. Many liver patients been previously diagnosed with "cryptogenic cirrhosis." Cirrhotic patients with ZZ alpha-1 phenotype who do have pulmonary issues have usually been cigarette smokers, a known factor to accelerate alpha-1 related emphysema.

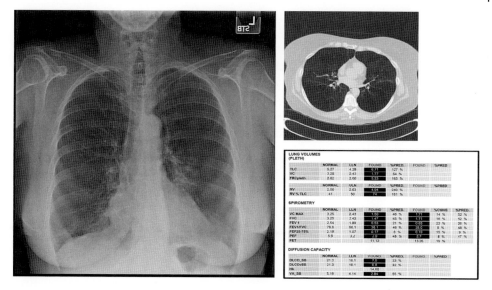

Figure 10.4 Chest x-ray showing severe emphysema and abnormal serum protein levels. Patient had ZZ alpha-1 antitrypsin deficiency.

Hereditary Hemorrhagic Telangiectasia

This autosomal dominant disorder presents as a triad of pulmonary arteriovenous malformations (PAVMs), epistasis, and skin telangiectasis, comprising the most common manifestations of hereditary hemorrhagic telangiectasia (HHT) seen by lung specialists [6]. CT of the chest and contrast-enhanced echocardiography best characterize the lung manifestations of HHT. The PAVMs documented by chest CT may or may not be associated with arterial hypoxemia but should be embolized to prevent stroke if the feeding vessel is greater than 3 mm in diameter. Arterial hypoxemia is treated with nasal cannula supplemental oxygen to keep oxygen saturations measured by finger pulse oximetry greater than 90%

Extension of the chest CT into the upper abdomen is routinely suggested as a liver screening study, since hepatic arteriovenous malformations (AVMs) are common in HHT. Confirmation of these AVMs can be made by abdominal CT with contrast. Three variants of hepatic AVMs exist: hepatic artery to hepatic vein, hepatic artery to portal vein, and portal vein to hepatic vein. These abnormalities may be clinically silent on one hand, they may manifest as mild liver enzyme elevations, or may appear as portal hypertensive complications, and rarely, biliary ischemia (with subsequent secondary sclerosing cholangitis), or most seriously, may present as a cause of high-output cardiac failure due to the excessive blood flow through the liver. The latter can be suggested by transthoracic echocardiography measurements (cardiac chamber enlargements) and confirmed by right-heart catheterization (elevated cardiac output which may be associated with increased pulmonary artery wedge pressure).

Patients with high-output heart failure should be seen by liver specialists to direct further management. Unfortunately, embolization of hepatic AVMs can lead to biliary tract necrosis and is therefore not advised. High-output heart failure due to hepatic AVMs can be ameliorated, but nor cured by intravenous octreotide or bevacizumab. If medical therapy fails to improve the high-output state, liver transplantation is a definitive therapy to reverse the associated heart failure. Recurrence of hepatic AVMs years after liver transplantation has been reported.

Cystic Fibrosis

Cystic fibrosis is a multisystem disorder caused by pathogenic mutations of the CFTR (cystic fibrosis transmembrane conductance regulator) gene [7]. Subsequent abnormalities in the CFTR protein, a complex chloride channel and regulatory protein found in all exocrine tissue, results in viscous secretions in the lungs liver and other organs.

Upper lung bronchiectasis and infiltrates are the common manifestations of children and adults. Targeted antibiotic therapy based upon bacterial cultures, as well as inhaled therapies with hypertonic saline, DNase, mannitol, and bronchodilators remain the mainstay for treating these lung issues. Recently, identifying specific genetic mutations has focused the therapeutic medical options directed toward improving airway hygiene and long-term survival. CFTR modulator therapy is recently available for selected cystic fibrosis mutations. Bilateral lung transplantation remains the ultimate therapy for the lung situation due to the bronchiectasis.

The hepatic manifestations of cystic fibrosis can be expected, occurring in 30–50% of patients with the disease. The most significant form of cystic fibrosis-related liver disease is a biliary cirrhosis with portal hypertension. Obstruction of the biliary ductules due to viscous bile leads to progressive fibrosis and cirrhosis. Referral to a hepatologist should be considered whenever liver manifestations appear, since there are a variety of therapeutic options including nutrition management, risk reductions, medication options such as ursodeoxycholic acid, and management of specific complications of portal hypertension. In addition to hepatomegaly and elevations of transaminases, there are characteristic findings on liver ultrasound (heterogeneous increased echogenicity) and liver biopsies (steatosis and fibrosis). Liver biopsy is generally not needed to manage cystic fibrosis.

The development of ascites is considered ominous in cystic fibrosis-related liver disease and should prompt referral for evaluation for liver transplantation. Other manifestations that may warrant liver transplantation consideration include hypoalbuminemia, coagulopathy, HPS, and severe malnutrition.

Deteriorating lung function due to HPS or hemoptysis, as a consequence of coagulopathy, may also benefit from liver transplantation. Rarely, the progressive deterioration of the liver and the lung merits consideration for combined liver and double lung transplant in highly selected patients at special transplant centers.

Immunologic/Inflammatory Lung Disorders with Liver Manifestations

Sarcoidosis

Sarcoidosis is a chronic granulomatous inflammatory disorder of unclear etiology, but which typically affects young adults [8]. Although sarcoidosis can affect any organ, the lung parenchyma and mediastinal lymph nodes are the most frequently affected areas.

Pulmonary sarcoid is incidentally detected is about 50% of patients via radiographic abnormalities such as bilateral hilar adenopathy and upper lung filed reticular opacifications. Sarcoid is more common and severe in Black Americans compared with white Americans.

Most patients with sarcoids have asymptomatic liver disease discovered in pursuit of abnormal biochemical tests, predominantly involving ALP and gamma-glutamyl transferase. Elevated transaminases are less common. Hypodense nodular lesions are the more common liver imaging abnormalities.

The relationship between sarcoidosis and primary sclerosing cholangitis is intriguing. Both entities can present with a cholestatic picture, and mediastinal adenopathy, and an immunologic mechanism is postulated in the pathogenesis of both entities. Radiographic imaging of the liver and mediastinum can be similar. Referral to a hepatologist would be appropriate for management in such cases, since the entities are distinct in terms of concomitant disease (irritable bowel disease– primary sclerosing cholangitis, PSC), response to corticosteroids (PSC insignificant), progression of diseases (PSC progressive), and biomarker assessments (PSC-positive anti-neutrophilic cytoplasmic antibody, negative angiotensin-converting enzyme).

Telomere Disorders

Short telomere syndromes (STS) promote cellular senescence and apoptosis leading to organ failure [9]. Genetic forms do exist in 70–80% of STS, with the most common gene mutation in telomerase reverse transcriptase (TERT) accounting for nearly 50% of those cases. Following bone marrow failure (most commonly aplastic anemia), idiopathic pulmonary fibrosis (IPF) is the most frequent pulmonary manifestation seen in STS and can occur in the setting of familial IPF. STS are suspected when patients present with, or have a strong family history of, premature graying of hair before the age of 30 years, IPF, and unexplained bone marrow failure. Patient characteristics of IPF include cough, dyspnea, impaired gas exchange, and reduced lung volumes. Chest imaging suggests a diffuse fibrosis predominantly in the subpleural region (Figure 10.5). IPF in the setting of is accelerated by cigarette smoking and often presents with an overlap of emphysema and IPF. It is believed that many more patients with IPF have short telomeres than identified mutations, suggesting as-yet-unidentified genetic abnormalities in a higher proportion of IPF patients. End-stage liver disease is the third most common complication of STS, presenting with signs and symptoms consistent with nodular regenerative hyperplasia leading to noncirrhotic portal hypertension or cryptogenic cirrhosis. The findings of IPF associated with STS should prompt an evaluation of the liver by ultrasound, magnetic resonance liver imaging (preferably with liver and spleen elastography) and referral to a hepatologist, as well as a referral to a hematologist.

Interstitial Lung Disease

Diffuse parenchymal lung disease, collectively referred to as interstitial lung disease (ILD) are a heterogenous group of disorders classified as idiopathic, related to occupational/environmental toxins, connective tissues disorders, and infectious/inflammatory/autoimmune disorders [10]. When autoimmune etiologies are considered in the differential diagnosis of ILD, the association with PBC should be considered in view of the connective tissue

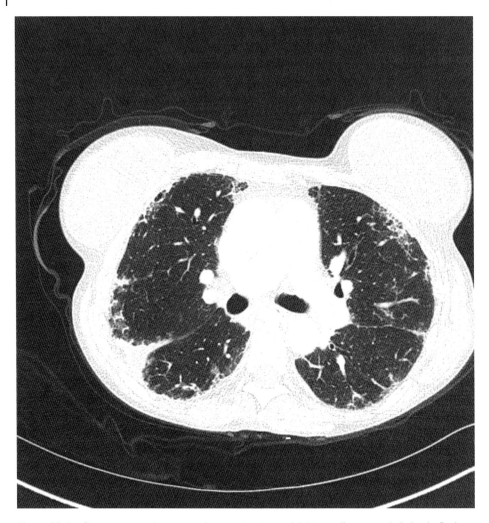

Figure 10.5 Chest computed tomography showing interstitial lung disease and cirrhosis. Patient had cryptogenic cirrhosis and telomere mutation.

overlap characteristics (limited scleroderma) that may be present. ILD associated with PBC may take the form of lymphoid interstitial pneumonia (especially in those with Sjogren syndrome), pulmonary fibrosis, and bronchiolitis obliterans with organizing pneumonitis, each with varying responses to therapies such as steroids and immunosuppressives. Autoimmune hepatitis and hepatis C infection have also been associated with ILD.

Table 10.1 provides a summary of the more common lung disorders that may have associated liver abnormalities. These liver abnormalities, although unexpected during initial lung evaluations, may be causative of the lung problems, or simply pathophysiologic associations. Important implications for liver transplantation are briefly addressed.

Table 10.2 summarizes the spectrum of the common liver diagnostics, beyond blood tests, that are available if there is a suspicion or unexpected finding of a liver abnormality in the setting of a respiratory problem.

Table 10.1 Selected lung disorders and associated liver considerations.

Lung presentation	Liver abnormality	Liver evaluation/transplant?
Lung disorders:		
Arterial hypoxemia	Liver cirrhosis	Enzymes/liver ultrasound/CT
		LT indicated (expedited priority)
		Expect resolution of hypoxemia with LT
Pulmonary artery hypertension	Portal hypertension ± cirrhosis	Enzymes/liver ultrasound/portal pressure measurements
		LT high risk
		50% resolve PAH with LT
Systemic liver–lung disorders:		
Alpha-1 antitrypsin deficiency	Hepatocyte alpha-1 antitrypsin engorgement/cirrhosis	Circulating alpha-1 level and phenotype/genotype
		LT can prevent further lung damage
Sarcoid	Non-caseating granulomas	LT unlikely to benefit lung abnormality
	Primary sclerosing cholangitis	
Interstitial lung disease	Primary biliary cholangitis	Anti-mitochondrial antibody
	Telomere abnormality	Assess for telomerase mutation
		LT unlikely to benefit lung abnormality
HHT	Common/hepatic AVMs	Liver ultrasound/CT
		LT can resolve the high-output right heart failure caused by hepatic AVMs
Cystic fibrosis	Hepatosplenomegaly/enzymes↑	LT alone unlikely to benefit lungs
	Bile duct inflammation/fibrosis	Combined liver/lung transplants reported

AVM, arteriovenous malformation; CT, computed tomography; LT, liver transplant; PAH, pulmonary arterial hypertension;

Table 10.2 Further studies to consider whether liver blood tests[a] and/or clinical examination are concerning.

Diagnostic test	Indication
Liver ultrasound	Non-invasive assessment for portal hypertension
Liver CT with intravenous contrast	Non-invasive assessment for hepatic AVMs/masses
Liver elastography (FibroScan®, Echosens, Paris, France; MRI)	Non-invasive assessment for fibrosis/cirrhosis
Portal pressure studies	Diagnose portal hypertension/hepatologist discretion
Liver biopsy	Hepatologist discretion

AVM, arteriovenous malformation; CT, computed tomography; MRI, magnetic resonance imaging.
[a] Bilirubin, transaminases (aspartate amino transferase, alanine amino transferase), alkaline phosphatase, hepatitis serologies.

References

1. Krowka, M.J., Fallon, M.B., Kawut, S.M. et al. (2016). International Liver Transplant Society practice guidelines: diagnosis and management of hepatopulmonary syndrome and portopulmonary hypertension. *Transplantation* 100: 1440–1452.
2. Rodriguez-Roisin, R. and Krowka, M.J. (2008). Hepatopulmonary syndrome: a liver-induced lung vascular disease. *N. Engl. J. Med.* 358: 2378–2387.
3. DuBrock, H. and Krowka, M.J. (2020). The myths and realities of portopulmonary hypertension. *Hepatology* 72: 1455–1460.
4. Garbuzenko, D.V. and Arefyev, N.O. (2017). Hepatic hydrothorax: an update and review of the literature. *World J. Hepatol.* 9: 1197–1204.
5. Strnad, P., McElvaney, N.G., and Lomas, D.A. (2020). Alpha-1 antitrypsin deficiency. *N. Engl. J. Med.* 382: 1443–1455.
6. Debray, D., Narkewicz, M.R., Bodewes, F.A.J.A. et al. (2017). Cystic fibrosis-related liver disease: research challenges and future perspectives. *J. Pediatr. Gastroenterol. Nutr.* 65: 443–448.
7. Garcia-Tsao, G. (2007). Liver involvement in hereditary hemorrhagic telangiectasia. *J. Hepatol.* 46: 499–507.
8. Patnaik, M.M., Kamath, P.S., and Simonetto, D.A. (2018). Hepatic manifestations of telomere biology disorders. *J. Hepatol.* 69: 736–743.
9. Ungprasert, P., Crowson, C.S., Simonetto, D.A., and Matteson, E.L. (2017). Clinical characteristics and outcome: of hepatic sarcoidosis: a population-based study 1976–2013. *Am. J. Gastroenterol.* 112: 1556–1563.
10. Koksal, D., Koksal, A.S., and Gurkar, A. (2016). Pulmonary manifestations among patients with primary biliary cirrhosis. *J. Clin. Transl. Hepatol.* 4: 258–262.

11

Gastroenterology

Kathleen Rooney[1] and Gerry MacQuillan[2]

[1] Department of Hepatology, Sir Charles Gairdner Hospital, Nedlands, Australia
[2] UWA Medical School, University of Western Australia, Nedlands, Australia

---

KEY POINTS

- Abnormal serum liver tests are frequently encountered in gastroenterology practice.
- A systematic approach is recommended to evaluation, with a focus on identifying relevant pancreatobiliary or luminal disease contributing to abnormal liver biochemistry.
- Appropriate use of screening blood tests, imaging, and liver histology can help to clarify the relevance and severity of any associated liver injury.
- Careful consideration to drug-induced liver injury is always important.
- Some liver diseases (primary sclerosing cholangitis in particular) are associated more frequently with luminal gastroenterology practice.

Hepatology is a subspecialty of gastroenterology, and as such, most gastroenterologists are familiar and experienced with interpreting a blood panel that suggests a sick liver. Acknowledging that this book is not a liver medicine textbook, that most hepatologists are by trade also gastroenterologists, and that gastroenterologists are well versed in liver conditions, the content provided here is aimed mostly toward those practicing internal medicine, to whom gastroenterological conditions frequently first come to attention.

Abnormal Liver Tests in Gastroenterological Disease

Routine initial workup of any patient with gastrointestinal (GI) symptoms invariably includes standard liver blood tests. With the organs being so intimately connected, it is unsurprising that abnormal liver tests are overwhelmingly common in gastroenterological disease, often raising unnecessary concern of a primary liver disorder. These can be thought of in two main categories:

1) Pancreatobiliary conditions.
2) Luminal conditions.

The Liver in Systemic Disease: A Clinician's Guide to Abnormal Liver Tests, First Edition.
Edited by Gideon M. Hirschfield, Paramjit Gill, and James Neuberger.
© 2023 John Wiley & Sons Ltd. Published 2023 by John Wiley & Sons Ltd.

Table 11.1 Liver test abnormality patterns in gastroenterological conditions.

Indication	Acute	Chronic
Hepatocellular	Choledocholithiasis	Inflammatory bowel disease
↑ ALT, AST	Pancreatitis	Celiac disease
Cholestatic	Choledocholithiasis	Malignant obstruction
↑ ALP ± GGT	Malignant obstruction	Chronic pancreatitis
		Inflammatory bowel disease
Mixed	Choledocholithiasis	Malignant obstruction

ALP, alkaline phosphatase; AST, aspartate amino transferase; GGT, gamma-glutamyl transferase.

These disorders can also be broadly considered according to the "pattern" of liver test abnormality they typically cause, and whether they present acutely or chronically (Table 11.1). Bear in mind that the pattern of abnormality does not always stand true; it can be dynamic, and should be interpreted in the context of the clinical picture. Diseases have not read medical textbooks and are not always aware of the strict expectations placed upon them.

Pancreatobiliary Conditions

The distinction between pancreatobiliary medicine and hepatology is sometimes blurred, but the concepts behind disease process and impact on liver biochemistry are the same. These conditions cause an abnormality in liver enzymes via biliary obstruction and resulting cholestasis; and depending on where this obstruction occurs, they are considered to be either intrahepatic or extrahepatic (Figure 11.1). Although the terms "obstruction" and "cholestasis" are often used synonymously in this setting, this use is not accurate. Indeed, intrahepatic biliary obstruction is perhaps better thought of only as *intrahepatic cholestasis* and further defined by its cause, as bile stasis can occur in the presence or absence of mechanical bile duct obstruction; it may be due to a functional impairment of hepatocytes in the excretion of bile constituents.

Conditions causing *intrahepatic cholestasis* range from any cause of acute or chronic hepatocyte injury, such as drug-induced liver injury (including alcohol), biliary conditions such as primary sclerosing cholangitis (PSC) and primary biliary cholangitis, and infiltrative diseases (sarcoidosis, amyloidosis, secondary malignancies).

Diseases that result in biliary obstruction (both intrahepatic and extrahepatic) are also frequently considered according to the site of obstruction, with specific reference to the bile duct wall (Box 11.1). Note that the conditions resulting from abnormalities of the biliary wall are, for the most part, also those generally considered to be primary liver disorders. This seems logical, given that the surface area of the intrahepatic biliary tree is far greater than the extrahepatic system; it follows, then, that any intrinsic disease of the bile duct wall has greater potential to affect the much smaller intrahepatic ducts and ductules, a process that tends to be more insidious and causes gradual destruction to the liver parenchyma.

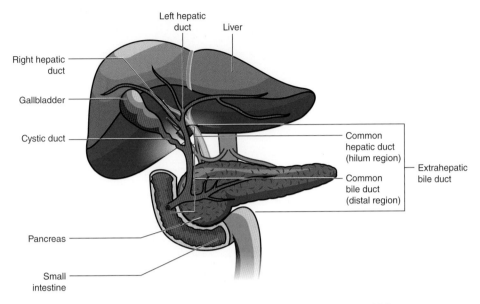

Figure 11.1 Biliary drainage system. Source: Modified from Terese Winslow LLC.

Pancreatobiliary conditions managed by gastroenterologists (and associated with abnormal liver tests), generally refer to those that cause *mechanical obstruction and blockage of the extrahepatic biliary tree.*

Unfortunately, elevation in cholestatic liver enzymes (ALP, gamma-glutamyl transferase, GGT) does not differentiate whether the disruption of bile flow is secondary to disease of the intrahepatic or extrahepatic biliary tree (or both), nor etiology. This can, however, be further delineated on imaging. Ultrasound is the first step in investigating cholestatic liver blood tests but may not always be diagnostic. Depending on clinical suspicion of malignancy versus stone, computed tomography (CT) of the abdomen, and magnetic resonance cholangiopancreatography (MRCP; or CT cholangiogram) are the most useful imaging modalities, respectively. Note that CT cholangiogram requires a normal serum bilirubin, as impaired contrast excretion in the bile will reduce opacification of the biliary tree and potentially result in a non-diagnostic study.

Biliary obstruction can have varied clinical presentations depending on the underlying etiology and degree of obstruction, but frequently presents with abdominal pain, jaundice, pale stools, dark urine, and pruritus. Fever may be present in the setting of infection.

Liver test derangement will frequently show a cholestatic pattern with variable degrees of conjugated hyperbilirubinemia. There will typically also be elevation of serum aminotransferases in cases of acute obstruction.

Of note, prothrombin time may be prolonged in the setting of biliary obstruction due to vitamin K-dependent clotting factor deficiency (factors II, VII, IX, X), as there is impaired absorption of fat-soluble vitamins (A, D, E, and K) in the absence of bile. This may initially raise concern for coagulopathy resulting from injured hepatocytes; however, the rapid normalization of prothrombin time with administration of parenteral vitamin K will reassure that hepatocyte function is normal.

Box 11.1   Causes of Intrahepatic and Extrahepatic Biliary Obstruction with Respect to Bile Duct Wall

Within the bile duct lumen:
- Stone
  - Gallstone
  - In situ ductal stone formation
- Sludge
- Parasite
  - Ascariasis
  - Liver flukes

Intrinsic: disease of the bile duct wall
Non-malignant:
- Primary sclerosing cholangitis
- Primary biliary cholangitis
- Secondary sclerosing cholangitis:
  - Iatrogenic – trauma, surgical anastomosis
  - Ischemia
  - AIDS cholangiopathy
  - Chronic or recurrent infective cholangitis
- IgG4-related disease

Malignant:
- Cholangiocarcinoma

Extrinsic: external compression on the bile duct wall
- Pancreas:
  - Pancreatitis
  - Cyst
  - Neoplasm
- Duodenum:
  - Ampullary neoplasm
  - Ulcer with periampullary edema
- Perihilar lymphadenopathy:
  - Lymphoma
  - Secondary metastasis
- Gallbladder:
  - Carcinoma
  - Mirizzi syndrome

Choledocholithiasis

Choledocholithiasis is the most common cause of biliary obstruction. A frequent misunderstanding based on traditional dogma is that the first abnormality seen in choledocholithiasis is an elevated ALP or GGT, the conventional "cholestatic" picture; it is in fact the alanine amino transferase (ALT) that will show the highest initial rise above reference range, subsequently followed by a rise in cholestatic enzymes and often, but not always, bilirubin. An elevated bilirubin represents the degree of biliary obstruction in this setting, and if rising precipitously must be acted on urgently to prevent the potential complications of acute pancreatitis, acute cholangitis, and sepsis. Depending on the clinical setting and the information gained from abdominal ultrasound, these patients need urgent MRCP potentially followed by endoscopic retrograde cholangiopancreatography (ERCP).

Following relief of the obstruction, either by intervention or spontaneously, the transaminases and bilirubin drop rapidly; cholestatic enzymes may take one to two weeks to normalize.

Pancreatitis

Patients with acute pancreatitis due to a biliary etiology may have elevated serum aminotransferases on liver blood tests, but levels can also be normal. Hyperbilirubinemia with corresponding obstructive jaundice can occur in gallstone pancreatitis, when a stone is impacted at the ampulla, or less commonly as a result of edema of the head of the pancreas in the setting of other causes of pancreatitis. The feature that differentiates pancreatitis from primary liver disease is the marked elevation in pancreatic enzymes (amylase and lipase).

Rarely, chronic pancreatitis (from any cause) may lead to fibrosis or pseudocyst formation causing compression of the distal common bile duct (CBD) as it traverses the pancreas, and subsequent features of biliary obstruction.

Secondary Sclerosing Cholangiopathy

Secondary sclerosing cholangitis can result from a number of different insults that eventually lead to chronic inflammation and fibrosis of the bile ducts in a manner resembling PSC, and which can usually be excluded based on the patient's history and radiological appearances. The more common causes include chronic bacterial cholangitis, choledocholithiasis (including conditions that predispose to in situ ductal stone formation), and surgical biliary trauma.

Steroid-Responsive Cholangiopathies

There are a few unusual types of cholangiopathies that are considered steroid responsive. Immunoglobulin (Ig) G4-related sclerosing cholangitis is perhaps the most increasingly recognized of these, seen to occur as one of the characteristic conditions of IgG4-related disease. Indeed, this is the most common extrapancreatic manifestation of type 1 (IgG4-related) autoimmune pancreatitis, occurring in around 70% of patients.

Malignant Obstruction

Malignant obstruction may be secondary to cholangiocarcinoma or extrinsic compression of the bile duct from any number of malignancies, but most commonly pancreatic cancer (usually involving the head of the pancreas where the CBD passes through to the ampulla). Although traditional teaching is that the classic presentation of pancreatic cancer is painless jaundice, roughly half of patients will in fact experience abdominal or back pain; if the tumor is in the tail of the pancreas, they may not develop jaundice until disease is advanced.

If malignancy is suspected clinically, tumor markers (e.g. CA 19-9, carcinoembryonic antigen, α-fetoprotein) and cross-sectional imaging (CT) may be useful in aiding diagnosis, but it must be recognized that tumor markers have low sensitivity and specificity. For example, CA 19-9 can be elevated in biliary obstruction of any etiology. Following relief of obstruction, however, the level will typically normalize; failure to do so may indicate underlying malignant pathology.

Luminal Conditions

Other GI disorders that can occasionally cause abnormal liver blood tests are those that primarily involve the gut lumen, such as inflammatory bowel disease (IBD) and celiac disease.

Inflammatory Bowel Disease

Transient or persistent elevation in liver blood tests are common in IBD; the majority of cases are mild and spontaneously return to normal. Non-alcohol-associated fatty liver disease is the most frequent cause of persistent transaminase elevation.

Patients with severe active IBD frequently have low albumin. This is not a reflection of synthetic function of the liver, but rather a result of protein-losing enteropathy secondary to mucosal inflammation.

It is important to note, that certain medications used to treat IBD can be hepatotoxic, and should be kept in mind as a potential cause of liver test abnormalities (discussed below).

Celiac Disease

Celiac disease may be associated with non-specific mild to moderate chronic elevation in transaminase levels, which is often seen to normalize following commencement of a gluten-free diet. It can also cause a protein-losing enteropathy, resulting in hypoalbuminemia, and can, albeit rarely, be associated with nodular regenerative hyperplasia.

Take-Home Messages

- Acute-onset severe abdominal pain in the setting of any abnormality of liver enzymes is most likely associated with extrahepatic biliary disease rather than a primary hepatic process.
- All patients with suspected biliary obstruction on clinical and biochemical grounds need further investigation with imaging of their biliary tree.
- Ultrasonography is the first diagnostic test, looking for the presence of a dilated intrahepatic or extrahepatic biliary tree suggestive of downstream obstruction, and to identify gallstones. Depending on resource availability, cross-sectional imaging with MRCP or CT cholangiogram will usually be required to further characterize the biliary tree and cause of obstruction.
- Patients who are unwell with continuing symptoms, or who are clearly cholangitic with worsening liver tests, should be managed in a center with endoscopic ultrasound/ERCP capability.

- Serum IgG4 levels should be measured in all those with recently diagnosed PSC, as clinical and radiographic features are similar; however, treatment notably differs. Glucocorticoids are the cornerstone of treatment for IgG4 disease, which could be potentially disastrous in PSC.
- IBD and celiac disease can be associated with mild transaminase elevations and occasionally hypoalbuminemia in the setting of active gut wall inflammation.

When to Refer

- Patients with persistent cholestatic liver blood tests in the absence of overt biliary disease on radiological investigation should be referred to a hepatologist for further workup of intrahepatic cholestasis.
- If biliary tract imaging demonstrates features consistent with PSC, referral to a hepatologist is indicated.

Liver Diseases that may Mimic Gastroenterological Diseases

In actuality, liver diseases that may mimic gastroenterological diseases are few and far between; the reverse is more common, with gastroenterological disease mimicking liver disease (e.g. choledocholithiasis). Notably, however, there are many forms of liver disease that may cause various GI symptoms and signs. These may be easiest to consider as either non-specific or specific.

Non-specific GI symptoms are those such as nausea, vomiting, abdominal pain, and diarrhea. Acute onset of these symptoms may suggest infective gastroenteritis, but can actually be associated manifestations of an acute infective hepatitis. These infections invariably cause jaundice, however, which differentiates them from straightforward gastroenteritis (Table 11.2).

Chronic non-specific GI symptoms can be seen in IBD, celiac disease, and even irritable bowel syndrome, but are also not uncommon in patients with liver cirrhosis. However, once again, there are usually discerning features in the history and examination, and a less pronounced or absent derangement in liver tests (including synthetic function tests) that will differentiate these from a primary liver disorder.

Similarly, liver disorders that result in cholestasis and reduced bile salt excretion, such as PSC or primary biliary cholangitis, may lead to steatorrhea, a feature also seen in malabsorptive conditions such as celiac disease and chronic pancreatitis.

Specific GI symptoms and signs are those of upper GI bleeding (hematemesis and melena). Although more commonly due to peptic ulcer disease, gastritis, or upper GI malignancy, this presentation warrants particular consideration for the potential of underlying liver disease and cirrhosis, with resultant gastroesophageal varices or portal gastropathy. Clinically, there will often be signs of chronic liver disease and ascites in the setting of portal hypertension. Ultimately, upper GI bleeding is investigated reasonably urgently with endoscopy, which will reveal the etiology of bleeding.

Note that non-cirrhotic portal hypertension can also lead to the development of gastroesophageal varices and portal gastropathy and their subsequent manifestation with upper GI bleeding.

Table 11.2 Non-specific symptoms in primary liver diseases compared with gastrointestinal diseases.

Disease	GI symptoms	GI disorder with similar symptoms	Discerning features of liver disease
Acute viral hepatitis: Hepatitis A/B/E	Nausea/vomiting Anorexia Abdominal pain ± Diarrhea	Infective gastroenteritis Irritable bowel disease Acute pancreatitis	Jaundice, hepatomegaly Relevant exposure risk Marked transaminitis (> 1000 iu/l)
Autoimmune hepatitis	Nausea Anorexia Abdominal pain	Irritable bowel disease Celiac disease Peptic ulcer disease Gastritis	Elevated ALT/AST ANA+ Elevated IgG
PBC/PSC	Steatorrhea	Celiac disease Chronic pancreatitis	Pruritus AMA+ Abnormal cholangiogram
Alcoholic hepatitis	Nausea/vomiting Anorexia Abdominal pain	Acute pancreatitis Peptic ulcer disease Gastritis	Jaundice, hepatomegaly Relevant alcohol history Modest transaminases (ALT often normal, AST < 300 iu/l)

ALP, alkaline phosphatase; ALT, alanine amino transferase; AMA, anti-mitochondrial antibody; AST, aspartate amino transferase PBC, primary biliary cholangitis; PSC, primary sclerosing cholangitis.

Primary Sclerosing Cholangitis

One liver disease that is worth mentioning in greater detail here is PSC. Patients are often asymptomatic and are diagnosed following evaluation of cholestatic derangement of liver biochemistry (often in the clinical setting of IBD). However, patients can occasionally present with symptoms of mechanical biliary obstruction from a dominant stricture (focal high-grade stricture), located in one of the main intrahepatic ducts or any point downstream to this. In those without a known diagnosis of PSC, this may be clinically mistaken for choledocholithiasis (although this may be present concurrently) or malignant obstruction. Ultimately, cholangiography is required to differentiate this condition. It is important, however, to recognize that a dominant biliary stricture, even in the setting of cholangiographically confirmed PSC, may still be secondary to cholangiocarcinoma; and every effort should be made to exclude this, usually on cytology from brushings performed during ERCP.

Take-Home Messages
Any patient with acute jaundice and elevated transaminases without radiographic evidence of biliary obstruction should be screened for viral hepatitis, autoimmune liver disease, and potential toxins (including alcohol). It is also essential to assess for coagulopathy and clinical signs of acute liver failure.

Liver Diseases Associated with Gastroenterological Diseases

When to Refer

- Acute jaundice and elevated aminotransferases, with or without coagulopathy, without radiographic evidence of obstruction.
- Any patient found to have gastroesophageal varices or portal gastropathy should be referred to a hepatologist for workup of underlying portal hypertension with or without cirrhosis and appropriate ongoing surveillance.

Primary Sclerosing Cholangitis: Inflammatory Bowel Disease

There is a strong one-way association between PSC and IBD, in that most patients with PSC have underlying ulcerative colitis (up to 90% in some series); however, only around 5% of patients with ulcerative colitis have PSC. The connection would suggest a common pathogenesis, for which there are multiple theorized mechanisms; however, the cause of PSC is ultimately unknown. Furthering its mysterious reputation, the onset of PSC has no regard for time, and may develop over a decade after ulcerative colitis is diagnosed, or may equally predate it.

Secondary Sclerosing Cholangitis/Secondary Biliary Cirrhosis

Secondary sclerosing cholangitis and secondary biliary cirrhosis are consequential conditions that may result from repeat instrumentation or overt iatrogenic injury to the CBD. Similarly, recurrent episodes of ascending cholangitis may result in extra- and intra-hepatic structuring, with chronic cholestasis and infection, eventually leading to progressive hepatic fibrosis and cirrhosis.

Take-Home Messages

- All patients with PSC should be evaluated for IBD with colonoscopy.
- Patients with IBD who have abnormal liver tests should be evaluated for PSC with cholangiography (MRCP).

Unexplained Abnormal Liver Tests in Patients with Known Gastroenterological Diseases

Care should be taken not to dismiss abnormal liver tests in those with gastroenterological diseases that are known to cause these abnormalities, especially if the derangement is new and/or worsening without any recent change in disease control or current treatment (Table 11.3). PSC among patients with IBD is an important consideration, although not the only one.

Table 11.3 Drugs commonly used for irritable bowel disease that may cause liver test abnormality.

Medication	Biochemical picture	Mechanism of injury	Result of injury	Typical severity/outcome
Aminosalicylates (SSZ, 5-ASAs)	Mixed hepatocellular Cholestatic	Hypersensitivity reaction	Immunoallergic hepatitis Granulomatous hepatitis Acute liver failure	Unpredictable, but usually resolves with drug cessation
Thiopurines (AZA, 6-MP)	Cholestatic hepatocellular (mild) Mixed	Toxic metabolites Hypersensitivity reaction	Cholestatic hepatitis NRH SOS (rare)	Improves with drug cessation, but can progress or cause chronic liver injury
Methotrexate	Hepatocellular	Direct hepatocyte injury Dose dependent	Steatohepatitis Fibrosis Cirrhosis (rare)	Often subclinical, seen in long-term use
Cyclosporin	Cholestatic Hyper-bilirubinemia	Bile acid accumulation Dose dependent	Cholestatic hepatitis	Mild, rapid recovery with dose reduction
Anti-TNF agents	Hepatocellular Cholestatic	Autoimmune Immunosuppression (HBV)	Autoimmune-like hepatitis (DI-AIH) Cholestasis Acute liver failure	DI-AIH: Mild, rapid recovery with drug cessation HBV reactivation may be fatal
Steroids	Variable	Steatosis Immunosuppression (HBV, HCV) Dose/duration dependent	Worsening NASH Worsening of chronic viral hepatitis Acute liver failure	Metabolic effects usually mild with recovery post-drug cessation HBV reactivation may be fatal

6-MP, 6-mercaptopurine; AZA, azathioprine; DI-AIH, drug-induced autoimmune hepatitis; HBV, hepatitis B virus; HCV, hepatitis C virus; NASH, non-alcoholic steatohepatitis; NRH, nodular regenerative hyperplasia; SOS, sinusoidal obstruction syndrome; SSZ, sulfasalazine; TNF, tumor necrosis factor.

One frequently encountered problem in patients with IBD is toxicity related to medications used to control their disease. These toxicities can be varied, both in regard to the organ involved and the severity, but not uncommonly will involve the liver. The injury to the liver can be a result of either the drug itself, which may or may not be dose dependent, or secondary to their immunosuppressive effects and potential reactivation of undiagnosed or overlooked hepatitis B infection, a complication that can lead to fulminant liver failure.

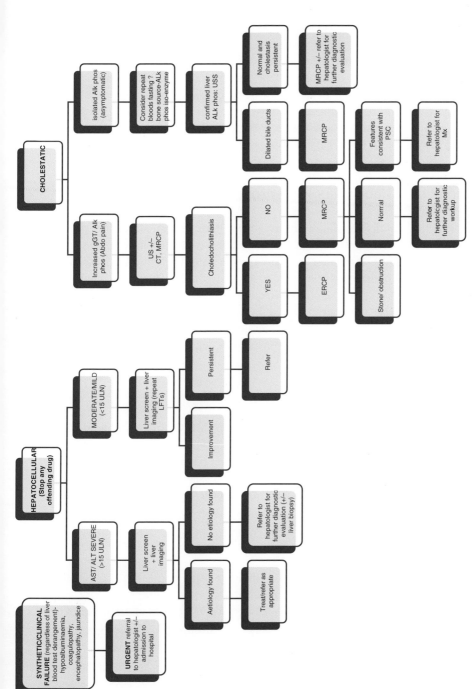

Figure 11.2 Algorithm for the approach to deranged liver blood tests in patients with no known primary liver disorder.

Key

ALP, alkaline phosphatase; AST, aspartate amino transferase; CT, computed tomography; ERCP, endoscopic retrograde cholangiopancrea-tography; GGT, gamma-glutamyl transferase; LFTs, liver function tests; MRCP, magnetic resonance cholangiopancreatography; PSC, primary sclerosing cholangitis; ULN, upper limit of normal; US, ultrasound.

Take-Home Messages

- Screen for chronic viral hepatitis (in addition to other relevant latent infections) prior to commencement of immunosuppressive therapy.
- Abnormal liver blood tests that occur shortly after commencement of a new immunomodulatory agent are likely drug-related; the offending drug should be dose adjusted or discontinued, as guided by the patient's gastroenterologist.
- Liver injury secondary to sulfasalazine is idiosyncratic; in this situation, sulfasalazine should be immediately stopped and not rechallenged. Likewise, care should be taken when using thiopurines if liver injury is suspected to be a hypersensitivity reaction.

Monitoring Liver Blood Tests in Gastroenterology

Most situations that require monitoring of liver blood tests in gastroenterology revolve around monitoring for adverse effects of medications. Every center will have its own protocol for how frequently to perform these tests, but the general rule of thumb is close monitoring for a short period of time post-commencement, and gradual reduction in monitoring with proof of tolerance (Figure 11.2). More frequent monitoring should be done in the setting of concurrent use of other potential hepatotoxic medications or substances. Ultimately, this will be guided by the gastroenterologist who prescribed the medication. Patients should be advised to report any new symptoms, which would of course prompt repeat liver blood tests.

Liver Screen

- Viral serology ± polymerase chain reaction: hepatitis A/B/C virus, cytomegalovirus, Epstein–Barr virus, herpes simplex virus, varicella zoster virus.
- Autoimmune screen: anti-nuclear antibodies, smooth-muscle antibodies, anti-neutrophil cytoplasmic autoantibodies, anti-mitochondrial antibodies, immunoglobulin levels.
- Iron studies, alpha1-AT level, ceruloplasmin ± genotype testing.

Further Reading

Mendes, F.D., Levy, C., Enders, F.B. et al. (2007). Abnormal hepatic biochemistries in patients with inflammatory bowel disease. *Am. J. Gastroenterol.* 102: 344–350.

Núñez, F.P., Quera, R., Bay, C. et al. (2022). Drug-induced liver injury used in the treatment of inflammatory bowel disease. *J. Crohns Colitis* jjac013. https://doi.org/10.1093/ecco-jcc/jjac013.

Restellini, S., Chazouillères, O., and Frossard, J.L. (2017). Hepatic manifestations of inflammatory bowel diseases. *Liver Int.* 37: 475–489.

12

Renal Medicine

Javeria Peracha and Graham Lipkin

Queen Elizabeth Hospital, Birmingham, UK

KEY POINTS

- Renal impairment in patients with liver disease is common, as is liver dysfunction in patients who have renal disease.
- Patients with advanced cirrhosis are vulnerable to episodes of acute kidney injury (AKI), usually pre-renal, precipitated by infections, hypovolaemia, or drugs. Treatment should center on withdrawal of nephrotoxic agents, treating infection and adequate volume resuscitation.
- Hepatorenal syndrome (HRS) is a diagnosis of exclusion, characterized by functional renal impairment, due to altered haemodynamics of cirrhosis. Patients may develop AKI-HRS or the more indolent chronic kidney disease (CKD) HRS, both of which are difficult to treat. Renal function should normalize following liver transplantation as there is usually no structural damage to kidneys.
- In patients with acute liver failure, development of renal dysfunction is an important prognostic indicator and forms part of commonly used scoring systems for liver transplantation.
- Liver transplant recipients are vulnerable to renal dysfunction in the perioperative period.
- Glomerulonephritis in patients with liver disease is uncommon; some known associations include immunoglobulin A nephropathy in patients with alcoholic cirrhosis and cryoglobulinemic vasculitis in patients with hepatitis C infection.
- Liver dysfunction is commonly seen in patients with AKI. Differential diagnoses in these cases are wide ranging, including sepsis/hypovolaemia, drug toxicity, or decompensated heart failure.
- Systemic disorders may affect both kidney and liver function, including genetic diseases.
- Hepatitis B and C infections are prevalent in hemodialysis populations; staff and patient safety can be maintained through vaccination policy, isolation of machines and regular screening programs.
- Liver dysfunction in renal transplant recipients may be linked to toxicity from medications, viral infections that may involve the liver and non-alcohol-associated fatty liver disease (NAFLD).

The Liver in Systemic Disease: A Clinician's Guide to Abnormal Liver Tests, First Edition.
Edited by Gideon M. Hirschfield, Paramjit Gill, and James Neuberger.
© 2023 John Wiley & Sons Ltd. Published 2023 by John Wiley & Sons Ltd.

Introduction

Patients with abnormal liver tests are commonly encountered by renal physicians across the breadth of clinical practice. Hepatic and renal function are closely intertwined through involvement in systemic disease processes, hemodynamic interrelationships, coexisting primary organ disorders, and drug toxicity.

This chapter starts by examining factors related to the assessment and management of AKI in patients with liver cirrhosis, one of the most frequently encountered scenarios in clinical practice. CKD in patients with cirrhosis is then be explored, alongside renal impairment in the context of acute liver failure (ALF) and liver transplantation. We then review common causes of abnormal elevations in liver enzymes among patients with renal disease, including AKI, CKD (including dialysis), and renal transplantation.

Each section in this chapter outlines key differential diagnoses relevant to the clinical settings and a framework that will allow further investigation and assessment of these conditions. We briefly touch on pathophysiology and management of some key conditions, including HRS, and the challenges surrounding viral hepatitis screening, diagnosis, and management amongst patients with AKI, CKD (including dialysis), and renal transplants.

Renal Impairment in Patients with Liver Disease

Measurement of Renal Function in Patients with Cirrhosis

Limitations of creatinine-based estimates of kidney function in patients with cirrhosis including calculated estimated glomerular filtration rate (eGFR) should be recognized, due to sarcopenia, altered tubular secretion of creatinine, and an increased volume of distribution (Box 12.1). Serum cystatin C level may provide a more sensitive and reliable marker of renal function in patients with cirrhosis, although laboratory measurement is not widely available. When accurate measurement of glomerular filtration rate (GFR) is required (e.g. for transplant assessment), isotopic clearance of 99Tc DTPA (diethylenetriaminepentaacetic acid) or iohexol overcomes some of the inaccuracies associated with creatinine-based measurement [1].

Box 12.1 Factors Contributing to Low Serum Creatinine (SCr) Values in Patients with Cirrhosis

- Reduced skeletal muscle mass.
- Reduced dietary protein intake.
- Reduced hepatic production of creatinine.
- Increased tubular secretion of creatinine.
- Increased volume of distribution leading to diluted SCr measurements.
- Interference in SCr measurement assays (colorimetric) due to hyperbilirubinemia.

Acute Kidney Injury in Patients with Liver Cirrhosis

AKI describes a sudden reduction in kidney function, observed in up to 50% of hospitalized patients with cirrhosis and is associated with substantial additional morbidity and mortality. The International Ascites Club standardized AKI diagnostic criteria for patients with cirrhosis is based on the Kidney Disease: Improving Global Outcomes (KDIGO) AKI clinical practice guidelines (Table 12.1) [2]. However, trends in serum creatinine predominate over urine output parameters, which can be unreliable in patients with cirrhosis, where avid sodium and water retention can cause oliguria, independent of true kidney function [2, 3].

Etiology of Acute Kidney Injury

Most cases of AKI in patients with cirrhosis are "pre-renal," due to reduced glomerular perfusion on top of reduced renal blood flow. This is frequently precipitated by infection (46%), including bacterial peritonitis or relative hypovolemia (32%), such as when there is variceal bleeding or paracentesis without adequate albumin replacement (Table 12.2). Prolonged or severe pre-renal AKI may progress to acute tubular necrosis (ATN). Less commonly, primary renal parenchymal disease may cause AKI. Associations of liver disease with glomerulonephritis are outlined in Table 12.3. Bile-cast nephropathy leading to AKI or a Fanconi-like proximal tubulopathy (characterized by low serum uric acid and phosphate) is associated with severe hyperbilirubinemia. Particular attention should be paid to management of medication as patients with cirrhosis are at risk from nephrotoxic medications.

Table 12.1 International Ascites Club acute kidney injury diagnostic criteria.

Subject	Definition
Baseline sCr	A value of sCr obtained in the previous three months
	In patients with more than one sCr, the one closest to the hospital admission should be used
	In patients with no previous sCr, the value on admission should be used
Definition of AKI	Increase in serum creatinine (sCr) of ≥ 0.3 mg/dl (≥ 26.5 µmol/l) within 48 hours or a > 50% rise in sCr from "baseline"
Staging:	
1a	Increase in sCr ≥ 1.5 to 2 fold from baseline[a]
	Or increase in sCr by ≥ 0.3 mg/dl (≥ 26.5 µmol/l) within 48 hours
2	Increase in sCr $\geq$ 2–3-fold from baseline[a]
	Increase in sCr $\geq$ 3-fold from baseline[a]
3	Or increase in sCr to ≥ 4.0 mg/dl (≥ 353.6 µmol/l)
	Or initiation of renal replacement therapy

AKI, acute kidney injury; SCr, serum creatinine.
[a] Stage 1 is divided further into stage 1a (sCr < 132.6 µmol/l or 1.5 mg/dl) and 1b (sCr > 132.6 µmol/l or 1.5 mg/dl) [2].

Table 12.2 Etiology of acute kidney injury in patients hospitalized with liver cirrhosis. Adapted from [4].

Cause	Frequency (%)	Precipitants
Infection associated	46	Sepsis
		Spontaneous bacterial peritonitis
Hypovolemia associated	32	Diuretic overuse
		Gastrointestinal bleeding (including variceal bleeds)
		Lactulose and infection-related diarrhea
		Large-volume paracentesis (without adequate albumin replacement)
Hepatorenal syndrome	13	Decompensated liver cirrhosis
Parenchymal renal disease	9	Acute tubular necrosis
		Interstitial nephritis
		Bile-cast nephropathy
		Glomerulonephritis

Table 12.3 Glomerulonephritis reported in association with chronic liver disease.

Disease	Association
Alcoholic cirrhosis	Immunoglobulin A nephropathy
Hepatitis B	Membranous nephropathy (most common)
	Polyarteritis nodosa
	Membranoproliferative glomerulonephritis
Hepatitis C	Membranoproliferative glomerulonephritis with or without cryoglobulins (most common)
	Membranous nephropathy
	Fibrillary glomerulonephritis
Primary biliary cholangitis	Membranous nephropathy
	Anti-neutrophilic cytoplasmic antibody vasculitis
Autoimmune hepatitis	Immune complex glomerulonephritis
	Membranous nephropathy
	Membranoproliferative glomerulonephritis
Alpha-1-antitrypsin deficiency	Membranoproliferative glomerulonephritis

Acute Kidney Injury Hepatorenal Syndrome "AKI HRS", previously referred to as "type 1 HRS," is a diagnosis of exclusion, resulting from the renal physiological changes seen in advanced liver cirrhosis, in the absence of structural or parenchymal renal disease (Figure 12.1).

Development of portal hypertension leads to increased release of vasodilatory mediators into the splanchnic arterial circulation (nitric oxide, prostacyclin, carbon monoxide, and endogenous cannabinoids). Pooling of blood within the splanchnic system causes "effective arterial hypovolemia" and reduced renal perfusion. The simultaneous release of damage-associated molecular patterns from cirrhotic liver tissue and pathogen-associated

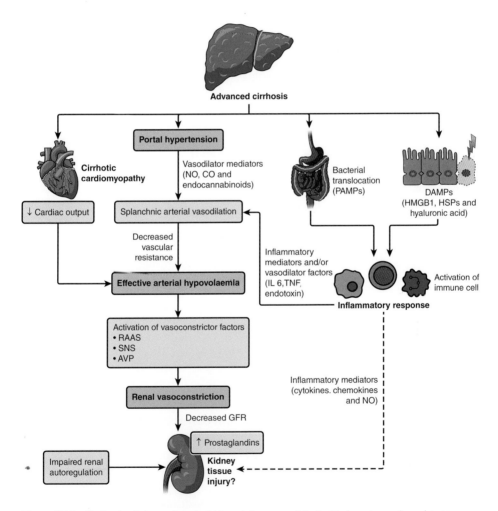

Figure 12.1 Pathophysiology of acute kidney injury associated with hepatorenal syndrome. AVP, arginine vasopressin; DAMPs, damage-associated molecular patterns; GFR, glomerular filtration rate; HMGB1, High mobility group box protein 1; HSPs, heat shock proteins; LI-6, interleukin-6; NO, nitric oxide; PAMPs, pathogen-associated molecular patterns; RAAS, renin–angiotensin–aldosterone system; SNS, sympathetic nervous system; TNF, tumor necrosis factor.

molecular patterns from bacterial translocation in the gut are thought to activate circulating innate immune cells, triggering a systemic inflammatory response and release of cytokines (including tumor necrosis factor alpha and interleukin-6) into the circulation, which may further exacerbate circulatory dysfunction.

In the earlier stages of chronic liver disease, a compensatory increase in cardiac output helps to maintain adequate renal perfusion. As hepatic dysfunction progresses, however, this compensatory mechanism is overwhelmed, exacerbated by the presence of "cirrhotic cardiomyopathy" (characterized by systolic and diastolic dysfunction, seen in up to 50% of patients with cirrhosis). Compensatory activation of the sympathetic nervous system, the renin–angiotensin–aldosterone system, and vasopressin release in addition may lead to intense renal vasoconstriction and a decline in GFR, alongside increased sodium and water retention, contributing to ascites formation.

Investigation

Initial evaluation to determine the underlying cause of AKI should include a detailed history and examination, including review of the drug treatment chart. Important investigations include:

- *Septic screen*, including C-reactive protein, blood and urine cultures, chest x-ray and ascitic tap to diagnose spontaneous bacterial peritonitis.
- *Endoscopy* in cases where gastrointestinal bleeding is suspected.
- *Urine analysis*: hematuria or proteinuria may suggest a glomerular pathology. Laboratory urine protein quantification (spot urine albumin : creatinine ratio or protein : creatinine ratio) is advised.

In patients where the cause of AKI remains unclear or if patients are slow to respond to initial resuscitation, the following additional investigations are suggested:

- *Ultrasound of the urinary tract* to define renal size, exclude obstructive uropathy or other structural urinary tract abnormalities.
- *Urine microscopy*: granular casts may be observed in patients with both AKI-HRS and ATN, but renal tubular epithelial cell casts are more specific to ATN. Red-cell casts can indicate active glomerulonephritis and bile acid casts may be associated with development of bile-cast nephropathy (Figure 12.2).
- *Urinary sodium*: in ATN, renal tubular function is impaired, leading to high urinary sodium concentration (>40 mEq/l), raised fractional sodium excretion ($>2\%$), and low urine osmolality (<350 mOsm/kg). Conversely, patients with AKI-HRS have low urinary sodium (<20 mEq/l), low fractional excretion of sodium ($<1\%$), and elevated urine osmolality (>500 mOsm/kg). Caution is advised, however, as these findings can frequently be misleading, especially when patients are receiving diuretic therapy.
- A *renal immunology screen* should be requested for all patients with proteinuria or hematoproteinuria, where glomerulonephritis is suspected from history or examination, or the cause of AKI remains unclear (Box 12.2; Figure 12.3; Table 12.4).
- *Renal biopsy* allows definitive histological diagnosis of AKI etiology, especially when intrinsic renal disease is suspected. It is important to note, however, that, due to coagulopathy, patients with cirrhosis are at especially high risk of bleeding complications and

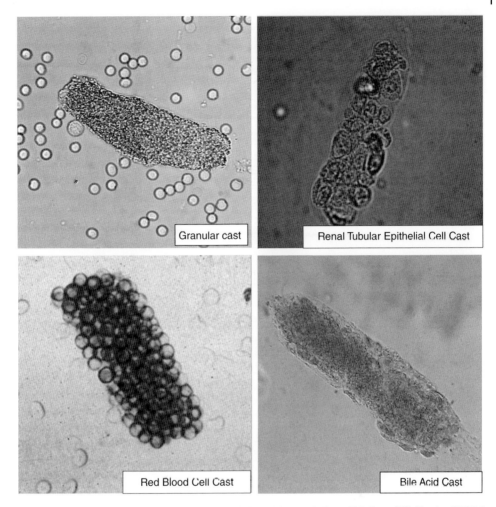

Figure 12.2   Urine microscopy. Source: Reilly 2013 / with permission of McGraw Hill. Usatine 2013 / with permission of McGraw-Hill. Mohapatra 2016 / Oxford University Press.

a decision to biopsy should only be made following careful risk–benefit assessment and correction of any ascites and coagulopathy.

Management

A step-by-step approach to management of AKI in patients with liver disease is outlined in (Figure 12.4). For patients with AKI, it is important stop any nephrotoxins such as non-steroidal anti-inflammatory drugs, aminoglycosides, or angiotensin-converting enzyme inhibitors/angiotensin receptor blockers. Vasodilator agents and laxatives should be discontinued in patients with severe diarrhea. Where intravascular volume depletion is present, diuretics should be withheld, and cautious fluid resuscitation, initiated with crystalloids or blood products (if hemoglobin <70 g/l), followed by volume expansion with albumin (1 g/kg/day for 48 hours) if renal impairment persists. There should be a low threshold for commencing

---

Box 12.2   Renal Involvement in Patients with Hepatitis C Virus-Associated Cryoglobulinemia

---

- Hepatitis C virus (HCV) is associated with type II (and to a lesser extent type III) mixed cryoglobulinemia.
- Patients are at risk of developing systemic vasculitis with multiorgan involvement.
- In patients with renal disease, histology typically demonstrates membranoproliferative glomerulonephritis with immune complex deposition.
- Other features include palpable purpura, usually over the lower limbs, which can ulcerate and progress to gangrene (Figure 12.3). Arthralgia/arthritis and peripheral neuropathy may also be observed.
- Treatment of HCV with direct antiviral agents is advised.
- In patients with nephrotic syndrome, declining kidney function, or systemic cyroglobulinemic flare; immunosuppression (e.g. rituximab ± plasmapheresis) should be considered.

Source: Based on Charles and Dustin (2009).

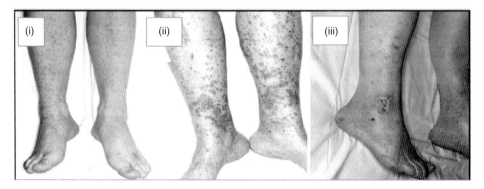

Figure 12.3   Cutaneous cryoglobulinemic vasculitis. Palpable purpura of the legs with (i) isolated, (ii) confluent lesions, and (ii) cutaneous perimalleolar ulcers. Source: Garini 2010 / with permission of Elsevier.

antibiotic therapy in cases of suspected infection. Assessment to guide continuing resuscitation is notoriously difficult, requiring regular clinical review in the setting of a high-dependency environment. Strict fluid balance, daily weight and measurement of postural blood pressure, hourly urine output, and central venous pressure may facilitate this process.

Key diagnostic criteria for AKI-HRS are outlined in (Box 12.3). Following albumin replacement, persistent AKI-HRS may be treated with splanchnic vasoconstriction using, for example, terlipressin. Terlipressin has been shown to reduce mortality risk in patients with AKI-HRS and to increase the proportion of patients who recover their renal function. Of note, terlipressin is not yet licensed for this indication in many countries, and caution is advised regarding its adverse effect profile, including severe abdominal pain and diarrhea, increased risk of cardiovascular events and respiratory failure. Alternative vasoconstrictors such as noradrenaline or midodrine/octreotide may be used, but there is increasing

Table 12.4 Renal screen – suggested immunology blood test panel.

Test	Associated conditions
Immunoglobulins A, G, M	IgA nephropathy, myeloma
Protein electrophoresis	Myeloma
Serum free light chains	Myeloma
ANA and dsDNA	SLE
Complement factors (C3 and C4)	SLE, cryoglobulinemic vasculitis
Anti-neutrophil cytoplasmic antibodies MPO and PR3	Vasculitis
Anti-glomerular basement membrane antibodies (GBM)	Goodpasture's syndrome
Anti-streptolysin O titer (ASOT)	Post-infectious glomerulonephritis
Angiotensin-converting enzyme (ACE)	Sarcoidosis
Cryoglobulins	Hepatitis C virus associated membranoproliferative glomerulonephritis
Phospholipase A2 receptor antibodies (PLA2R)	Idiopathic membranous nephropathy
Rheumatoid factor	Cryoglobulinaemic vasculitis

Ig, immunoglobulin; MPO, myeloperoxidase; PR3, proteinase 3; SLE, systemic lupus erythematosus.

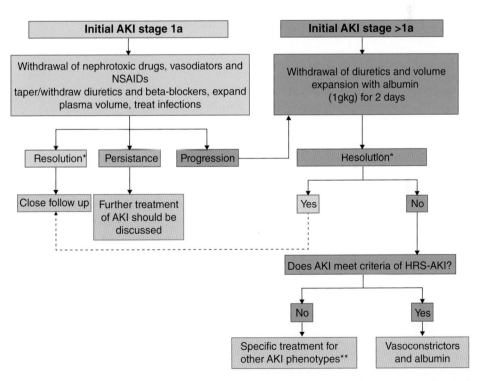

Figure 12.4 International Club of Ascites algorithm for the management of acute kidney injury (AKI) in patients with cirrhosis. Source: Sanchez and Francoz. [3] /with Permission of John Wiley & Sons. * Return of serum creatinine to a value within 0.3 mg/ml (26.5 μmol/l) from baseline. ** Specific diseases such as acute glomerulopathies or acute vascular diseases may require specific treatments discussed with nephrologist; in contrast, there is no specific treatment for acute tubular necrosis. HRS, hepatorenal syndrome; NSAIDs, non-steroidal anti-inflammatory drugs.

Box 12.3   Diagnostic Criteria for Acute Kidney Injury Hepatorenal Syndrome [2]

- Cirrhosis with ascites.
- Acute kidney injury: defined as increase in serum creatinine (sCr) $\geq$ 0.3 mg/dl ($\geq$ 26.5 µmol/l) within 48 hours; or > 50% rise in sCr from "baseline" in three months.
- No current or recent use of nephrotoxic drugs (non-steroidal anti-inflammatory drugs, diuretics).
- Absence of shock.
- No response after volume expansion with albumin 1 g/kg/day for 48 hours.
- Absence of parenchymal kidney disease:
  - no proteinuria (> 500 mg/day)
  - no hematuria (> 50 red blood cells/high-power field)
  - normal kidney ultrasonography.

---

evidence to suggest that the latter are less effective therapies. Patients with AKI-HRS require close monitoring to prevent fluid overload and progressive hyponatremia [5, 6].

Renal Replacement Therapy   Standard indications for initiating renal replacement therapy (RRT) in patients with AKI include intractable hyperkalemia, diuretic-unresponsive fluid overload, severe acidosis, and uremic complications. Careful consideration is required in patient selection, as RRT may be futile and burdensome in patients with advanced liver cirrhosis who have been deemed unsuitable for liver transplantation. It can be difficult to distinguish patients with potentially reversible ATN from those with AKI-HRS at presentation, and in selected cases a trial period of RRT while the clinical course and prognosis is clarified may be appropriate. There is inadequate high-quality evidence to support selection of any one RRT modality over another in this population, although continuous RRT may be better tolerated in patients with hemodynamic instability and/or cerebral edema.

Extracorporeal Liver Support Devices   Examples of extracorporeal albumin dialysis systems include the Molecular Adsorbent Recirculating System (MARS®), the Prometheus® Fractionated Plasma Separation and Adsorption System, and the Single-Pass Albumin Dialysis (SPAD®) systems. These systems allow removal of albumin-bound toxins from blood alongside RRT. Extracorporeal liver support devices may improve patient biochemistry profiles and symptoms of hepatic encephalopathy, and may reduce albumin-bound vasoactive agents, toxins, and proinflammatory cytokines, which contribute to splanchnic vasodilation in AKI-HRS. Evidence of survival benefit from such support devices is conflicting and, given their high costs, they are not currently part of routine clinical practice.

Transjugular Intrahepatic Portosystemic Shunt   In carefully selected cases, transjugular intrahepatic portosystemic shunt (TIPS) can reduce portal hypertension, improve kidney function, and relieve ascites. It may be less effective in AKI-HRS than in CKD associated with HRS (CKD-HRS). Unfortunately, TIPS can also precipitate hepatic encephalopathy (in up to 50% of cases), limiting its use in this setting [7].

Liver Transplantation   Given the high mortality risk for patients with cirrhosis who develop AKI, many of the prognostic indicators used to prioritize patients for liver transplantation, such as the Model for End-stage Liver Disease Score [8] and the UK Model for End-stage Liver Disease score incorporate serum creatinine measurements [9].

As AKI-HRS is characterized by functional renal impairment and structurally normal kidneys, AKI usually improves following liver transplantation. For this reason, a liver-only transplant with temporary RRT support would be appropriate for most patients. In some patients where there is severe AKI, in whom a prolonged period of RRT was required (over eight weeks), there may be irreversible renal injury, and a combined or sequential liver–kidney transplant may need to be considered (discussed further below).

Biomarkers   A critical issue in the diagnosis of AKI-HRS is differentiating it from other forms of AKI, particularly ATN. Biomarkers, including urinary neutrophil gelatinase-associated lipocalin and interleukin-18, are higher in patients with ATN compared with patients with AKI-HRS. The role of these biomarkers in clinical practice will likely continue to evolve.

Chronic Kidney Disease in Patients with Liver Cirrhosis

CKD is defined by KDIGO as "abnormalities of kidney structure or function, present for over three months." It requires one of two criteria documented or inferred for over three months: either GFR less than 60 ml/minute/1.73 m^2 or markers of kidney damage, including albuminuria. This definition encompasses CKD as a result of renal parenchymal damage, as well as due to functional renal impairment (e.g. from the altered hemodynamic in cirrhosis "CKD-HRS", previously "type 2 hepatorenal syndrome").

The true prevalence of CKD in cirrhotic patients is unknown. Studies have reported hugely varying prevalence and inadequacies of serum creatinine in this cohort likely leads to significant underrecognition. Patients with CKD in conjunction with cirrhosis appear to be at significant additional risk of morbidity and mortality, however, including inferior outcomes after liver transplantation.

Non-Alcohol-Associated Fatty Liver Disease

Owing to shared risk factors, CKD is common in patients with NAFLD, likely due to hypertensive and/or diabetic nephropathy. It is important to improve testing and early recognition of renal impairment in this high-risk population, to try to limit disease progression. Clinical management should center on optimization of risk factors including weight loss and better blood pressure and glycemic control. Early introduction of angiotensin receptor blockers or angiotensin-converting enzyme inhibitors can help reduce proteinuria (if tolerated), which is important to minimise risk of kidney disease progression and cardiovascular risk.

Other Causes

There is a high prevalence of diabetic nephropathy in patients with chronic hepatitis C virus (HCV) and these patients appear to be at high risk of progression to end-stage renal disease. Other causes include chronic glomerulonephritis (often in association with viral hepatitis or immunoglobulin A (IgA) nephropathy, particularly in patients with alcohol-use associated cirrhosis).

Chronic Kidney Disease Associated with Hepatorenal Syndrome

CKD-HRS is observed in patients with cirrhosis and ascites, characterized by a persistent eGFR less than 60 ml/minute/m^2, with no other cause of kidney disease found. Differences in mechanisms underlying the development of functional renal impairment in patients with AKI-HRS compared with CKD-HRS are not fully understood. Clinically, CKD-HRS tends be more gradual in onset and is often associated with refractory ascites. Untreated, patients with CKD-HRS tend to have longer median survival than patients with AKI-HRS (six months vs one to two months, respectively). CKD-HRS does not appear to respond to vasopressor therapy (e.g. terlipressin/norepinephrine). TIPS procedures, however, may be more effective at improving refractory ascites and renal dysfunction in CKD-HRS compared with AKI-HRS, albeit with a risk of encephalopathy.

For patients with CKD-HRS that require RRT, peritoneal dialysis may be considered, as it allows frequent drainage of ascites and may provide patients with symptomatic relief (although this benefit needs to be offset against the risk of additional protein wasting via peritoneal dialysis membranes and possible peritoneal infection). Liver transplantation for patients with CKD-HRS is discussed further below.

Renal Impairment in Patients with Acute Liver Failure

Approximately 70% of patients with ALF will develop AKI (30% requiring RRT). The incidence of AKI is highest in patients with ALF due to toxic paracetamol ingestion, compared to other etiologies. Most patients with ALF require early referral to specialist liver units for high-dependency care and monitoring. In cases where organ damage is potentially reversible, the underlying cause should be treated promptly (e.g. timely administration of N-acetylcysteine in patients who have taken a toxic paracetamol overdose). For the majority of patients, supportive therapy forms the mainstay of treatment. This includes restoration of circulatory volume and vasopressor support to maintain mean arterial pressure and renal perfusion. If there is limited response to initial resuscitation and oliguria persists, a low threshold to commence RRT is advised. Rising serum ammonia levels (greater than 150–200 µmol/l) and/or development of cerebral edema are independent clinical indications to commence RRT, regardless of serum creatinine values. Continuous RRT is usually preferred over intermittent hemodialysis in this setting to avoid rapid change in mean arterial pressure and biochemistry, which may adversely affect cerebral perfusion and lead to cerebral edema. Liver transplantation remains the definitive treatment for patients that do not respond to medical management.

Prognosis

Patients who have AKI at the time of emergency liver transplantation have not been found to have an increased risk of developing CKD during future follow-up. Despite this, patients with ALF who develop AKI still tend to have longer hospitalizations and reduced survival rates compared with patients without AKI.

Renal Impairment in Liver Transplant Recipients

Renal impairment is common among liver transplant recipients and associated with an increased risk of adverse patient outcomes, including reduced patient and graft survival.

Table 12.5 Spectrum of renal dysfunction in liver transplantation.

Period	Renal dysfunction
Before transplantation:	Hemodynamic-related GFR decline:
	Gastrointestinal bleed
	Lactulose
	Diuretics
	Infection
	Hepatorenal syndrome
	Pre-existing chronic kidney disease
	Parenchymal renal disease associated with liver disease:
	Immunoglobulin A nephropathy
	Membranoproliferative glomerulonephritis
	Membranous nephropathy
	Bilirubin cast nephropathy
At time of transplantation	Acute tubular necrosis
	Residual pretransplant renal dysfunction
	CNI-related acute hemodynamic decline in GFR
After transplantation	Acute tubular necrosis[a]
	CNI-related chronic toxicity
	Post-transplant diabetes
	Post-transplant hypertension

[a] Can be prolonged, lasting up to three months.
CNI, calcineurin inhibitor.

Patients may have pre-existing renal impairment or alternatively, they may develop AKI or CKD in the immediate postoperative period or during longer-term follow-up (Table 12.5).

Pre-Transplant Renal Dysfunction

Pre-liver transplant renal dysfunction (AKI or CKD) is associated with increased recipient morbidity and mortality, and increased costs to the healthcare system. Liver transplantation can trigger an accelerated decline in renal function due to a combination of factors, including perioperative AKI and calcineurin inhibitor toxicity. Although a combined liver–kidney transplant may be considered in some cases, for example in patients with end-stage renal failure, advanced CKD and/or with significant chronic damage on kidney biopsy, a liver transplant followed by a staged kidney transplant (at a later date) has some advantages, especially if there is a suitable live kidney donor. In this setting, the renal graft is implanted in a less toxic environment without the need for vasopressor support and has a higher rate of primary function.

Postoperative Acute Kidney Injury

AKI is commonly observed in the acute setting following liver transplantation, with the reported incidence as high as 95% (25% of patients requiring postoperative RRT). Risk factors for postoperative AKI include pre-transplant renal dysfunction, HCV infection and long-standing diabetes. Acute changes in kidney function are usually due to pre-renal AKI, ATN, hemodynamic changes associated with calcineurin inhibitor use or residual pre-transplant renal dysfunction.

Chronic Kidney Disease in Liver Transplant Recipients

CKD rates among liver transplant recipients are also high, with a reported five-year cumulative incidence of around 20%, increasing to around 50% at 10 years (CKD defined as eGFR $< 30\,\text{ml/minute/1.73}\,\text{m}^2$, persisting for more than three months). The most common cause for CKD is toxicity from calcineurin inhibitors. Other reported causes include hypertensive vascular changes, diabetic nephropathy, prolonged ATN, viral hepatitis-related glomerulonephritis, IgA nephropathy, and rarely proliferative glomerulonephritis.

Abnormal Liver Enzymes in Patients with Kidney Disease

Abnormal Liver Enzymes in Patients with Acute Kidney Injury

Abnormal liver enzymes are frequently observed in patients with AKI. Ischemic hepatitis in association with arterial hypotension or systemic inflammation is common. An extensive list of differential diagnoses to consider are outlined in Table 12.6, many of these conditions and their management have already been discussed across other specialty chapters.

Meticulous history taking and examination is essential to narrow down diagnoses and some key investigations to consider include:

- hepatitis viral serology
- blood film and hemolysis screen
- toxicology screen
- renal immunology screen (Table 12.4)
- urine dipstick and urine protein quantification (albumin : creatinine ratio)
- renal and liver ultrasound scan
- transthoracic echocardiography.

Abnormal Liver Enzymes in Patients with Chronic Kidney Disease

Elevated liver enzymes are commonly observed in patients with CKD, owing to systemic diseases that involve both the kidneys and the liver, hepatic congestion from fluid overload in patients with advanced CKD, or conditions such as viral hepatitis B (HBV) and HCV, that are prevalent among patients on dialysis. Figure 12.5 outlines a pathway for initial assessment of elevated liver enzymes among patients with CKD.

Systemic Diseases with Kidney and Liver Involvement

Systemic diseases can frequently involve both the kidneys and the liver, including metabolic, genetic, and autoimmune conditions (Table 12.7).

Table 12.6 Differential diagnoses for patients presenting with acute kidney injury and elevated liver enzymes.

Condition	Examples
Systemic conditions	Shock
	Congestive cardiac failure
	Thrombotic microangiopathies
	Hemophagocytosis lymphohistiocytosis
Infections	Viral hepatitis
	Leptospirosis
	Herpes simplex virus
	Varicella zoster virus
	Viral hemorrhagic fevers
	Toxoplasmosis
	Typhoid
	Borreliosis
	Rickettsioses
	Cytomegalovirus
Drugs/poisons	Paracetamol
	Amanita phalloides
	Isoniazid
	Halothane
Autoimmune	Glomerulonephritis (Table 12.4)

Polycystic Kidney Disease

Autosomal dominant polycystic kidney disease (ADPKD) is the most common inherited kidney disease worldwide and one of the leading causes of end-stage kidney disease (ESKD). In ADPKD, polycystic liver disease occurs in 75–95% of cases. Liver cysts are rare in children but their frequency increases with age, especially in women, under hormonal influences (e.g. pregnancy and/or use of estrogen replacement therapies). Synthetic liver function is usually unaffected in patients with polycystic liver disease, but many patients experience symptoms and discomfort related to "mass effect" from the enlarging liver and vena caval obstruction may develop in those with massive hepatomegaly. While tolvaptan (a vasopressin 2 receptor antagonist) therapy is increasingly used to delay CKD progression of ADPKD, it has little impact on hepatic cyst growth and is contraindicated in patients with liver dysfunction, requiring close monitoring of liver enzymes during therapy. There are, however, emerging data demonstrating the efficacy of the long-acting somatostatin analog, lanreotide, in reducing growth of liver cysts [10].

In autosomal recessive polycystic kidney disease, mutation of the *PKHD1* (fibrocystin) gene, leads to impaired development of the biliary tract. This is associated with congenital hepatic fibrosis, resulting in portal hypertension. Clinical phenotype and disease severity is

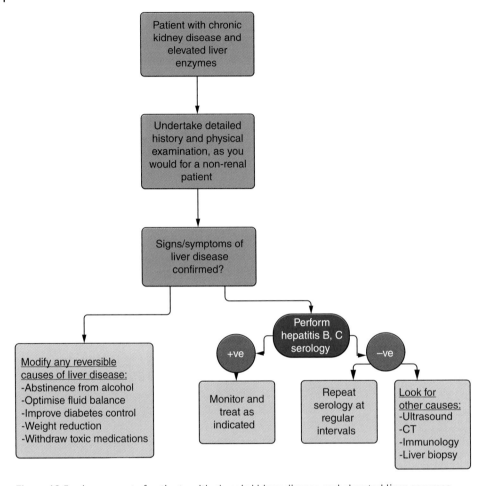

Figure 12.5   Assessment of patients with chronic kidney disease and elevated liver enzymes.

Table 12.7   Systemic conditions with liver and kidney involvement.

Grouping	Conditions
Metabolic	Diabetes
	Hereditary, primary, or secondary amyloidosis
Genetic	Autosomal dominant or recessive polycystic kidney disease
	Sickle cell disease
	Primary hyperoxaluria (liver function normal)
	Cystinosis
	Alagille syndrome
	Alpha-1-antitrypsin deficiency
	Wilson's disease
	Glycogen storage disease 1
Autoimmune	Sarcoidosis

highly variable, but clinical liver disease tends to become an increasing concern as patients age. Patients may develop recurrent cholangitis due to biliary tract dilatation, and/or complications of portal hypertension (occasionally requiring liver transplantation).

Primary Hyperoxaluria

Primary hyperoxaluria (PH) types 1–3 are metabolic disorders with autosomal recessive inheritance, leading to hepatic oxalate overproduction. Increased urinary excretion of oxalate can lead to formation of lithiasis and the development of nephrocalcinosis, associated with progressive CKD. Diagnosis is through genetic molecular analysis after finding of raised urinary oxalate. Type 1 often presents in childhood due to a deficiency in the alanine-glycolate aminotransferase enzyme, usually found in hepatic peroxisomes, whereas type 2 and 3 present later in life with renal calculi. Recent advances in management include development of RNA interference therapies which substantially reduce hepatic oxalate production in PH1 and 2. In PH1, liver–kidney transplantation is considered to be the definitive management, with best results when performed pre-dialysis in CKD stage 4/5.

Cystinosis

Cystinosis is a rare, autosomal recessive lysosomal storage disorder caused by mutations in the *CTNS* gene. Defective clearance of cystine from lysosomes leads to accumulation of cystine crystals in every tissue of the body, including the kidneys, eyes, muscles, liver, pancreas, and brain. Proximal tubules in the kidney are often affected first, leading to renal Fanconi syndrome. This is responsible for many of the early manifestations of disease (e.g. polyuria, polydipsia, rickets, feeding difficulties, and growth restriction). A late complication of hepatic cystine crystal accumulation in the liver involves activation of Kupffer cells, rarely leading to development of non-cirrhotic portal hypertension, usually with preserved liver function. Life-long regular oral cysteamine, ideally started in infancy, reduces the concentration of lysosomal cysteine in cells and reduces secondary organ dysfunction.

Alagille Syndrome

Alagille syndrome is a rare inherited disease, usually linked to gene mutations in *JAG1* or *NOTCH2*. The disease is characterized by a paucity of bile ducts in the liver, leading to jaundice, cholestasis, and associated complications. Extrahepatic manifestations of disease may include cardiac, ocular, and renal malformations, although clinical phenotype, disease severity, and age at presentation can vary considerably. Renal disease appears to be more common in patients with the *NOTCH2* mutations, and may include abnormalities of glomerular vasculature, podocytes, proximal tubules, renal dysplasia, and/or renal cysts. In addition, known alterations in lipid metabolism in Alagille syndrome can cause mesangial lipidosis in the kidney. Treatment is mainly supportive with a small proportion (10–30%) of patients requiring liver or combined liver–kidney transplants.

Dialysis

For patients with ESKD receiving dialysis, development of liver cirrhosis is associated with a 30–40% increased risk of mortality. Management of cirrhosis in patients with ESKD should typically follow the same principles as in patients without CKD. Reversible factors such as abstinence from alcohol, weight loss in NAFLD, and treatment of hepatitis should be addressed. It is important to note, however, that the use of dialysis is associated with lower transaminase levels and hepatitis viral counts, which should be taken into account during clinical assessment.

Viral Hepatitis in Patients on Dialysis

Viral hepatitis is a particular challenge in patients on dialysis, owing to the immunosuppressive effect of kidney disease, increased patient susceptibility to de novo bloodborne infections and risk of nosocomial transmission.

Hepatitis B Infection   Despite the availability of effective vaccines, HBV remains endemic in many countries worldwide. To reduce the risk of nosocomial transmission on dialysis units, robust infection control practice is essential. Expert international guidance underlies this. Patients with chronic HBV infection must be segregated from other patients during hemodialysis and necessitate dedicated hemodialysis machines. HBV vaccination response is reduced in patients with advanced CKD and vaccination programs optimized for patients receiving dialysis are required in addition to vaccination of staff members. It is essential this be combined with a rigorous screening policy for hepatitis B surface antigen (HBsAg) and hepatitis B surface antibody (HBsAb) antibody response to vaccine.

The natural history of HBV infection in patients on dialysis will vary according to the timing of infection, genotype, and locality. In endemic areas, most adult patients on dialysis with HBV infection are chronic carriers who acquired HBV infection during early childhood. By comparison, HBV infection in non-endemic areas is often acquired during adulthood. The majority of patients on dialysis who are newly HBV infected have a relatively mild clinical course, often asymptomatic with normal or only slightly elevated serum transaminase levels. Approximately 80% of patients will go on to develop chronic HBV infection, however. Some patients may have inactive disease, but others may experience intermittent disease flares, contributing to the development of cirrhosis or low-grade chronic hepatitis.

Once diagnosed, regular three- to six-monthly monitoring is required to assess for progression of HBV-related liver disease and for the development of hepatocellular carcinoma. The majority of studies to date have shown no convincing evidence of increased mortality or morbidity in patients on dialysis who are HBsAg positive compared with those who are HBsAg negative, with only 5% of patients dying from their liver problems. Despite a mild clinical course, treatment is still indicated in patients who are HBsAg positive with evidence of disease activity, as indicated by viral replication (with or without abnormal transaminase levels). Importantly, relying on hepatitis B e antigen (HBeAg) positivity alone to make decisions regarding treatment can be misleading, as it can be negative in patients with precore or core promotor-mutant infection, despite active disease. In view of the adverse effects of interferon in patients on dialysis, nucleotide, or nucleoside analogs are better choices, with entecavir or tenofovir the recommended first-line oral agents.

Hepatitis C Infection   HCV infections is also seen more commonly in patients on dialysis than in the general population. Infected patients demonstrate reduced survival compared to those without HCV. Risk factors include dialysis vintage, hemodialysis (compared with peritoneal dialysis), a high local prevalence of HCV infection and understaffing in individual dialysis units. Routine HCV screening of all patients on dialysis is recommended, followed by nucleic acid tests if the immunoassay is positive. Although standard infection prevention measures should always be followed, most guidelines recommend cohort dialysis of patients with HCV. Successful treatment of HCV infection (prior to the development of decompensated cirrhosis), can lead to decreased all-cause mortality and liver-related mortality, reduced need for liver transplantation and reduced incidence of hepatocellular carcinoma. Interferon-based therapies have demonstrated frequent and severe adverse effects, but the availability of direct-acting antiviral agents (DAAs) suitable for use with reduced renal clearance has revolutionized the management of these patients with excellent virus eradication seen in those with ESKD [11].

Hepatitis E Infection   Hepatitis E virus (HEV) is the most common cause of acute viral hepatitis worldwide. The prevalence of antibodies against HEV is higher among dialysis patients and staff, compared with the general population in parts of the world, suggesting possible nosocomial or parenteral transmission, alongside the fecal–oral route. Disease is mild and self-limiting in most cases, but it is important to remain vigilant over water sanitation and hygiene to reduce the risk of outbreaks. In immunosuppressed patients, HEV infection may become chronic and lead to cirrhosis, as discussed below.

Nephrogenic Ascites

Nephrogenic ascites is a rare condition, seen in ESKD. Patients present with refractory ascites of unknown cause after exclusion of infection, malignancy, cardiac, or liver failure. The ascitic fluid is characteristically high in protein, with a low leukocyte count (Box 12.4). It is a poorly understood condition, but contributing factors are likely to include altered permeability of the peritoneal membrane, hypoalbuminemia/poor nutrition, and impaired reabsorption of peritoneal fluid via the lymphatic system. Progressive cachexia occurs from the early satiety and poor appetite associated with large-volume ascites. Measures such as fluid and sodium restriction, albumin infusions, and repeat large-volume paracentesis usually provide only temporary relief. Improved uremic toxin clearance with daily hemodialysis or continuous ambulatory peritoneal dialysis have both been advocated, believed to alter the permeability of the peritoneal membrane. Kidney transplantation remains the most effective treatment however, with complete resolution of ascites noted within two to six weeks of transplantation in most cases.

Liver Disease in Kidney Transplant Recipients

Worldwide, elevated liver enzymes are seen in up to one third of renal transplant recipients. Possible reasons for this include:

- Pre-existing liver disease:
  - *Viral hepatitis*: there is a high prevalence of viral hepatitis among hemodialysis patients worldwide. Following transplantation, immunosuppressants may enhance the ability of HBV, for example to evade host immune response and replicate freely.
  - *Genetic diseases*: concomitant liver and renal dysfunction may develop in transplanted patients with inherited liver–kidney syndromes (e.g. polycystic kidney disease; Table 12.7).

Box 12.4   Nephrogenic Ascites

- Clinical features:
  - Ascites
  - End-stage renal disease
  - Anorexia, early satiety, cachexia
- Ascitic fluid analysis:
  - Straw-colored fluid
  - Low leukocyte count
  - High protein level
  - High albumin level
  - Low serum ascites albumin gradient
  - Negative culture and cytology
- Exclusions:
  - Congestive cardiac failure
  - Pericarditis
  - Liver cirrhosis
  - Budd–Chiari syndrome
  - Pancreatic pseudocyst
  - Peritoneal infection or malignancy
  - Hypothyroidism

- Post-transplant liver disease:
  - *Drug-induced liver injury*: potentially hepatotoxic drugs commonly used in the setting of kidney transplantation include antimetabolites (azathioprine) as well as ciclosporin. Idiosyncratic drug reactions are also frequently observed, including with antimicrobials (e.g. beta-lactam antibiotics, co-trimoxazole, isoniazid, and statins).
  - *NAFLD*: post-transplant metabolic syndrome and NAFLD are common among kidney transplant recipients, exacerbated by the association of calcineurin inhibitors and steroids with weight gain, diabetes, hypertension, and hyperlipidemia.
  - *Infections*: immunosuppressed kidney transplant recipients are vulnerable to a multitude of viral infections that frequently involve the liver, some of which are discussed in more detail below.

Viral Hepatitis in Kidney Transplant Recipients

Hepatitis C Virus

Chronic HCV infection in renal transplant recipients is associated with reduced graft and patient survival and an increased risk of developing systemic complications, such as:

- immune-mediated nephropathies (e.g. membranoproliferative glomerulonephritis)
- post-transplantation diabetes mellitus
- hepatocellular carcinoma.

HCV infection should not be considered a contraindication to kidney transplantation as transplant patients maintain a survival advantage over those who remain on dialysis. Whenever possible, patients should receive eradication treatment for HCV infection prior to transplant listing. The advent of new DAA has revolutionized treatment of HCV for patients with renal impairment, as DAAs appear to be relatively well tolerated in this cohort and are also extremely effective, with more than 95% of patients "cured" (demonstrating sustained viral response following 12 weeks of treatment). For patients infected in the post-transplantation period, it is important to remember to minimize immunosuppression as much as possible alongside DAA therapy.

HCV-Infected Organ Donors Owing to a shortage of organs worldwide, extended criteria kidneys from HCV-positive donors are increasingly being used for transplantation in HCV-positive recipients. Use of these kidneys can substantially reduce transplant waiting time, with no difference in short-term mortality compared with recipients of conventional donor criteria organs in initial studies. There is also now evolving experience of using HCV-positive donor kidneys to transplant HCV-negative recipients, treated post-transplant with a 12-week course of DAA therapy administered concurrently. This appears to be successful in curing HCV in organ recipients, with excellent short-term allograft outcomes observed thus far.

Hepatitis B Virus

Renal transplant recipients with chronic HBV infection are known to have significantly reduced graft and patient survival rates. Patients may have chronic HBV infection prior to transplantation or alternatively may develop HBV infection post-transplantation (donor-derived transmission). The highest risk for transmission occurs when the donor is HBsAg positive, with risk increasing if HBeAg is also detected. The risk from donors who are HBcAb positive (negative HBsAg and HBV DNA) is less than 5% in non-immune recipients and lower in those with post-vaccination therapeutic antibody levels. Anti-viral prophylaxis should be offered to naïve recipients of HBcAb-positive donor kidneys. Treatment regimens center on antiviral therapy and minimization of immunosuppression.

Hepatitis E Virus

HEV infection acquired via the facel–oral route has increased, and HEV infection can persist in immunosuppressed individuals, leading to chronic hepatitis and significant liver fibrosis if untreated. HEV screening is recommended for all potential organ donors. Transplant recipients should also be specifically advised against the risk of consuming undercooked meat (particularly processed pork). Transplant recipients do not need to be routinely screened for HEV, but testing should be undertaken in any patient with an unexplained elevation in liver enzymes or cirrhosis. Virus specific tests, including HEV RNA detection, must be used to diagnose HEV infection, as antibody detection is unreliable in immunosuppressed individuals.

The initial management of newly diagnosed or acute HEV infection includes monitoring of HEV RNA levels and liver enzymes, as more than 30% will spontaneously clear infection within three months. A strategic reduction in immunosuppression may be considered in patients with acute or persistent HEV as this may facilitate viral clearance, but the risk of rejection must be carefully balanced. Individuals with persistent HEV infection (documented or estimated duration of infection of more than three months) should be considered for treatment with ribavirin, with the aim of achieving sustained virological response (HEV RNA not detected in plasma and stool six months after completion of treatment) [12].

Other Infections

Cytomegalovirus   In immunocompetent patients, cytomegalovirus (CMV) is typically a self-limiting and mild disease. However, in kidney transplant recipients, new infection with or reactivation of CMV is a significant source of patient morbidity. Guidelines recommend 100–200 days of valganciclovir prophylaxis for CMV immunoglobulin G-negative recipients of a positive kidney, although frequent early monitoring of CMV via polymerase chain reaction (PCR), with treatment of positives is advocated by some. Roughly 50% of patients who develop systemic CMV disease will have hepatitis, which is typically worse in primary infection than reactivation. Diagnosis may be made using CMV PCR tests on blood in association with abnormal transaminase values. Liver biopsy is rarely required but, when performed, shows typical histology with intracellular CMV inclusions. Treatment is with oral or intravenous antivirals (ganciclovir and valganciclovir).

Herpes Simplex Virus   Primary herpes simplex virus (HSV) infection tends to be more severe in renal transplant recipients and reactivation is also more common. The risk of HSV reactivation is closely related to the level of immunosuppression and as such is highest within the first three months following transplantation. HSV hepatitis is associated with a high mortality rate (67%) and classically presents fever, herpetic stomatitis, abdominal pain, and may be associated with elevated transaminases. Risk factors for death include concomitant bacteremia, hypotension, disseminated intravascular coagulation or gastrointestinal bleeding. Owing to the high mortality risk, there should be a low threshold for commencing intravenous acyclovir therapy in the presence of suggestive symptoms.

Varicella Zoster Virus   The most common features of varicella zoster virus infection in renal transplant recipients include fever, cutaneous vesicles, abdominal pain, and diarrhea. In disseminated varicella zoster virus disease, however, there is often visceral involvement, including hepatitis, pneumonitis, and encephalitis. The clinical course is usually prolonged, with high patient morbidity and mortality rates, and treatment should include high-dose intravenous acyclovir therapy. Pre-transplantation zoster vaccination is recommended.

Liver Abscess   Pyogenic liver abscesses are extremely rare. The majority are polymicrobial, involving enteric bacteria, but up to 22% may be from *Candida* species. Immunosuppressed kidney transplant recipients traveling outside of the United States and Western Europe are also at risk of developing amoebic abscesses, as a result of ingesting contaminated food washed with fresh water. *Entamoeba histolytica* cysts can only be destroyed by boiling water, not iodine tablets or ultraviolet light. Clinical presentation is classically with right upper-quadrant pain, fever, and jaundice. Liver enzymes tend to be only modestly elevated, with abscesses detected via imaging. Treatment includes percutaneous drainage and antimicrobial therapy. Occasionally, surgical drainage or resection will be required, for example when there are multifocal abscesses or when abscesses are loculated.

Mycobacterium Infection The rate of active tuberculosis is 50-fold higher in kidney transplant recipients than the general population, with the bulk of disease attributed to reactivation within the first year after transplant. In many centers, tuberculosis prophylaxis is recommended post-transplant for those patients at high risk for 6–12 months postoperatively. Liver involvement is generally concurrent with pulmonary or gastrointestinal disease. Patients will usually present with constitutional symptoms, such as fever and modestly abnormal liver chemistries, in a hepatocellular or infiltrative pattern. Imaging and tissue sampling with acid fast staining and mycobacterial culture are required to make the diagnosis.

References

1. Yoo, J.-J., Kim, S.G., Kim, Y.S. et al. (2019). Estimation of renal function in patients with liver cirrhosis: impact of muscle mass and sex. *J. Hepatol.* 70 (5): 847–854.
2. Kidney Disease: Improving Global Outcomes (2012). Clinical practice guideline for acute kidney injury (AKI). *Kidney Int. Suppl.* 2 (4): 1–138.
3. Sanchez, L.O. and Francoz, C. (2021). Global strategy for the diagnosis and management of acute kidney injury in patients with liver cirrhosis. *United European. Gastroenterol J.* 9 (2): 220–228.
4. Martín-Llahí, M., Guevara, M., Torre, A. et al. (2011). Prognostic importance of the cause of renal failure in patients with cirrhosis. *Gastroenterol.* 140 (2): 488–496.e4.
5. Gluud, L.L., Christensen, K., Christensen, E., and Krag, A. (2012). Terlipressin for hepatorenal syndrome. *Cochrane Database Syst. Rev.* (9): CD005162.
6. Wong, F., Pappas, S.C., Curry, M.P. et al. (2021). Terlipressin plus albumin for the treatment of type 1 hepatorenal syndrome. *N. Engl. J. Med.* 384 (9): 818–828.
7. Aggarwal, A., Mitchell, J.E., Hanouneh, I.A. et al. (2011). The effect of transjugular intrahepatic portosystemic shunt on renal function in patients with liver cirrhosis. *Gastroenterol* 5 (140): S-958.
8. Singal, A.K. and Kamath, P.S. (2013). Model for End-stage Liver Disease. *J. Clin. Exp. Hepatol.* 3 (19): 50–60.
9. Wong, F., O'Leary, J.G., Reddy, K.R. et al. (2013). New consensus definition of acute kidney injury accurately predicts 30-day mortality in patients with cirrhosis and infection. *Gastroenterol.* 145 (6): 1280–1288.e1. https://doi.org/10.1053/j.gastro.2013.08.051.
10. van Aerts, R.M.M., Kievit, W., D'Agnolo, H.M.A. et al. (2019). Lanreotide reduces liver growth in patients with autosomal dominant polycystic liver and kidney disease. *Gastroenterol.* 157 (2): 481–491.e7.
11. Kidney Disease: Improving Global Outcomes (2018). KDIGO 2018 Clinical Practice Guideline for the Prevention, Diagnosis, Evaluation, and Treatment of Hepatitis C in Chronic Kidney Disease. *Kidney Int. Suppl.* 8 (3): 1–165.
12. British Transplantation Society (2017). *Guidelines for Hepatitis E and Solid Organ Transplantation.* St. Albans: BTS.
13. Charles, E.D. and Dustin, L.B. (2009). Hepatitis C virus–induced cryoglobulinemia. *Kidney Int.* 76 (8): 818–824.

13

Dermatology

Jennifer A. Scott and Peter C. Hayes

Royal Infirmary of Edinburgh, Edinburgh, UK

KEY POINTS

- Transient changes in liver function tests (LFTs) are frequently observed after commencing new drug therapies and are often improved when the medication is stopped.
- The risk of methotrexate-induced liver fibrosis is heightened by the presence of obesity, diabetes, increased age, and intake of more than 10 units of alcohol per week.
- Alcohol misuse is seen in up to 40% of patients with psoriasis and it can exacerbate a psoriatic flare.
- Patients with a detectable hepatitis B surface antigen (HBsAg) should be reviewed by a gastro-enterologist/hepatologist; they are usually treated with antivirals when immunosuppressed.

Introduction

Abnormal LFTs could be identified in dermatology as part of new patient assessment either in an acute setting or outpatient appointment, or during routine monitoring of drug therapies. Further investigation and management of abnormal LFTs are summarized in Figure 13.1.

Dermatological Drugs and Liver Function Tests

Transient changes in LFTs are frequently observed after commencing new drug therapies and are often improved when the medication is stopped. Some drugs, including methotrexate, can cause liver fibrosis. These drugs require regular monitoring of LFTs while on treatment. Table 13.1 summarizes the impact that common dermatological therapies may have on LFTs, discussed in more detail below.

The Liver in Systemic Disease: A Clinician's Guide to Abnormal Liver Tests, First Edition.
Edited by Gideon M. Hirschfield, Paramjit Gill, and James Neuberger.

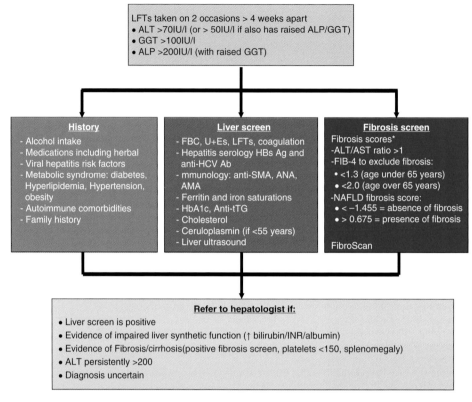

Figure 13.1 Flowchart to investigate abnormal liver function tests (LFTs) in dermatology setting. Ab, antibodies; ALP (IU/l), alkaline phosphatase; ALT (IU/l), alanine amino transferase; AMA, anti-mitochondrial antibody; AST (IU/l), aspartate amino transferase; FBC, full blood count; FIB-4, Fibrosis-4 Index for Liver Fibrosis; GGT, gamma-glutamyl transferase; HbA1c, hemoglobin A1c; HBsAg, hepatitis B surface antigen; HCV, hepatitis C virus; INR, international normalized ratio; NAFLD, non-alcoholic fatty liver disease; SMA, smooth muscle antibody; tTG, tissue transglutaminase; U+Es, urea and electrolytes;

* Fibrosis scores:
- ALT/AST ratio > 1 (in the absence of alcohol-related liver disease),
- FIB-4
  - excluding advanced fibrosis was < 1.3 for patients ≤ 65 years and < 2.0 for age > 65 years
  - to predict advanced fibrosis was > 3.25 for both age groups
- NAFLD fibrosis score:
  - < −1.455: predictor of absence of significant fibrosis (F0–F2 fibrosis)
  - ≥ −1.455 to ≤ 0.675: indeterminate score
  - > 0.675: predictor of presence of significant fibrosis (F3–F4 fibrosis)

Methotrexate

Methotrexate is used in the treatment of severe psoriasis [1–3]. It is an antifolate and anti-metabolite drug that blocks dihydrofolic acid reductase, inhibiting purine and pyrimidines synthesis, and depleting intracellular stores of folate reducing synthesis of DNA and RNA causing cellular arrest. Moreover, there are increased levels of intracellular adenosine

Table 13.1 Drugs used in dermatology and patterns of LFTs.

Pattern	Drug
Cholestatic (↑ ALP/GGT)	Co-amoxiclav
	Erythromycin
	Estrogen (oral contraceptives)
	Flucloxacillin
	Terbinafine
	6-Mercaptopurine
	Phenytoin
	Rifampicin
	Sulfonamides
	Terinabine
	Tetracyclines
	Tricyclics
Cholestatic pattern (↑ALP/GGT)	Cytotoxic pattern (↑ ALT)
	Allopurinol
	Azathioprine/6-mercaptopurine
	Etretinate
	Ketoconazole/fluconazole
	Methotrexate

ALP, alkaline phosphatase; ALT, alanine amino transferase; GGT, gamma-glutamyl transferase.

secondary to 5-aminoimidazole-4-carboxamide ribonucleotide formyltransferase inhibition. Adenosine stimulates hepatic stellate cells (liver-specific mesenchymal cells) to release pathological collagen fibers promoting liver fibrosis. Methotrexate has also been shown to promote proliferation of hepatic stellate cells.

The resultant liver damage can range from mild hepatitis to, very rarely, fulminant hepatic failure. Elevation in serum aminotransferase is common. High-dose methotrexate can increase alanine amino transferase (ALT) to 10–20 times the upper limit of normal (ULN). These levels often improve within 12–48 hours of treatment. Moderate methotrexate doses can cause elevation in serum aminotransferase in 15–50% of the population, but this is often mild and self-limiting. The fluctuation seen in LFTs could also be dependent on timings of blood tests taken before or after the dose of methotrexate. Studies have demonstrated that concurrent folic acid replacement reduces the rate of ALT elevation in patients on low-dose methotrexate. Acute jaundice or liver failure secondary to drug induce liver injury with methotrexate is very rare. With high rates of coexistent fatty liver, low level changes in serum liver tests are very commonly encountered coincidentally.

Hepatitis B can be reactivated by low-dose methotrexate, even in those with normal ALT, no detectable hepatitis B virus (HBV) DNA and no hepatitis B e antigen. This acute reactivation can result in hepatic failure, liver transplantation, and death. It is therefore important to complete a viral hepatology screen prior to methotrexate therapy. Patients with detectable HBsAg should be reviewed by a gastroenterologist/hepatologist, and are usually treated with antivirals when immunosuppressed. Patients with prior exposure to hepatitis B (cAb positive, sAg negative) are usually monitored every three months.

Liver fibrosis is the result of deposition of pathologic collagen-rich extracellular matrix, in response to continuing chronic liver injury. End-stage liver disease or cirrhosis causes portal hypertension, resulting in varices, ascites, and encephalopathy, for which the only curative therapy is liver transplantation. The risk of methotrexate-induced liver fibrosis is heightened by the presence of obesity, diabetes, increased age, and intake of more than 10 units of alcohol per week. With such a high prevalence of fatty liver, methotrexate is not usually the culprit.

Around 30% of patients treated with methotrexate will develop mild to moderate histological changes, including fatty deposition and mild inflammation. Up to 15% of patients treated with methotrexate will develop mild fibrosis and 1% will have moderate fibrosis or cirrhosis often within 2–10 years of commencing therapy. Some patients will develop portal hypertension without significant fibrosis, suggesting that methotrexate could result in nodular regeneration of the liver. Hepatocellular carcinoma in patients treated with methotrexate is rare and the evidence is limited to case reports.

Liver biopsy has been considered the gold standard to diagnose liver fibrosis. Previously, patients would undergo biopsy after 1, 4, and 8 g of cumulative methotrexate. However, diagnostic accuracy is impeded by sampling error and inter-pathologist variation in interpretation. Moreover, liver biopsy is invasive and associated with morbidity including pain, bleeding, infection, and damage to nearby organs.

In modern hepatic clinical practice fibrosis scores and measurement of transient elastography (TE) using a FibroScan® (Echosens) have become well established for diagnosing liver fibrosis without biopsy. Box 13.1 shows our recommendations for their use in patients on methotrexate.

Retinoids

Retinoids are used in the management of acne, psoriasis, and Darier's disease. A rise in serum aminotransferases is seen in around 20% of patients but its significance is uncertain. Retinoids can cause acute hepatitis but rarely cause chronic liver disease. Monitoring for retinoids [5] consists of monitoring LFTs at the start of therapy. If they are persistently abnormal, reduce and potentially stop treatment.

Azathioprine

Azathioprine is used to treat various dermatological conditions including pemphigus, pemphigoid, eczema, systemic lupus erythematosus, and dermatomyositis. Elevation of liver enzymes and cholestasis are not uncommon, but are usually reversible on withdrawal of azathioprine. A hypersensitivity reaction to azathioprine is rare, but can result in cholestatic jaundice, portal fibrosis, nodular regenerative hyperplasia, hepatocellular necrosis, fever, and shock. LFTs should be monitored every three months.

Box 13.1 Recommendations for The Use of Transient Elastography in Patients on Methotrexate

---

- Advice to patients on methotrexate:
  - Avoid alcohol
  - Weight loss to achieve a body mass index within normal range
  - Good diabetic control
  - Concurrent folic acid
- Monitoring blood tests in patients on methotrexate [4]:
  - Three-monthly LFTs
  - ± procollagen III N-terminal peptide (PIIINP) levels (for patients with psoriasis only)
  - Refer to hepatologist if:
    - ○ Persistently abnormal LFTs on two separate occasions (Figure 13.1)
    - ○ PIIINP > 8 g/l on two occasions
    - ○ PIIINP > 4.2 g/l on three occasions in a 12-month period
    - ○ PIIINP > 10 g/l on a single occasion
- Measurement of fibrosis in patients on methotrexate:
  - In patients at high risk, consider fibrosis assessment prior to commencing methotrexate
  - Assess for evidence of fibrosis using one of the following fibrosis scores
    - ○ Elevated hyaluronic acid or Enhanced Liver Fibrosis score
    - ○ Non-alcoholic fatty liver disease fibrosis score ≥ −1.455: request TE
    - ○ Fibrosis-4 Index for Liver Fibrosis > 1.3: request TE
  - Interpretation of FibroScan® or TE [1]
    - ○ TE < 7.5 kPa: repeat in three years
    - ○ TE 7.5–9.5 kPa: repeat in one year
    - ○ TE > 9.5 kPa: stop methotrexate and refer to hepatologist

---

Cyclosporin

Cyclosporin is used to treat a large range or conditions in dermatology, including psoriasis, eczema, pyoderma gangrenosum, Behçet's disease, lichen planus, pemphigus, and pemphigoid. Metabolism of cyclosporin is controlled primarily by the liver; it should be given cautiously to people with pre-existing liver disease.

Asymptomatic hyperbilirubinemia occurs in up to 50% of those taking cyclosporin, and withdrawal of treatment results in normalization of bilirubin levels.

Antifungal Medication

Itraconazole has a low risk of causing hepatic injury and therefore LFTs should be monitored regularly while on treatment. Terbinafine, which is used to treat toenail and skin infections, can cause intrahepatic cholestasis.

Chinese Herbal Medication

Chinese herbal medications are taken for a variety of conditions and contain a mixture of unregulated products. LFTs are commonly elevated as a result of these medication and can take between one and six months to normalize after stopping treatment. Chinese herbal medicine can result in both acute hepatitis and chronic liver damage.

When is Further Investigation Required?

If patients are asymptomatic with deranged LFTs on drug monitoring or patient review, LFTs should be repeated four weeks later. Further investigation is required if LFTs are persistently abnormal on two separate occasions greater than four weeks apart (Figure 13.1):

- ALT > 70 IU/l or >50 IU/l if also has raised alkaline phosphatase (ALP)/gamma-glutamyl transferase (GGT)
- GGT > 100 IU/l
- ALP > 200 IU/l (with raised GGT).

Liver Disease that Mimics Dermatological Diseases

Several conditions in hepatology may present initially with skin changes.

Primary Biliary Cholangitis

Xanthelasmas are fatty deposits found on the upper and lower eyelids. Together with cutaneous xanthomas, they are seen in around 5% of patients with primary biliary cholangitis (PBC) [6]. Less frequently, patients with PBC can also develop sicca syndrome and vitiligo. More rarely, PBC has been associated with cutaneous vasculitis, polyarteritis nodosa, and pustular vasculitis.

Alcohol-Related Liver Disease

Porphyria cutanea tarda occurs as a result of uroporphyrinogen decarboxylase deficiency. It causes a purple blistering rash in sun-exposed areas. Alcohol is the most common trigger for this, exacerbated by concurrent hepatitis C infection.

Hepatitis C

Hepatitis C viral infection can exacerbate porphyria cutanea tarda rash. It is also associated with several other dermatological conditions including cryoglobulinemia, polyarteritis nodosa, leukocytoclastic vasculitis, and an urticarial rash.

Hemochromatosis

Haemochromatosis causes iron levels to build up in the body, which can result in liver cirrhosis. A "slate gray" skin has been described as the classic skin manifestation.

Liver Disease Associated with Dermatological Disease

There are several conditions in hepatology that are associated with dermatological disease.

Psoriasis

- Non-alcoholic fatty liver disease is seen in 50% of patients with psoriasis, with increased rates in those with higher psoriasis area and severity index scores.
- Alcohol misuse is seen in up to 40% of patients with psoriasis; it can exacerbate a psoriatic flare.
- PBC has been identified in up to 13% of patients with psoriasis [7].
- Hepatitis C can be a late trigger for psoriasis; several treatments for psoriasis could potentially reactivate previous hepatitis B and C.
- A raised bilirubin or hypoalbuminemia may occur as a result of general toxicity in erythrodermic psoriasis.

Sarcoidosis

- Sarcoidosis of the skin occurs in many forms, including erythema nodosum (30%) or lupus pernio.
- Hepatic granulomas are found in two thirds of liver biopsies performed on patients with sarcoidosis. These rarely result in fibrosis and often causes no symptoms or complications.
- The hepatic complication rate is less than 1% and typically affects black male patients with severe fibrotic sarcoidosis of the lungs and eyes with symptoms of:
  - cholestatic form: jaundice, pruritis, and hepatosplenomegaly
  - portal hypertension: presinusoidal due to narrowing of smaller portal venous radicles.
- Treatment is with corticosteroids, which can improve LFTs but no not reduce portal hypertension.

Lichen Planus

Up to 50% of patients with lichen planus have been found to have raised LFTs. Although the exact cause is unclear, lichen planus has been associated with PBC and hepatitis C.

Dermatitis Herpetiformis

- Patients with celiac disease can develop multiple pruritic vesiculobullous lesions; around 17% of these patients have abnormal LFTs.
- Most LFTs will normalize following withdrawal of gluten, although a raised bilirubin can be due to dapsone, a treatment for dermatitis herpetiformis.

Mastocytosis

- Mastocytosis is the result of mast cell proliferation in one or more organ systems; it has four different dermatological presentations.

- Around 40% of patients will have hepatomegaly and a raised ALP.
- Complications of hepatic mastocytosis include liver fibrosis, nodular regenerative hyperplasia, and portal veno-occlusive disease.

Dermatological Malignancies

- Basal-cell carcinoma: rarely metastasises.
- Squamous cell carcinoma: metastases are rare and unpredictable.
- Malignant melanoma: metastasises widely to liver, lungs, bone, and brain.
- Primary sarcomas do have metastatic potential, but rare.
- Merkel cell tumor has a high incidence of secondary spread, including the liver.
- Kaposi sarcoma is related to HIV, and may have co-infection with hepatitis B and C.

Neurofibromatosis

Type 1 neurofibromatosis is an autosomal dominant condition affecting 1 : 2500 people:

- Cutaneous lesions include café au lait spots, axillary freckling, and cutaneous neurofibromas.
- Plexiform neurofibromas can involve the liver, infiltrating the porta hepatis, and intrahepatic portal branches of the liver causing hepatomegaly and abdominal pain. Moreover, jaundice can result from extrahepatic biliary obstruction.

Type 2 neurofibromatosis is an autosomal dominant condition affecting 1 : 30000 people:

- It is associated with bilateral acoustic neuroma.
- Skin lesions are rare and liver lesions even more so.

Other Dermatology Conditions

- *Toxic epidermal necrolysis*: elevated aminotransferases may occur as a result of the severe systemic impact of this condition.
- *Dermatomyositis*: transaminases aspartate amino transferase and ALT levels can be elevated but as a result of muscle fiber damage, not liver disease.
- *Kawasaki disease*: occasionally associated with hepatomegaly and non-specific elevation of ALT. Few cases of intrahepatic cholangitis have been reported.

Unexplained Abnormal Liver Function Tests in Patients with Known Dermatological Disease

Once abnormal LFTs have been identified, further investigations are needed and the diagnostic steps for this are detailed in Figure 13.1. These investigations will help to identify the cause of abnormal LFTs and assess for evidence of organ damage and fibrosis.

References

1. Cheng, H.S. and Rademaker, M. (2018). Monitoring methotrexate-induced liver fibrosis in patients with psoriasis: utility of transient elastography. *Psoriasis (Auckl.)* 8: 21–29.
2. National Institute of Diabetes and Digestive and Kidney Diseases (2020). Methotrexte. In: *LiverTox: Clinical and Research Information on Drug-Induced Liver Injury*. Bethesda, MD: https://www.ncbi.nlm.nih.gov/books/NBK548219. Accessed 1 May 2022.
3. Zachariae, H. (1990). Methotrexate side-effects. *Br. J. Dermatol.* 122 (s36): 127–133.
4. Potts, J.R., Maybury, C.M., Salam, A. et al. (2017). Diagnosing liver fibrosis: a narrative review of current literature for dermatologists. *Br. J. Dermatol.* 177 (3): 637–644.
5. Shalita, A.R. (1992). Introduction: retinoids: present and future. *J. Am. Acad. Dermatol.* 27 (6, Part 2): S1.
6. Koulaouzidis, A., Bhat, S., and Moschos, J. (2007). Skin manifestations of liver diseases. *Ann. Hepatol.* 6 (3): 181–184.
7. Howel, D., Fischbacher, C.M., Bhopal, R.S. et al. (2000). An exploratory population-based case-control study of primary biliary cirrhosis. *Hepatology* 31 (5): 1055–1060.

14

Oncology

Mai Kilany and Morven Cunningham

Toronto General Hospital, Toronto, Ontario, Canada

KEY POINTS

- Abnormal serum liver tests are common in patients with oncologic disease.
- Differential diagnosis may vary according to treatment status, primary cancer, and type of oncologic therapy.
- Abnormal serum liver tests identified at any stage should be fully evaluated, to identify any pre-existing or de novo causes unrelated to oncologic disease or its treatment.
- Situations to consider hepatology referral include:
  - identification of a coexistent primary liver disease during investigation of abnormal serum liver tests
  - persistent, unexplained abnormal serum liver tests
  - on-treatment abnormal serum liver tests that do not resolve after stopping treatment
  - any signs or symptoms of liver dysfunction (e.g. elevated bilirubin; elevated international normalized ratio (INR); ascites; hepatic encephalopathy).

Liver Diseases That May Mimic Oncologic Diseases

Primary liver disease that mimics oncologic disease is relatively uncommon. Benign liver lesions, such as hemangiomas, focal nodular hyperplasia, or adenomas are common incidental radiological findings, affecting around 7–10% of the general population [1]. Occasionally, benign liver lesions may be identified for the first time in patient undergoing abdominal imaging following a new diagnosis of malignancy, or in follow- up after previous cancer treatment, causing diagnostic confusion over the possibility of metastatic disease. Focal nodular hyperplasia can develop following vascular injury to the liver, which may occur after some systemic chemotherapies or radiation therapy. Dedicated contrast imaging in experienced hands is often diagnostic, although in some cases a biopsy may be required for confirmation of the nature of the lesion. Imaging diagnosis may be preferable to avoid the potential for tumor seeding after biopsy, although with modern techniques and limited sampling, this risk appears to be very low.

The Liver in Systemic Disease: A Clinician's Guide to Abnormal Liver Tests, First Edition.
Edited by Gideon M. Hirschfield, Paramjit Gill, and James Neuberger.
© 2023 John Wiley & Sons Ltd. Published 2023 by John Wiley & Sons Ltd.

Liver Diseases Associated with Oncologic Diseases

With the exception of hepatocellular carcinoma (HCC), liver disease associated with primary oncologic disease is rare. HCC occurs almost exclusively in patients with underlying chronic liver disease, usually either cirrhosis or chronic hepatitis B virus (HBV) infection. If HCC is diagnosed in a patient not previously known to have liver disease, screening for viral hepatitis, and other causes of liver disease should be performed.

Although not common, chronic hepatitis C virus (HCV) infection may be associated with a range of extrahepatic manifestations, including B-cell lymphoproliferative disorders. These manifestations range from mixed cryoglobulinemia and monoclonal gammopathies to B-cell non-Hodgkin's lymphoma, especially lymphoplasmacytic, marginal zone, and diffuse large B-cell lymphomas. Clinical remission of low-grade B-cell lymphomas following successful antiviral therapy has been reported, especially in patients with splenic lymphoma [2].

Rarely, paraneoplastic syndromes may cause abnormal liver tests. Stauffer syndrome is a paraneoplastic disorder, originally described as a combination of hypoalbuminemia, hypergammaglobulinemia, elevated alkaline phosphatase (ALP), and prolonged prothrombin time in association with renal cell carcinoma, with normalization of liver enzymes and function after tumor resection. This syndrome has also been reported in association with other malignancies including soft tissue sarcomas, prostate cancer, and lymphoproliferative diseases. Since the original description, cases including jaundice and transaminase elevation have also been reported. The pathophysiology of Stauffer syndrome remains uncertain, but may involve pro-inflammatory activity of the cytokine interleukin-6. This syndrome should be considered in patients with oncologic disease presenting with liver dysfunction and cholestatic liver enzyme elevations, especially if more common caused have been ruled out [3].

Many instances of liver test abnormalities seen in patients with oncologic disease represent consequences or complications of cancer treatment. Almost all antineoplastic drugs are associated with some risk for hepatotoxicity, and host factors that may predispose to drug-induced liver injury (DILI; such as age, sex, nutritional status, combination therapies, concomitant medications, genetic susceptibility, hepatic metastases, radiation, and pre-existing liver disease) may also be prevalent in patients with oncologic disease. However, such is the unmet health need in cancer therapeutics that new therapies known to cause significant liver injury may be approved for use in circumstances where the potential benefit in cancer outcome outweighs the recognized risk for liver injury. Antineoplastic drugs are associated with a broad spectrum of liver injury, although some specific associations are recognized (Table 14.1) [4].

Liver Enzyme Elevations

Some degree of liver enzyme elevation is often seen after initiation of an antineoplastic therapy, and the pattern of enzyme elevation may be hepatocellular, cholestatic, or mixed. It is important to distinguish mild enzyme elevations, which may represent an adaptive response in the liver and may normalize even without dose adjustment, from more significant enzyme elevations, which indicate a more significant liver injury and necessitate drug

Table 14.1 Characteristic patterns of drug-induced liver injuries associated with cancer therapies.[a]

Pattern of injury/ phenotype	Description	Examples of typical associated drugs	Postulated mechanism(s)
Hepatitis	Hepatocellular pattern of injury; time to onset often – 12 weeks	Fluorouracil, cytarabine, doxorubicin	Production of toxic intermediates during metabolism in the liver
Cholestasis/ mixed	Liver injury with ALP elevation ≥ ALT elevation; time to onset usually 2–12 weeks, may be associated with jaundice	Temozolomide, cyclophosphamide, melphalan, chlorambucil, tamoxifen	Idiosyncratic; mechanism unclear
Hepatic steatosis	Micro- or macrovesicular steatosis ± inflammation and fibrosis	Fluorouracil, irinotecan, etoposide; tamoxifen	Inhibition of mitochondrial function; estrogenic effects on fat metabolism
Sinusoidal obstruction syndrome	Hepatic endothelial cell injury	Busulphan, cyclophosphamide, oxaliplatin, dacarbazine	Damage to hepatic sinusoidal endothelium
Nodular regenerative hyperplasia	Benign small regenerative nodules	Busulphan, oxaliplatin, trastuzumab emtansine	Damage to portal venules
Immune-mediated hepatitis	Hepatocellular pattern of injury (rarely cholestatic); typically 6–14 weeks after starting immune checkpoint inhibitor	Immune checkpoint inhibitors (e.g. ipilimumab; pembrolizumab; nivolumab)	Seronegative immune-mediated liver injury

ALP, alkaline phosphatase; ALT, alanine amino transferase.
[a] This table gives typical examples but does not include every class of oncologic treatment. The list of associated drugs is not exhaustive.
Source: Based on [4].

hold or dose adjustment. Biochemical criteria to identify potential cases of DILI have been defined by consensus expert opinion, such as those described by the Drug-Induced Liver Injury Network [5]:

- Alanine amino transferase (ALT) or aspartate amino transferase (AST) greater than five times the upper limit of normal (ULN), or ALP greater than twice the ULN on two consecutive occasions.
- Total bilirubin greater than 2.5 mg/dl (43 μmol/l) and elevated ALT, AST, or ALP.
- INR greater than 1.5 and elevated ALT, AST, or ALP.

Liver injury will usually normalize after the causative drug is held, although this is not always the case and it can evolve into a chronic injury. Although relatively rare, severe liver injury leading to liver failure has been reported with several antineoplastic agents, emphasizing the importance of close monitoring. DILI causing hepatocellular pattern enzyme elevation associated with jaundice carries a 10% risk of death or need for liver transplant.

Chemotherapy-Associated Steatohepatitis

Non-alcoholic fatty liver disease (NAFLD), comprising steatosis (accumulation of fat in hepatocytes), and steatohepatitis (NASH; steatosis associated with hepatocyte ballooning and inflammation) is common, with a prevalence of 20–30% in many countries worldwide. Common risks for NAFLD include obesity and metabolic syndrome (abdominal adiposity, diabetes, hypertension, dyslipidemia). Development of hepatic steatosis and steatohepatitis, histologically identical to NAFLD/NASH, has also been associated with chemotherapeutic agents including 5-flurouracil, irinotecan, L-asparaginase, methotrexate, and tamoxifen, through mechanisms leading to mitochondrial toxicity and dysfunction. Patients with coexisting metabolic risks appear to be at higher risk for chemotherapy-associated steatohepatitis (CASH), which usually presents with elevated liver enzymes and hepatic steatosis on imaging. To distinguish steatosis from steatohepatitis requires a liver biopsy, although in practice this is rarely necessary.

In patients with metastatic colorectal cancer receiving chemotherapy prior to resection of hepatic metastases, CASH forms part of a spectrum of chemotherapy-associated liver injury (CALI), which also includes vascular injury, specifically sinusoidal injury and nodular regenerative hyperplasia (NRH) [6]. Patients with CALI who undergo surgical resection of hepatic metastases may have an increased risk of postoperative morbidity and possibly mortality [6]. The relative impact of different patterns of liver injury remains unclear, although the presence of steatohepatitis (as opposed to simple steatosis) may be associated with increased mortality after surgical resection of hepatic metastases [7]. Shorter durations of chemotherapy may optimize anti-cancer effects while minimizing toxicity, with several reports indicating that administration of up to six cycles of neoadjuvant chemotherapy has minimal impact on risk of morbidity and mortality after subsequent liver resection, while patients receiving more than 12 cycles of preoperative chemotherapy had higher rates of reoperation and longer hospital stay [6, 8].

CASH is usually reversible upon completion of chemotherapy. In patients who will require long-term treatment (e.g. patients treated with tamoxifen), benefits of treatment need to be weighed against potential risks for progressive liver disease. Large case series have shown that tamoxifen-related fatty liver disease occurs predominantly in women who are overweight or obese with other metabolic risks, indicating the importance of host factors on risk for CASH. Management of other metabolic risks should be optimized, and patients should be advised on lifestyle management of fatty liver disease (including gradual, sustainable loss of 7–10% of body weight, through increased physical activity and adoption of a "Mediterranean style" diet). Risk for progression to advanced fibrosis/cirrhosis appears low. Therefore, the balance of risk and benefit is usually in favor of continuing treatment and optimizing the management of other metabolic risk factors. However, referral to a hepatologist for risk assessment, particularly fibrosis assessment, should be considered.

Hepatic Sinusoidal Injury

Hepatic sinusoidal injury can range from asymptomatic sinusoidal dilatation to sinusoidal obstruction syndrome (SOS; previously termed veno-occlusive disease). SOS is most frequently seen in the setting of conditioning treatment prior to hematopoietic cell transplant, where combination myeloablative treatments (such as busulfan, cyclophosphamide, melphalan, carmustine, and whole-body irradiation) may be used. However, SOS has also been described after single-agent treatment with other agents, including dacarbazine, gemtuzumab, oxaliplatin, and carboplatin [9]. Aggregation of endothelial cells and erythrocytes causes occlusion of the small hepatic veins and eventually resulting in hepatic congestion and sinusoidal dilatation. This may trigger activation of stellate cells and a fibrotic reaction in the sinusoids, leading to obliteration of the central venules. SOS is associated with severe congestion, and potentially fatal centrilobular hepatocyte necrosis.

Mild hepatic sinusoidal injury is often asymptomatic, although is recognized as part of the spectrum of CALI reported in patients with metastatic colorectal cancer undergoing liver resection. Oxaliplatin-based combination regimens are particularly associated with vascular injury, with background liver in resection specimens from just over 50% of oxaliplatin-treated patients showing pathological changes of SOS [10]. Interestingly, combination treatment with the anti-vascular endothelial growth factor A antibody bevacizumab appears protective against oxaliplatin-associated vascular injury [11].

The clinical presentation of symptomatic SOS is classified as acute, subacute, and chronic. Acute SOS presents with abdominal pain, ascites, and edema, with or without jaundice and elevated liver enzymes, usually within one to three weeks of drug exposure. Subacute or chronic SOS usually presents with fatigue, weakness, ascites, and other symptoms of portal hypertension, and may present months or even years after exposure [12]. Imaging may demonstrate perfusion abnormalities although with patent portal and hepatic veins.

The diagnosis of SOS can usually be made on clinical grounds, with biopsy reserved for atypical presentations. Clinical criteria such as the modified Seattle, Baltimore, or European Society for Blood and Marrow Transplantation criteria, can be used for diagnosis and staging severity [12, 13].

Treatment of SOS depends on severity. Mild to moderate cases are managed supportively and the condition is usually self-limiting. In severe cases, defibrotide, a mixture of porcine oligodeoxyribonucleotides with antithrombotic, and profibrinolytic properties, may be beneficial. While most patients with SOS will recover, severe disease with multiorgan involvement is associated with mortality of over 80% [13].

Nodular Regenerative Hyperplasia

NRH is another consequence of vascular injury, specifically obliterative changes to the portal venules. Affected areas of hepatic parenchyma atrophy, with the nodular areas representing a hypertrophic response to normal or slightly increased portal blood flow in areas where the portal venules are preserved. NRH is characterized by diffuse, small (<0.5 cm) nodules throughout the hepatic parenchyma, with little to no fibrosis. Several antineoplastic agents have been associated with development of NRH, including oxaliplatin, busulfan, daunorubicin, chlorambucil, cyclophosphamide, bleomycin, and trastuzumab emtansine. NRH has also been reported to occur as a consequence of certain malignancies, including metastatic breast cancer, carcinoid, lymphoproliferative and myeloproliferative disorders, and Castelman's disease [14].

The natural history of NRH is variable, and there is likely a significant reporting bias toward symptomatic disease which presents with clinical features of non-cirrhotic portal hypertension, most often variceal bleeding. Ascites can occur but is less common [14]. Both progression and regression of portal hypertension have been described after cessation of the causative drug [15]. Patients usually have normal or at most trivially elevated liver enzymes, although ALP elevation can develop in chronic disease. Liver synthetic function is preserved. Tiny nodules are usually not visible discretely on imaging, although the liver parenchyma may appear heterogeneous and a nodular contour may be seen, leading to an erroneous radiological diagnosis of cirrhosis. Other clinical features of portal hypertension (splenomegaly, low platelet count) may develop. Treatment involves identification and withdrawal of the causative agent, and monitoring/treating complications of portal hypertension. Prognosis is related to the underlying cause, rather than the severity of portal hypertension.

Immune-Mediated Hepatitis

Immune checkpoint inhibitors (ICI) are a novel class of anticancer therapy which effectively enhance the immune response against tumor cells in several cancer types, and are now approved for treatment of a broad range of malignancies. Just as ICI can activate tumor-specific immunity, they can also promote autoimmunity by removing the protective inhibitors of immune activation against self-antigens. Their use is associated with a distinct profile of adverse effects termed immune-related adverse events, which lead to immune-mediated organ damage. Liver toxicity, manifesting as liver enzyme elevation, is well recognized with use of ICI, with varying incidence reported by drug class. A higher incidence has been reported with anti-CTLA-4 drugs (3–9%) than with PD-1 or PD-L1 inhibitors (1.8–7.1% and 0.9–4.0%, respectively), and combination therapy may have a synergistic effect on the risk of hepatotoxicity [16, 17].

The typical presentation of ICI-associated liver injury is with hepatitis, with predominant ALT/AST elevations. Distinct from other forms of DILI, assessment and management of ICI-associated hepatitis is based on the severity of hepatoxicity as per National Cancer Institute Common Terminology Criteria for Adverse Events (CTCAE). These criteria are used to grade severity of liver injury in oncology clinical trials, and as many management algorithms for immune-related adverse events have been developed from trial protocols and early experience reported in case series, their use has extended into societal practice guidelines [16, 17]. It is important to recognize that hepatotoxicity with a high CTCAE severity grade based on elevation of ALT/AST, without elevation of bilirubin or impairment of liver synthetic function, does not necessarily signify a more clinically severe liver injury than lower CTCAE grades.

Most cases of ICI-associated hepatitis resolve with holding the checkpoint inhibitor. If liver enzymes remain elevated, high-dose corticosteroid treatment is recommended. Rarely, additional treatment with second- or even third-line immunosuppressive drugs may be required, in which case mycophenolate mofetil, tacrolimus, or infliximab have shown efficacy in case reports or case series [16, 17].

Radiation-Associated Liver Injury

Radiation-induced liver injury (RILD) is a common complication of radiation therapy and a major limitation to radiation for primary liver cancer. It typically occurs four to eight weeks after completion of radiation therapy, although it can appear as early as two weeks or as late as seven months after treatment [18]. Radiation injury to the sinusoidal endothelial cells is thought to initiate the coagulation cascade, leading to accumulation of fibrin, clot formation, and occlusion of the central veins and hepatic sinusoids, resulting in histopathological changes of SOS [19].

Reported incidence of RILD varies widely (6–66% of patients treated with hepatic radiation of 30–35 Gy), likely influenced by the volume of radiation, as well as underlying liver reserve, with a higher risk of injury in those with pre-existing liver disease or cirrhosis [18]. Stereotactic body radiation therapy delivers precisely targeted external beam radiation to small, well-defined targets, and is therefore associated with a lower risk of adverse effects. Radioembolization is a relatively novel treatment for primary and secondary liver malignancies, delivering targeted radioactive particles through the hepatic artery. Although the majority of the radiation is directed to the tumor, some radiation may be delivered to the non-tumor-containing liver tissues, leading to a radioembolization-induced liver disease. The risk is increased in patients with poor hepatic reserve, and possibly prior treatment with chemotherapy.

Classic RILD usually presents clinically with fatigue, hepatomegaly, and anicteric ascites one to three months after radiation therapy. Elevation in ALP may be out of proportion to other liver enzymes. Non-classic clinical presentations of RILD may be seen in patients with underlying chronic liver disease, such as cirrhosis or viral hepatitis, and present with significantly elevated serum transaminases ($> 5 \times$ ULN) and/or jaundice. The exact mechanism of injury in non-classic RILD is not fully understood but may involve loss of regenerating hepatocytes [19].

No specific treatments are available for RILD, and management is purely supportive, including low sodium diet and diuretics for fluid retention, analgesics for pain, paracentesis for tense ascites, and correction of coagulopathy.

Hepatitis B Virus Reactivation

An indirect impact of cancer therapy on the liver is a risk of reactivation of HBV in patients with current or past HBV infection. It is important to recognize that patients with prior, resolved HBV infection can be at risk of viral reactivation, as well as patients with current, chronic infection. HBV DNA can persist in a latent form with hepatocytes of patients with previous HBV exposure for decades after apparent resolution of infection, and has the potential to act as a reservoir for HBV reactivation. This is usually controlled by host immunity but in the event of treatment with immunosuppressive therapies, HBV reactivation may occur.

Definitions of HBV reactivation vary, but generally this refers to an increase in circulating HBV DNA in a patient with chronic HBV infection, or to newly detectable HBV DNA and/or reversion of HBV surface antigen (HBsAg) from negative to positive in a patient with prior, resolved HBV. The clinical presentation of HBV reactivation is very variable, ranging from asymptomatic abnormal liver enzymes to acute hepatitis or even fulminant liver failure.

Considering that an estimated one in every three people worldwide may have been exposed to HBV infection, all patients with oncologic disease should be screened for current or previous HBV infection, prior to commencing any treatment. Serologic tests recommended for screening, and their interpretation, are summarized in Table 14.2. In general, patients with current HBV infection (HBsAg positive) have a high risk for reactivation with immunosuppressive treatments, including antineoplastic therapies, and should receive

Table 14.2 Recommended serologic tests for screening for current or prior, resolved hepatitis B virus infection, and their interpretation.

HBsAg	HBcAb	HBsAb	Interpretation
+	+	−	HBV positive (current infection)
−	+	+/−	Prior resolved HBV infection, with/without immunity
−	−	+	Immunity to HBV through prior vaccination
−	−	−	HBV negative, non-immune

HBcAb, anti-HBV core antibody; HBsAb, anti-HBV surface antibody; HBsAg, HBV surface antigen; HBV, hepatitis B virus.

antiviral prophylaxis. This treatment should be continued for the duration of immune-suppressing treatment, and for at least 6–12 months after. Patients should be referred to a hepatologist for supervision of treatment and ongoing management.

The risk for HBV reactivation in patients with prior resolved HBV varies according to the immunosuppressive therapy used. B-cell depleting agents (such as rituximab, ofatum-amab, or natalizumab), and stem-cell transplants are associated with a relatively high risk for HBV reactivation in patients with prior resolved HBV, and prophylactic antiviral therapy is recommended during and for at least 6–12 months after therapy.

Patients who are treated with other immunosuppressive drugs can usually be monitored closely with ALT, HBsAg, and HBV DNA (if available) checked every one to three months while on treatment, and for 12 months after, with on-demand antiviral therapy if required. However, depending on patient preference, clinical scenario, and feasibility of close monitoring, this group could also be treated with prophylactic antiviral therapy [20]. The preferred choice of prophylaxis is with a high-potency antiviral (tenofovir or entecavir) which have a much lower association with viral resistance than other antivirals.

Unexplained Abnormal Liver Tests in Patients with Known Oncologic Disease

Abnormal liver tests in patients with oncologic disease may pose a challenge to clinicians due to the broad differential diagnosis. However, likelihood of different causes for enzyme elevation will often vary according to treatment status, so a systematic approach to evaluation of causes, appropriate to the clinical context, is recommended.

At Diagnosis

All patients with a new cancer diagnosis should have baseline liver enzyme measurements taken and tests of liver synthetic function. Any derangement of liver function (elevated bilirubin, elevated INR, low albumin) usually warrants urgent referral for further assessment. Prior HBV infection is relatively common, and liver enzymes may be normal in patients with current HBV or HCV infection, so all patients should also be screened for past/present HBV or HCV infection. If screening tests suggest current or prior HBV infection, the patient should be referred for further assessment and management recommendations. A positive anti-HCV antibody should be followed up with testing for HCV RNA, to confirm whether this is a current or prior, resolved, infection. If HCV RNA is negative, no further action is required. Unlike HBV, HCV does not establish latency so there is no risk of reactivation with cancer therapy. If HCV RNA is positive, this indicates current HCV infection. The patient should be referred to a hepatologist for further evaluation, risk stratification with a fibrosis assessment and to discuss the need for, and timing of HCV treatment. Unlike chronic HBV infection, chronic HCV infection does not "flare" with immunosuppressive therapies, and so in most cases, cancer therapy can proceed prior to initiation of any specific treatment for HCV.

Patients with elevated liver enzymes at initial evaluation should be investigated to identify the cause and severity of any underlying liver disease. A suggested initial evaluation is summarized in Figure 14.1. Some causes may be easily identifiable from history/initial screening investigations. If a potential cause for chronic liver disease is positively identified (such as fatty liver disease or viral hepatitis) then referral to a hepatologist should be considered, for risk stratification through fibrosis assessment as well as specific management. Patients with advanced fibrosis/cirrhosis may be more prone to complications from certain cancer treatments, and early identification may guide further management decisions. Conversely, if enzyme elevation is persistent and no apparent cause is identified on initial investigation, referral for further assessment would be appropriate.

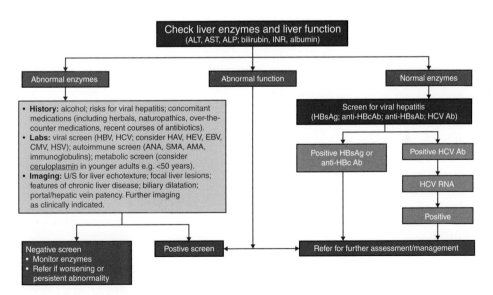

Figure 14.1 Suggested initial evaluation of liver enzymes and function in a patient with oncologic disease. Ab, antibody; AMA, anti-mitochondrial antibody; ANA, anti-nuclear antibody; anti-HBcAb, hepatitis B core antibody; anti-HBsAb, hepatitis B surface antibody; CMV, cytomegalovirus; EBV, Epstein–Barr virus; HAV, hepatitis A virus; HBsAg, hepatitis B surface antigen; HBV, hepatitis B virus; HCV, hepatitis C virus; HEV, hepatitis E virus; HSV, herpes simplex virus; SMA, smooth muscle antibody.

Metastatic disease to the liver is common, and often occurs without liver enzyme elevations. Where liver enzyme elevation does occur, ALP/gamma-glutamyl transferase (GGT) elevation is more frequent than ALT/AST elevation, although the extent of elevation does not correlate with the degree of liver involvement. In a patient with isolated ALP elevation, the serum GGT may help distinguish between a liver and bone source. Alternatively, ALP isoenzymes could be performed to confirm the source of elevated ALP.

During Therapy

Liver enzymes are usually checked regularly during cancer therapy. This is important for identification of any new changes, which may represent treatment-related toxicity. Patients remain at risk for acquisition of other causes for elevated liver enzymes, such as alcohol, other drugs/toxins, new viral hepatitis, and a thorough history to screen for these possibilities remains an important part of the evaluation. If any risks for acquisition of new viral hepatitis are identified, repeat testing for HCV/HBV is warranted. In this case, direct testing for HCV RNA or HBV DNA by polymerase chain reaction may be appropriate, given the window period from infection to seroconversion and development of antibodies. In immunosuppressed patients, other viral infections may cause hepatitis and specific testing for Epstein–Barr virus, cytomegalovirus, and possibly herpes simplex virus, is also recommended.

After Therapy

Some hepatic complications of cancer therapy, particularly vascular injury, may present weeks or even months after completion of therapy. Risk of HBV reactivation persists after completion of immunosuppressive treatment, so monitoring of HBsAg and liver enzymes should be continued for six months after completing cancer therapy (12–18 months in the case of B-cell depleting therapies). Similarly, if prophylactic antiviral therapy was prescribed, this should be continued for at least six months after completing cancer therapy (12–18 months in the case of B-cell depleting therapies). Again, patients remain susceptible to development of liver disease unrelated to their cancer or associated therapy, and so full consideration should be given to other potential causes for abnormal liver enzymes.

Summary

Abnormal liver tests are common in patients with oncologic disease. Often, this will be related to either the underlying disease or its treatment. Cancer therapies may be associated with some unique patterns of DILI, which may manifest during, or sometimes after treatment. Evaluating patients for pre-existing liver disease or viral hepatitis before commencing therapy is important to treat any pre-existing disease, to modify cancer therapy if needed (e.g. in patients with underlying cirrhosis), and to minimize the risk of avoidable interruptions to cancer therapy.

References

1. European Association for the Study of the Liver (2016). EASL Clinical Practice Guidelines on the management of benign liver tumours. *J. Hepatol.* 65 (2): 386–398.
2. Zignego, A.L., Giannini, C., and Gragnani, L. (2012). HCV and lymphoproliferation. *Clin. Dev. Immunol.* 2012: 980942.
3. Chavarriaga, J., Fakih, N., Cataño, J. et al. (2020). Stauffer syndrome, clinical implications and knowledge gaps, does size matter? Case report. *BMC Urol.* 20 (1): 105.
4. Council for International Organizations of Medical Sciences (2020). Drug induced liver injury (DILI): Current status and future directions for drug development and the post-market setting. A consensus by a CIOMS Working Group. Geneva, Switzerland: CIOMS.
5. Chalasani, N., Bonkovsky, H.L., Fontana, R. et al. (2015). Features and outcomes of 899 patients with drug-induced liver injury: the DILIN prospective study. *Gastroenterology* 148 (7): 1340–1352.e7.
6. Benoist, S. and Nordlinger, B. (2009). The role of preoperative chemotherapy in patients with resectable colorectal liver metastases. *Ann. Surg. Oncol.* 16 (9): 2385–2390.
7. Vauthey, J.N., Pawlik, T.M., Ribero, D. et al. (2006). Chemotherapy regimen predicts steatohepatitis and an increase in 90-day mortality after surgery for hepatic colorectal metastases. *J. Clin. Oncol.* 24 (13): 2065–2072.
8. Meunier, L. and Larrey, D. (2020). Chemotherapy-associated steatohepatitis. *Ann. Hepatol.* 19 (6): 597–601.
9. Bahirwani, R. and Reddy, K.R. (2014). Drug-induced liver injury due to cancer chemotherapeutic agents. *Semin. Liver Dis.* 34 (2): 162–171.
10. Rubbia-Brandt, L., Audard, V., Sartoretti, P. et al. (2004). Severe hepatic sinusoidal obstruction associated with oxaliplatin-based chemotherapy in patients with metastatic colorectal cancer. *Ann. Oncol.* 15 (3): 460–466.
11. Rubbia-Brandt, L., Lauwers, G.Y., Wang, H. et al. (2010). Sinusoidal obstruction syndrome and nodular regenerative hyperplasia are frequent oxaliplatin-associated liver lesions and partially prevented by bevacizumab in patients with hepatic colorectal metastasis. *Histopathology* 56 (4): 430–439.
12. Mohty, M., Malard, F., Abecassis, M. et al. (2016). Revised diagnosis and severity criteria for sinusoidal obstruction syndrome/veno-occlusive disease in adult patients: a new classification from the European Society for Blood and Marrow Transplantation. *Bone Marrow Transplant.* 51 (7): 906–912.
13. Bonifazi, F., Barbato, F., Ravaioli, F. et al. (2020). Diagnosis and treatment of VOD/SOS after allogeneic hematopoietic stem cell transplantation. *Front. Immunol.* 11: 489.
14. Reshamwala, P.A., Kleiner, D.E., and Heller, T. (2006). Nodular regenerative hyperplasia: not all nodules are created equal. *Hepatology* 44 (1): 7–14.
15. Ghabril, M. and Vuppalanchi, R. (2014). Drug-induced nodular regenerative hyperplasia. *Semin. Liver Dis.* 34 (2): 240–245.
16. Brahmer, J.R., Lacchetti, C., and Thompson, J.A. (2018). Management of immune-related adverse events in patients treated with immune checkpoint inhibitor therapy: American Society of Clinical Oncology Clinical Practice Guideline Summary. *J. Oncol. Pract.* 14: 247–249.

17. Haanen, J.B.A.G., Carbonnel, F., Robert, C. et al. (2017). Management of toxicities from immunotherapy: ESMO Clinical Practice Guidelines for diagnosis, treatment and follow-up. *Ann. Oncol.* 28 (suppl_4): iv119–iv142.

18. Kim, J. and Jung, Y. (2017). Radiation-induced liver disease: current understanding and future perspectives. *Exp. Mol. Med.* 49 (7): e359.

19. Guha, C. and Kavanagh, B.D. (2011). Hepatic radiation toxicity: avoidance and amelioration. *Semin. Radiat. Oncol.* 21 (4): 256–263.

20. Terrault, N.A., Lok, A.S.F., McMahon, B.J. et al. (2018). Update on prevention, diagnosis, and treatment of chronic hepatitis B: AASLD 2018 hepatitis B guidance. *Hepatology* 67 (4): 1560–1599.

15

Hematology
Navjyot K. Hansi[1] and Abid R. Suddle[2]

[1]*Addenbrooke's Hospital, Cambridge, UK*
[2]*Institute of Liver Studies, King's College Hospital, London, UK*

KEY POINTS

- Myeloproliferative disorders are strongly associated with splanchnic vein thrombosis.
- Patients with Budd–Chiari syndrome and non-cirrhotic portal vein thrombosis should be screened for prothrombotic disorders.
- Hepatitis B reactivation can cause acute liver failure. Screening and prophylaxis are often indicated in patients who are hepatitis B surface antigen-positive as they are at highest risk of reactivation, especially when exposed to immunosuppressive drugs or chemotherapy.
- Sinusoidal obstruction syndrome (SOS) primarily affects the hepatic sinusoids, as well as the hepatic veins, and the agents implicated are those commonly used prior to hematopoietic stem-cell transplant (HSCT).
- Graft versus host disease (GVHD) can mimic other causes of liver dysfunction both clinically and histologically, often presenting as cholestasis or acute hepatitis.
- Sickle-cell hepatopathy is a spectrum of disease manifestations with subtle differences and overlap in clinical presentation and biochemical features.
- Liver biopsy often adds clinical information where there is diagnostic uncertainty but there is a higher risk of bleeding in sickle-cell anemia (SCA).

Introduction

Abnormalities in liver tests are common in hematologic practice and it is therefore important to develop a systematic approach to investigation and management (Box 15.1). Liver abnormalities can be caused by (i) liver involvement by the hematologic condition, (ii) as a consequence of treatment of the hematologic condition, or (iii) concurrent or independent disease. Initial investigations can guide a clinician as to severity of a pre-existing liver condition and this may influence hematology assessment and treatment. As a general consideration, patients with advanced-stage liver disease can be well compensated with no symptoms, so incidental findings such as thrombocytopenia (more than 70% of cirrhotic

The Liver in Systemic Disease: A Clinician's Guide to Abnormal Liver Tests, First Edition.
Edited by Gideon M. Hirschfeld, Paramjit Gill, and James Neuberger.

Box 15.1   Initial Evaluation for Abnormal Liver Blood Tests

- History:
  - Risk factors for pre-existing liver condition
  - Timing of liver abnormality
  - Focus on medications (including non-prescription and recreational drugs)
- Examination:
  - Stigmata of chronic liver disease or signs of acute liver decompensation (jaundice, ascites, asterixis)
  - Full liver enzyme panel (aspartate amino transferase, alanine amino transferase, gamma-glutamyl transferase, and prothrombin time/international normalized ratio)
  - Serum ferritin and transferrin saturation
  - Viral screen: hepatitis B surface antigen, hepatitis C antibody, antibodies to hepatitis A and E, cytomegalovirus, and Epstein–Barr virus
  - Immunology: anti-mitochondrial antibody, anti-smooth muscle antibody, anti-nuclear antibody, serum immunoglobulins
  - Imaging: ultrasound of the abdomen (Doppler of portal and hepatic vein)
  - Liver elastography
  - Liver biopsy ± portal pressure studies

---

patients have some degree of thrombocytopenia) on routine blood tests can be a prompt to screen for underlying chronic liver disease, even in the context of normal liver function tests.

Primary hematologic conditions such as primary myelofibrosis can mirror liver disease symptoms and clinical signs such as jaundice and hepatosplenomegaly, and lymphoma can present, albeit rarely, with acute liver failure. Liver diseases can mimic features of hematologic diseases (Table 15.1) and can be associated concurrently with hematologic conditions (Table 15.2).

Unexplained Abnormal Liver Tests in Patients with Known Hematologic Disease

Figure 15.1 is a flow chart to work through initial management and investigations if a patient has a known underlying hematologic condition. The severity of liver dysfunction will identify those patients who need to be admitted for further investigations, such as liver biopsy and portal pressure studies. Imaging is essential to demonstrate whether the patient has ascites, patent portal and hepatic vasculature, liver volume, and signs of chronic liver disease or cirrhosis with portal hypertension radiologically. Features radiologically may include a shrunken, irregular contoured, and nodular liver, with established variceal bed and splenomegaly. Often, the liver biopsy will need to be performed via a transjugular approach to reduce the risk of bleeding if there is coagulopathy or jaundice. While patients with known underlying chronic liver disease have a prothrombotic

Table 15.1 Liver diseases that may mimic hematologic diseases.

Liver disease	Clinical feature	
Non-cirrhotic portal hypertension and cirrhosis	Thrombocytopenia ± hepatosplenomegaly	Hypersplenism resulting from: • platelet sequestration • bone marrow suppression • reduction in thrombopoietin levels (normally produced by liver) Platelet destruction: • in autoimmune liver disease may be immunologically mediated • HCV antibodies are positive in up to one third of patients with chronic ITP
HELLP syndrome (1–2%/1000 pregnancies)	Hemolysis	Abdominal pain and nausea; hypertension and proteinuria may be associated Bloods tests: hemolytic anemia, elevated liver enzymes, low platelet count
Alcoholic hepatitis (Zieve syndrome[a])	Hemolysis	History of alcohol excess; fatty liver/cirrhosis, severe right upper-quadrant pain, jaundice Blood tests: jaundice, hyperlipidemia, and hemolytic anemia
Wilson's disease	Hemolysis	May be associated with a hemolytic anemia in 1–12% Typically present as fulminant hepatic failure with hemolysis Blood tests: DAT negative hemolytic anemia A, low serum uric acid levels, low serum alkaline phosphatase activity and increased AST:ALT ratios
Autoimmune liver disease	Hemolysis	AIHA can be seen in association with autoimmune liver disease Blood tests: raised ALT, DAT-positive hemolytic anemia, haptoglobin reduced, reticulocyte increased

AIHA, autoimmune hemolytic anemia; ALT, alanine amino transferase; AST, aspartate aminotransferase; DAT, direct antiglobulin testing; HCV, hepatitis C virus; HELLP, hemolysis, elevated liver enzymes, low platelets; ITP, immune thrombocytopenic purpura.
[a] Mechanism poorly understood.

tendency, so do those with known hematologic disease. Myeloproliferative disorders, particularly Philadelphia chromosome-negative, including polycythemia vera, essential thrombocythemia, and primary myelofibrosis, are strongly associated with splanchnic vein thrombosis [1]. Of note, peripheral blood counts may be abnormal due to hypersplenism, iron deficiency, and hemodilution. The causes of Budd–Chiari syndrome, which is a blockage of hepatic venous outflow, can have a spectrum of both acute, acute on chronic,

Table 15.2 Liver diseases associated with hematologic disease.

Disease	Clinical features
Lymphoma	Hodgkin's lymphoma: • Liver involvement in 50–60% of those with Hodgkin's lymphoma • Hepatomegaly common • Jaundice rare • May have cholestasis and ductopenia on liver biopsy Non-Hodgkin's lymphoma: • Clinically silent • Mild to moderate rise in ALP • Jaundice uncommon • Acute liver failure rare Primary liver lymphoma: • Abdominal pain and B-type symptoms • ALP raised • Jaundice and ascites rare
Chronic hepatitis C	Cryoglobulinemia associated Higher incidence of non-Hodgkin's lymphoma: • Palpable purpura • Arthralgia • Myalgia
Budd–Chiari syndrome and portal vein thrombosis	Acute and chronic presentations: • Abdominal pain ± ascites Causes: • Genetic (protein C, protein S deficiency, antithrombin III deficiency, factor V Leiden mutation, prothrombin gene mutation) • Acquired thrombophilic conditions (myeloproliferative disorders, antiphospholipid syndrome, lupus)
Hemophagocytic syndrome or hemophagocytic lymphohistiocytosis	Clinical presentation: • Acute unremitting fever • Lymphadenopathy • Hepatosplenomegaly • Multiorgan failure Investigations: • Cytopenia, hyperferritinemia, hypertriglycemia, and/or hypofibrinogenemia • Hemophagocytosis in bone marrow, spleen, or lymph nodes • Low natural killer cell activity, high soluble CD15 (sIL-2Rα)

ALP, alkaline phosphatase; sIL-2Rα, soluble interleukin-2 receptor alpha.

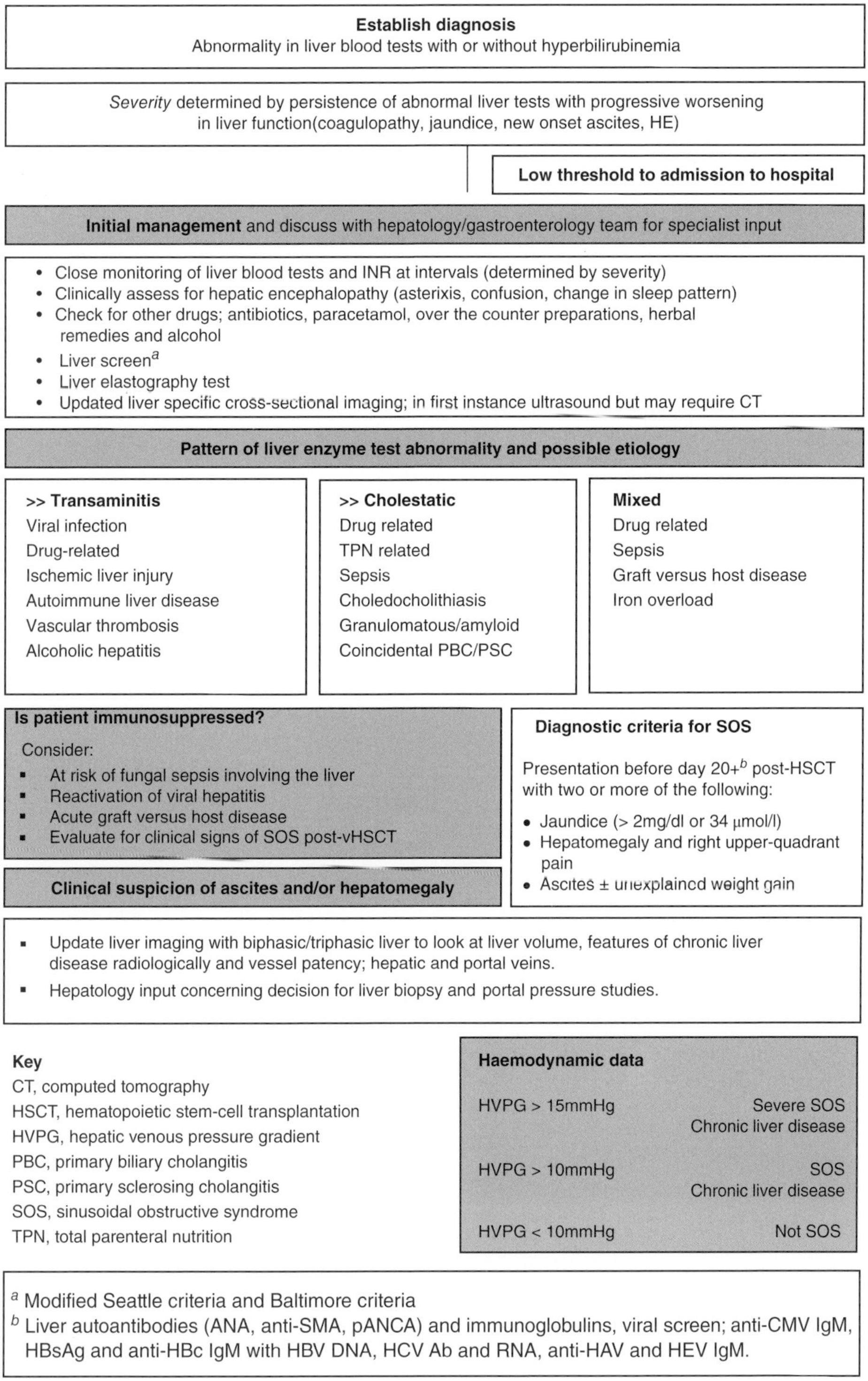

Establish diagnosis
Abnormality in liver blood tests with or without hyperbilirubinemia

---

Severity determined by persistence of abnormal liver tests with progressive worsening
in liver function(coagulopathy, jaundice, new onset ascites, HE)

Low threshold to admission to hospital

Initial management and discuss with hepatology/gastroenterology team for specialist input

- Close monitoring of liver blood tests and INR at intervals (determined by severity)
- Clinically assess for hepatic encephalopathy (asterixis, confusion, change in sleep pattern)
- Check for other drugs; antibiotics, paracetamol, over the counter preparations, herbal remedies and alcohol
- Liver screen[a]
- Liver elastography test
- Updated liver specific cross-sectional imaging; in first instance ultrasound but may require CT

Pattern of liver enzyme test abnormality and possible etiology

>> **Transaminitis**	>> **Cholestatic**	**Mixed**
Viral infection	Drug related	Drug related
Drug-related	TPN related	Sepsis
Ischemic liver injury	Sepsis	Graft versus host disease
Autoimmune liver disease	Choledocholithiasis	Iron overload
Vascular thrombosis	Granulomatous/amyloid	
Alcoholic hepatitis	Coincidental PBC/PSC	

Is patient immunosuppressed?

Consider:
- At risk of fungal sepsis involving the liver
- Reactivation of viral hepatitis
- Acute graft versus host disease
- Evaluate for clinical signs of SOS post-vHSCT

Clinical suspicion of ascites and/or hepatomegaly

Diagnostic criteria for SOS

Presentation before day 20+[b] post-HSCT
with two or more of the following:

- Jaundice (> 2mg/dl or 34 μmol/l)
- Hepatomegaly and right upper-quadrant pain
- Ascites ± unexplained weight gain

- Update liver imaging with biphasic/triphasic liver to look at liver volume, features of chronic liver disease radiologically and vessel patency; hepatic and portal veins.
- Hepatology input concerning decision for liver biopsy and portal pressure studies.

Key

CT, computed tomography
HSCT, hematopoietic stem-cell transplantation
HVPG, hepatic venous pressure gradient
PBC, primary biliary cholangitis
PSC, primary sclerosing cholangitis
SOS, sinusoidal obstructive syndrome
TPN, total parenteral nutrition

Haemodynamic data

HVPG > 15mmHg	Severe SOS Chronic liver disease
HVPG > 10mmHg	SOS Chronic liver disease
HVPG < 10mmHg	Not SOS

---

[a] Modified Seattle criteria and Baltimore criteria
[b] Liver autoantibodies (ANA, anti-SMA, pANCA) and immunoglobulins, viral screen; anti-CMV IgM, HBsAg and anti-HBc IgM with HBV DNA, HCV Ab and RNA, anti-HAV and HEV IgM.

Figure 15.1   The investigation and differential diagnosis of abnormal liver function tests with underlying hematological condition.

and chronic presentations. In the acute setting, irrespective of etiology, early anticoagulation therapy and discussion with tertiary hepatology centers are needed. Paroxysmal nocturnal hemoglobinuria is a possibility when a patient presents with Budd–Chiari syndrome associated with pancytopenia.

Importantly, patients with underlying hematologic conditions who are to start on immunosuppression, such as high-dose oral steroids (such as prednisolone > 20 mg daily for four weeks or longer), B-cell depleting therapies, HSCT or anthracyclines (such as doxorubicin), should be screened for viral hepatitis to reduce the risk of reactivation. Guidelines generally agree that patients with resolved hepatitis B virus (HBV) on high-potency immunosuppression regimens should be treated similarly to immunosuppressed patients with chronic HBV (Table 15.3), with oral antiviral drugs starting before immunosuppression, and continued 12–18 months after cessation, together with monitoring of liver function tests and HBV DNA levels for 12 months after antiviral withdrawal [2, 3]. Studies have shown that tenofovir and entecavir have lower HBV reactivation rates compared with lamivudine [4].

If a patient has had HSCT, there are key differential diagnoses of abnormal liver function with some central clinical and laboratory features (Table 15.4). Sinusoidal obstruction syndrome (SOS), also known as veno-occlusive disease, usually occurs early (within the first 21 days) but cases have been reported after day 30 and the diagnosis should be suspected where jaundice, painful hepatomegaly, or unexplained weight gain with or without ascites occurs after HSCT. Differentiation between SOS and acute GVHD can be challenging, especially as they can co-exist; however, the presence of ascites and fluid retention, and absence of evidence for GVHD affecting other organs, helps to exclude GVHD. Severe SOS is

Table 15.3 Reactivation of chronic hepatitis B with immunosuppression regimens.

	High risk	Medium risk	Low risk
Anticipated incidence of HBVr	> 10%	1–10%	< 1%
HBsAg+ and anti-HBc+ or HBsAg− and anti-HBc+	HSCT recipients	Tumor necrosis factor inhibitors	Azathioprine
	B-cell-depleting therapies	Cytokine or integrin inhibitors	6-MP
	Anthracyclines	Tyrosine kinase inhibitor	Methotrexate
			Intraarticular corticosteroids
			Oral steroids < 1 week
HBsAg+ and anti-HBc +	10–20 mg or > 20 mg of daily prednisolone or equivalent for > 4 weeks	<10 mg prednisolone or equivalent for >4 week	
HBsAg− and anti-HBc+		Moderate or high-dose steroids for > 4 weeks	Steroids (low dose) for > 4 weeks

6-MP, 6-mercaptopurine; anti-HBc, anti-hepatitis B core antigen-positive; HBsAg−, hepatitis B surface antigen negative; HBsAg+, hepatitis B surface antigen-positive; HBVr, hepatitis B virus reactivation; HSCT, hematopoietic stem-cell transplantation.

Table 15.4 Differential diagnoses of abnormal liver function after hematopoietic stem-cell transplantation and key clinical and laboratory features.

Timing post-HSCT (day of HSCT = day 0)	Differential diagnoses to consider	Clinical features	Laboratory features
Within 5 days Immediate	Drug toxicity Severe SOS	Weight gain, edema, ascites, painful hepatomegaly	
Day +5 to engraftment Early	Sepsis Hemolysis Mild to moderate SOS	Fever, neutropenia	↑↑↑ bilirubin, ↑ALP
After engraftment: day +15 to +50	Acute GVHD Infection (fungal or viral) Total parenteral nutrition Biliary sludge	Skin rash, diarrhea	↑↑bilirubin ↑ALP
Days +60 to +100	Acute GVHD Infection (fungal or viral) Early chronic GVHD	Skin lesions, Sicca syndrome	
After day +100 Late	Infection (fungal or viral) Nodular regenerative hyperplasia Biliary obstruction Chronic GVHD	Pain, dilated ducts on imaging	↑↑bilirubin ↑ALP ↑GGT

ALP, alkaline phosphatase; GGT, gamma-glutamyl transferase; GVHD, graft versus host disease; HSCT, hematopoietic stem-cell transplantation; SOS, sinusoidal obstruction syndrome.

associated with high morbidity and mortality [5]. Management includes supportive measures for fluid overload and defibrotide (25 mg/kg/day). Defibrotide is a mixture of oligonucleotides derived from porcine intestinal mucosal DNA and is an approved treatment for severe SOS in patients undergoing stem-cell transplantation [6].

In patients with SCA, the umbrella term "sickle hepatopathy" is used to describe sickle-related liver disease incorporating a wide differential and clinical phenotype of hepatic pathology with management measures that are broadly supportive (Figure 15.2) [7]. Patients with SCA may often exhibit transiently raised liver enzyme tests due to hemolysis, and while SCA patients are at risk of chronic liver disease (with a 30% prevalence of cirrhosis in an autopsy series) [8], it is not clear which group of patients are at particular risk of chronic liver disease. Acute liver syndromes such as sickle intrahepatic cholestasis (associated with the more severe clinical phenotype), hepatic sequestration, and acute sickle hepatic crisis are often related to an acute vasoactive crisis. We rarely biopsy the liver in patients with SCA because of the higher risk of bleeding, but it

---

Establish diagnosis
Abnormality in liver blood tests with or without hyperbilirubinemia

---

Severity determined by persistence of abnormal liver tests with progressive worsening in liver function (coagulopathy, jaundice, new-onset ascites, hepatic encephalopathy)

Low threshold for admission to hospital

- Close monitoring of liver blood tests and INR at intervals (determined by severity)
- Clinically assess for hepatic encephalopathy (asterixis, confusion, change in sleep pattern)
- Check for other drugs; paracetamol, over-the-counter preparations, herbal remedies and alcohol
- Liver screen[a]
- Updated liver-specific cross-sectional imaging; in first instance ultrasound

---

Acute

Acute sickle hepatic crisis:
- Right upper-quadrant pain
- leucocytosis, bilirubin <15mg/dL, ALT rarely higher than 300 iu/l

Sickle intrahepatic cholestasis :
- Right upper-quadrant pain, fever, jaundice
- Leukocytosis, very high bilirubin ALT can be in 1000s, coagulopathy, renal failure

Hepatic sequestration:
- Right upper-quadrant pain
- Anemia, enlarging liver, reticulocytosis

Viral hepatitis
Choledocholithiasis
Budd-Chiari syndrome
Hepatic abscess/biloma

Chronic
Chronic cholestasis
Biliary-type cirrhosis
Chronic viral hepatitis
Choledocholithiasis
Coincidental chronic liver disease

Key
Ab, antibodies
ALT, alanine amino transferase
ANA, anti-nuclear antibodies
anti-HBc, antibody to hepatitis B core antigen
CMV, cytomegalovirus
HBsAG, hepatitis B surface antigen
HAV, hepatitis A virus
HBV, hepatitis B virus
HCV,hepatitis C virus
HEV,hepatitis E virus
IgM, immunoglobulin M
INR, international normalized ratio
pANCA, perinuclear anti-neutrophilic cytoplasmic antibodies
SMA, smooth-muscle antibodies

Refer for specialist hepatology input
Initial management (supportive measures but no strong evidence base):
- Ursodeoxycholic acid
- Hydroxyurea
- Exchange transfusion (HbS percentage target of < 30% to 40%)
- Liver biopsy (risk/benefit of bleeding)
- Oral antiviral therapy
- Iron chelation (when liver iron concentration >7 mg Fe/g dry weight)
- Endoscopic retrograde cholangiopancreatography
- May refer for liver transplant assessment if young patient with advanced-stage chronic liver disease and predominant end-organ damage is liver

[a]Liver autoantibodies (ANA, anti-SMA, pANCA) and immunoglobulins, viral screen; anti-CMV IgM, HBsAg and anti-HBc IgM with HBV DNA, HCV Ab and RNA, anti-HAV and HEV IgM.

Figure 15.2 The investigation and management of abnormal liver tests in patient with known sickle-cell disease. Based on [7].

can be considered if there is a strong indication such as co-existing autoimmune liver disease with positive serology.

Liver transplant assessment can be considered in those with advanced-stage chronic liver disease, depending on the projected mortality from liver disease and absence of other end organ damage [9, 10].

In assessing the patient with abnormal liver blood tests, the first step is to determine acute or chronic pathology, and certain clinical, laboratory, and imaging data can be helpful in the diagnostic evaluation. Early discussion with hepatology and gastroenterology colleagues is helpful and a liver biopsy may be required to make a definitive diagnosis.

References

1. Pieri, G., Theocharidou, E., and Burroughs, A.K. (2013). Liver in haematological disorders. *Best Pract. Res. Clin. Gastroenterol.* 27 (4): 513–530.
2. European Association for the Study of the Liver (2017). EASL 2017 clinical practice guidelines on the management of hepatitis B virus infection. *J. Hepatol.* 67 (2): 370–398.
3. Terrault, N.A., Lok, A.S.F., McMahon, B.J. et al. (2018). Update on prevention, diagnosis, and treatment of chronic hepatitis B: AASLD 2018 hepatitis B guidance. *Hepatology* 67 (4): 1560–1599.
4. Picardi, M., Della Pepa, R., Giordano, C. et al. (2019). Tenofovir vs lamivudine for the prevention of hepatitis B virus reactivation in advanced-stage DLBCL. *Blood* 133 (5): 498–501.
5. Coppell, J.A., Richardson, P.G., Soiffer, R. et al. (2010). Hepatic veno-occlusive disease following stem cell transplantation: incidence, clinical course, and outcome. *Biol. Blood Marrow Transplant.* 16 (2): 157–168.
6. Mohty, M., Malard, F., Abecasis, M. et al. (2020). Prophylactic, preemptive, and curative treatment for sinusoidal obstruction syndrome/veno-occlusive disease in adult patients: a position statement from an international expert group. *Bone Marrow Transplant.* 55 (3): 485–495.
7. Banerjee, S., Owen, C., and Chopra, S. (2001). Sickle cell hepatopathy. *Hepatology* 33 (5): 1021–1028.
8. Berry, P.A., Cross, T.J., Thein, S.L. et al. (2007). Hepatic dysfunction in sickle cell disease: a new system of classification based on global assessment. *Clin. Gastroenterol. Hepatol.* 5 (12): 1469–1476.
9. Gardner, K., Suddle, A., Kane, P. et al. (2014). How we treat sickle hepatopathy and liver transplantation in adults. *Blood* 123 (15): 2302–2307.
10. Hurtova, M., Bachir, D., Lee, K. et al. (2011). Transplantation for liver failure in patients with sickle cell disease: challenging but feasible. *Liver Transpl.* 17 (4): 381–392.

16

Mental Health and Neurology

Fiona M. Thompson

Institute for Translational Medicine, University Hospitals Birmingham, Birmingham, UK

KEY POINTS

- Liver function tests (LFTs) in patients with mental illness are common.
- Legal and illegal drugs are common causes of abnormal LFTs.
- Rare liver disorders, such as Wilson's disease, may present with psychiatric symptoms.

Introduction

Mental health facilities care for patients with a wide variety of conditions that may affect the liver, from patients with alcohol use disorders and acute delirium secondary to withdrawal, to those with body dysmorphic syndromes and eating disorders such as anorexia nervosa. Some liver diseases may present with psychiatric features; classically, Wilson's disease but also hepatic encephalopathy. Many medications used for mental health indications may cause abnormalities of liver function or liver disease, and this can be made more complicated by polypharmacy and coexisting substance misuse.

LFTs are better considered as markers of liver inflammation, the liver enzymes, alanine amino transferase (ALT), aspartate amino transferase (AST), alkaline phosphatase (ALP), and gamma-glutamyl transferase (GGT) are all characteristically raised in the presence of hepatocyte damage and loss (AST and ALT are considered hepatocyte markers, while ALP and GGT are cholestatic markers, derived from cholangiocytes that line the bile ducts). Thus, they provide a snapshot of liver inflammation on the day the sample is taken, and do not necessarily provide any information about liver function or chronic liver disease. The serum bilirubin, albumin, and international normalized ratio (INR) may give more information about the synthetic capacity of the liver and therefore about underlying liver function. Abnormal LFTs therefore represent episodes of inflammation within the liver.

There are many potential causes of abnormal liver function (including a significant proportion where no clear cause can be found). The importance of evaluating patients with

The Liver in Systemic Disease: A Clinician's Guide to Abnormal Liver Tests, First Edition.
Edited by Gideon M. Hirschfield, Paramjit Gill, and James Neuberger.
© 2023 John Wiley & Sons Ltd. Published 2023 by John Wiley & Sons Ltd.

abnormal LFTs is to try and identify those that may already have undiagnosed liver disease and those at risk of developing chronic liver disease, to enable appropriate treatment or lifestyle changes to be made to prevent further progression of disease and appropriate management of potential complications of chronic liver disease.

Unexplained Abnormal Liver Function Tests in Mental Health and Neurology Settings

Mental health practitioners may not consider requesting LFTs in many of their patients. However, routine tests should be performed for those who have a history of alcohol or substance misuse, particularly those with risk factors for viral hepatitis. If these patients are found to have abnormal liver function, they should be referred for further assessment.

In addition, a number of commonly prescribed medications are metabolized in the liver and their use can be limited in the context of impaired liver function, while others require monitoring of LFTs as a precaution for use. Serum LFTs are likely to be requested in patients for whom these medications are considered. The most common drug-induced liver injury (DILI) is idiosyncratic, dose independent, and not predictable.

Drugs used in mental health that are commonly associated with abnormal liver function include antidepressants and atypical/typical antipsychotics.

Antidepressants

All antidepressants can cause liver injury. Mild abnormalities of liver function are reported in up to 3% of patients on antidepressants. However, liver toxicity requiring hospital admission is rare, with an estimated incidence of 1.28–4 cases/100 000 patient-years. Risk factors for liver injury appear to include age, polypharmacy, and obesity. Pre-existing liver damage may also play a role in some cases. Data are sparse and these may be underestimates; for older drugs, this information can only be found in case reports, while for newer medications the results of clinical trials as well as case reports are available. Life-threatening or severe DILI has been reported for the monoamine-oxidase inhibitor phenelzine, the tricyclic antidepressant imipramine, the selective serotonin reuptake inhibitor (SSRI) sertraline, the serotonin noradrenaline reuptake inhibitors venlafaxine and duloxetine, and serotonin-2 antagonist/reuptake inhibitor trazodone, while the SSRIs citalopram and fluvoxamine are characterized by lower risk.

Anti-depressant-associated liver injury can occur from several days up to six months after the beginning of treatment. It is generally hepatocellular rather than cholestatic, characterized by an increase in aminotransferase levels that normalize on drug withdrawal. In more severe cases, patients can also become jaundiced with synthetic dysfunction (prolonged INR) and there is a risk of fulminant hepatitis and acute liver failure. A cholestatic pattern of injury is more commonly associated with specific drugs (phenelzine, moclobemide, amitriptyline, mianserin, mirtazapine, and tianeptine), and tends to be slower to resolve. There are occasional reports of amitriptyline and imipramine causing prolonged cholestasis and vanishing bile-duct syndrome.

Table 16.1 Commonly used antidepressants and the patterns and proposed mechanisms of liver injury.

Drug	Class	Type of injury	Mechanism	Risk of liver injury
Phenelzine	MAOI	Cholestatic/hepatocellular	Metabolic	+++
Moclobemide	MAOI	Cholestatic/hepatocellular	Metabolic	++
Imipramine	TCA	Cholestatic/hepatocellular/ vanishing bile-duct syndrome	Direct toxicity or hypersensitivity	+++
Amitriptyline	TCA	Fulminant hepatitis/cholestasis	Immunoallergic	+++
Clomipramine	TCA	Hepatocellular	Immunoallergic	+
Fluoxctine	SSRI	Hepatocellular/cholestatic/mixed	Metabolic/idiosyncratic	+
Paroxetine	SSRI	Hepatocellular/cholestatic	Metabolic	+
Sertraline	SSRI	Hepatocellular/cholestatic/mixed	Immunoallergic	++
Citalopram, Escitalopram	SSRI	hepatocellular	Metabolic	+
Fluvoxamine	SSRI	Hepatocellular	Metabolic	+
Venlafaxine	SNRI	Hepatocellular, cholestatic	Idiosyncratic	++
Duloxetine	SNRI	Hepatocellular, cholestatic	Idiosyncratic	+++
Trazodone	SARI	Hepatocellular, mixed, cholestatic	Idiosyncratic	++
Mirtazapine	–	Hepatocellular, mixed	Metabolic	++
Lithium	–	Hepatocellular	?	+

MAOI, monoamine-oxidase inhibitor; SARI, serotonin-2 antagonist/reuptake inhibitor; SNRI, serotonin noradrenaline reuptake inhibitors; SSRI, selective serotonin reuptake inhibitor; TCA, tricyclic antidepressant.

Co-prescription of more than one drug targeting the same cytochrome P450 (CYP450) isoenzyme pathway may increase the risk of hepatotoxicity. Anti-depressants may inhibit or induce the CYP450 pathway, thereby affecting serum concentrations of the drugs or their metabolites and potentially increasing the risk of hepatotoxicity, alternatively antidepressants may compete with other drugs for the same pathway (Table 16.1). In an age of increasing polypharmacy therefore, care must be taken to review the potential for drug–drug interactions to reduce this risk.

Generally, antidepressants with a higher risk of hepatotoxicity should be used with caution in elderly patients, in those on multiple other medications, and those with substantial alcohol use, or possible underlying liver disease, as a severe DILI in these patients could have devastating consequences. Prescription of the lowest effective dose is recommended to reduce the risk of liver injury. It is useful to perform baseline LFTs followed by routine reassessment while on treatment. There is a significant physiological variation in ALT levels, so a single reading may not be that informative; however, it may be used as a reference to look for significant changes in levels on treatment. An elevated ALT in a patient on antidepressants may be related to an underlying liver disease (such as untreated hepatitis C virus infection or excess alcohol intake) that does not contraindicate antidepressant treatment, or it may represent a DILI. Baseline ALT results may help in the interpretation of abnormal liver results on anti-depressant treatment and aid in the decision to continue treatment or stop.

If serum ALT reaches more than three times the baseline value (or more than five times the upper limit of normal) treatment should be discontinued and the patient referred for further investigation to identify potential causes. If a DILI is confirmed then any drug from the same class should be avoided thereafter.

Antipsychotics

First-generation, typical, or classical antipsychotics (including chlorpromazine and haloperidol) were first introduced over 60 years ago and are effective against hallucination and delusions, but are associated with significant extrapyramidal adverse effects, they are also commonly associated with abnormal LFTs and significant liver damage as a consequence. Second-generation or atypical agents (clozapine, olanzapine, and risperidone) were introduced more recently. They are much less frequently associated with extrapyramidal adverse effects, but have significant metabolic effects with weight gain, obesity, hyperlipidemia insulin resistance, and diabetes (Table 16.2).

Abnormal liver function can also be seen in patients with conditions that affect their body weight. Antipsychotic medications (particularly olanzapine and clozapine) are associated with significant weight gain, and can impair glucose metabolism, increase cholesterol and triglyceride levels, and cause arterial hypertension, leading to the metabolic syndrome. The prevalence of metabolic syndrome is high in patients with schizophrenia, and is commonly associated with abnormal liver function, denoting the effect of metabolic syndrome on the liver in the form of non-alcoholic fatty liver disease.

Patients who are underweight may also have abnormal LFTs, specifically those with eating disorders such as anorexia nervosa or bulimia. Weight loss and starvation can cause

Table 16.2 Commonly used antipsychotic medications and the patterns and proposed mechanisms of liver injury.

Drug	Class	Type of injury	Mechanism	Risk of liver injury
Chlorpromazine	FGA	Cholestasis	? Hypersensitivity	+++
Haloperidol	FGA	Hepatitis	? Toxic intermediate	+
Clozapine	SGA	Hepatocellular/mixed	? Toxic intermediate	+++
Olanzapine	SGA	Hepatocellular/mixed/ cholestatic	? Toxic intermediate/ metabolic	+
Risperidone	SGA	Cholestatic/mixed/ hepatocellular	Immunoallergic	++
Quetiapine	SGA	Hepatocellular	? Toxic intermediate/ metabolic	
Aripiprazole	SGA	Not reported		+

FGA, first-generation antipsychotic; SGA, second-generation antipsychotic.

elevated serum transaminases as a direct result of hepatocyte injury and cell death, and malnutrition-induced hepatitis is more common as body mass index decreases. Rarely, it can cause acute liver failure, when elevated transaminases are associated with coagulopathy and encephalopathy. This can be a sign of serious multiorgan failure and requires prompt nutritional rehabilitation. Patients with severe anorexia and abnormal liver function require assessment by a specialist for this reason.

Refeeding can also lead to elevated transaminases, often due to steatosis. It can be useful to try and distinguish the causes as abnormal transaminases related to fasting are caused by hepatocyte apoptosis, and will improve with nutrition, while abnormal liver function related to refeeding and steatosis may improve if the rate of nutrition is reduced. Usually, these abnormalities are not clinically significant and supervised nutritional intake leading to return to a healthy bodyweight will lead to normalization of liver enzymes.

Liver Diseases that May Mimic Psychiatric Conditions

There are some liver diseases that can present with psychiatric symptoms. Wilson's disease: the classic example of liver disease presenting with psychiatric symptoms is Wilson's disease. Wilson's disease is a disorder of copper transport caused by mutations in the *ATP7B* gene, which encodes an intracellular protein responsible for mediating transport of copper in hepatocytes. Excess copper is usually excreted in bile, but in Wilson's disease it accumulates in the liver leading to liver injury and hepatocyte loss. As a result, free serum copper is increased, which in turn leads to accumulation in other tissues such as the brain where it is directly toxic.

Patients presenting with Wilson's disease may have a wide variety of symptoms and they may therefore be encountered by psychiatrists, but also neurologists and gastroenterologists. Psychiatric symptoms may precede the recognition of hepatic or neurologic Wilson's disease by a significant amount of time. The most commonly reported symptoms are depression, personality change, incongruous behavior, and irritability. A decline in school performance, impulsive behavior, labile mood, and psychosis are also reported. Behavioral and psychiatric symptoms can present during adolescence and therefore may be wrongly attributed to puberty. It is relatively uncommon for patients presenting with only psychiatric symptoms to be diagnosed with Wilson's disease, and it is only when these patients subsequently develop neurological symptoms or liver dysfunction that a diagnosis is made. Abnormal liver function in patients presenting with any of these features should therefore prompt further investigation, although of course, Wilson's disease is rare (one in 30 000 live births) and many of those psychiatric features are found very commonly.

Alcohol: Alcohol withdrawal may precipitate and acute delirium or psychosis and patients may therefore present to psychiatric services. For this reason, patients with acute psychosis should have an alcohol history taken and their liver enzymes should be evaluated. Any with a significant alcohol history and abnormal liver enzymes should be referred for further assessment.

Hepatic encephalopathy: People with underlying liver disease may develop hepatic encephalopathy, a reversible brain dysfunction, and this is reported to cause a wide variety of mental disturbances. The mechanisms causing brain dysfunction in advanced liver disease are not well understood, but it is associated with poor quality of life and often suggests a poor prognosis. Patients with undiagnosed liver disease presenting with encephalopathy can be thought to be manifesting psychiatric disease.

Hepatic encephalopathy classically presents with fluctuating symptoms, and this may be a clue to the underlying diagnosis. Typical symptoms range in severity from a mild alteration in mental state through to coma, additional neuromuscular symptoms can occasionally be seen. Minimal hepatic encephalopathy may result in alteration of attention, working memory, psychomotor speed, and visuospatial ability. As it progresses, it may be associated with reversal of the sleep–wake cycle, and may manifest with personality changes leading to apathy, irritability, and disinhibition, and excessive daytime somnolence.

More severe encephalopathy may cause progressive disorientation to time and place, inappropriate or aggressive behavior, acute confusion with agitation, and eventually coma. Neurological signs such as hypertonia, hyperreflexia, and upgoing plantars may be seen alongside a flapping tremor (asterixis). Extrapyramidal dysfunction such as loss of facial expression, rigidity, bradykinesia, monotonous, and slowed speech, and occasionally parkinsonian-like tremor may be found. Hepatic encephalopathy is found in patients with chronic liver disease; however, it may also be due to acute liver failure or to extensive port-systemic shunting without significant liver disease. The diagnosis of hepatic encephalopathy needs to be considered in patients presenting with fluctuating conscious levels, even those not known to have underlying chronic liver disease.

Wernicke's encephalopathy: Wernicke's encephalopathy is an acute syndrome arising from thiamine deficiency. It is characterized by encephalopathy, oculomotor dysfunction, and ataxia. It is underdiagnosed in clinical practice and is a neurological emergency, as untreated it may lead to permanent neurological injury. Neuropsychiatric symptoms are varied but typically include alteration in conscious level, mental slowing, impaired concentration and gait, and eye movement abnormalities. Risk factors for the development of Wernicke's include alcohol dependence, malnutrition (including patients with hyperemesis, anorexia, bulimia, or restricted diets), untreated HIV infection, treatment with chemotherapeutic agents for cancer, or gastrointestinal surgery, particularly bariatric surgery, which may predispose to thiamine malabsorption. Untreated Wernicke's can lead to Korsakoff syndrome, which is characterized by anterograde and retrograde amnesia and confabulation.

Liver Diseases Associated with Psychiatric Disease

Liver disease related to alcohol is clearly commonly associated with alcohol use disorder, characterized by an impaired ability to stop or control alcohol use despite adverse social, occupational, or health consequences. If a patient has a significant alcohol history it may be appropriate to perform routine blood tests (full blood count, INR, urea and electrolytes, LFTs) and in the presence of abnormal results to consider referring on for further assessment.

As described above, psychiatric medications and conditions are often associated with weight gain and the presence of the metabolic syndrome. Patients are at risk of developing non-alcoholic fatty liver disease (NAFLD) and should be assessed with a set of routine bloods and ideally performing a non-invasive assessment of fibrosis (NAFLD fibrosis, serum Enhanced Liver Fibrosis, or Fibrosis-4 Index for Liver Fibrosis score). If the results of these scores suggest the presence of any degree of fibrosis then the patient should be referred on for further assessment.

The acute porphyrias are rare metabolic conditions caused by mutations in the various enzymes involved in the haem biosynthesis pathway. The liver and bone marrow are the main sites for heme biosynthesis, and porphyria is associated with the accumulation of one or more of the heme pathway intermediates. They are classified as hepatic or erythropoietic, depending on the tissue the intermediates first accumulate. There are three main clinical categories of porphyria based on the predominant clinical features: acute neurovisceral symptoms, chronic blistering cutaneous, and acute non-blistering cutaneous. Those presenting with acute neurovisceral symptoms are the only ones that are likely to present to mental health practitioners. Clinical features include acute abdominal pain and neurovisceral features including psychiatric symptoms. Patients often present on multiple occasions with severe unexplained abdominal pain, weakness or peripheral neuropathy, and sensory loss. They may also present with acute confusion or psychosis, hallucinations, anxiety, or depression. Attacks may be precipitated by stress, or exposure to certain drugs or steroid hormones. Diagnosis of these conditions is often delayed because the non-specific nature of the presenting symptoms and failure to consider porphyria as a cause. This is unfortunate, as first-line biochemical screening tests are sensitive for the diagnosis of these disorders and effective treatment is also readily available. This diagnosis should therefore be considered in any patient presenting with unexplained abdominal pain and neuropsychiatric symptoms, and an initial screening test of a spot urine sample sent for urine porphobilinogen, total porphyrins, and creatinine. If urine porphobilinogen is normal and porphyrins are not elevated, this effectively rules out porphyria as a cause of symptoms.

Unexplained Abnormal Liver Function Tests in Patients with Known Psychiatric Disease

Any patient may present with abnormal liver function tests. As described above, a number of commonly used antidepressant and antipsychotic medications may be responsible for abnormal LFTs, and if there is a clear temporal association of abnormal liver function with the introduction of a drug then it is easier to be more confident of an association. Where liver enzymes are raised within two to three times the ULN, many mediations can be continued, with monitoring of LFTs.

If, however, there is no clear drug precipitant for abnormal liver function, further investigation is required. Abnormal liver enzymes are a marker of liver inflammatory changes and continuing liver inflammation is a risk factor for the development of significant chronic liver disease. It is important therefore to understand the etiology of abnormal liver enzymes, as it may be possible to prevent the development of chronic liver disease by appropriate intervention. In a patient with known psychiatric disease who develops abnormal liver function, the important considerations would include identifying any risk factors for liver disease:

- Ethnicity (? chronic hepatitis B)
- Weight: recent gain or loss? Metabolic syndrome?

- Alcohol history
- Drug history (including medication but also illegal drug use? Intravenous use is suggestive of viral hepatitis).

The patient should then be evaluated with a non-invasive liver screen and ultrasound of the liver. A non-invasive liver screen includes:

- Full blood count
- Urea and electrolytes
- LFTs
- INR
- Ferritin transferrin saturations
- Alpha 1 antitrypsin levels and phenotype
- Ceruloplasmin (in patients < 50 years)
- Viral serology (hepatitis B surface antibodies, anti-hepatitis C antibodies, hepatitis A)
- Autoimmune profile: anti-smooth muscle antibodies, anti-mitochondrial antibodies, anti-liver kidney microsomal antibodies, tissue transglutaminase, serum immunoglobulins, and electrophoresis.

If the results of this screen point to an underlying cause, the patient may require referral for specific treatment, but if there is continuing uncertainty about the cause of abnormal LFTs, the patient should be referred for further evaluation.

17

Non-Alcoholic Fatty Liver Disease

Matthew Collins[1,3] and Keyur Patel[2]

[1]*McMaster University, Hamilton, Ontario, Canada*
[2]*Toronto General Hospital, Toronto, Ontario, Canada*
[3]*Liver Care Canada, Hamilton, Ontario, Canada*

KEY POINTS

- Prevalence of obesity and metabolic diseases such as type 2 diabetes mellitus (T2DM) is rising globally.
- Non-alcoholic fatty liver disease (NAFLD) is associated with obesity and metabolic disorders.
- NAFLD is the most common chronic liver disease and second most indication for liver transplantation in high income countries.

Introduction

The term NAFLD and its clinical spectrum was first used 20 years ago and has since been accepted and increasingly referenced in clinical practice. NAFLD has been found to be strongly associated with metabolic disease, and rising prevalence parallels global increased rates of obesity and coinciding metabolic disease. NAFLD is now the most common chronic liver disease and the second most common indication for liver transplantation in developed nations.

Definition

NAFLD is defined as hepatic steatosis, as evidenced by radiologic or histologic examination, in the absence of secondary causes of hepatic fat accumulation (Box 17.1). The definition of significant alcohol consumption varies between different society guidelines. The American Association for the Study of Liver Diseases defines significant alcohol consumption per consensus meeting recommendations for clinical trial candidate eligibility.

The Liver in Systemic Disease: A Clinician's Guide to Abnormal Liver Tests, First Edition.
Edited by Gideon M. Hirschfield, Paramjit Gill, and James Neuberger.
© 2023 John Wiley & Sons Ltd. Published 2023 by John Wiley & Sons Ltd.

Box 17.1 Common Causes of Hepatic Steatosis

- Macrovesicular
  - Excessive ethanol consumption
  - Hepatitis C (genotype 3 in particular)
  - Wilson's disease
  - Hemochromatosis
  - Celiac disease
  - Autoimmune hepatitis
  - Lipodystrophy
  - Starvation
  - Total parenteral nutrition
  - Abetalipoproteinemia
  - Medications (i.e. corticosteroids, tamoxifen, methotrexate, amiodarone)
- Microvesicular
  - Reye's syndrome
  - Acute fatty liver of pregnancy
  - HELLP syndrome (hemolysis, elevated liver enzymes, low platelets)
  - Inborn errors of metabolism
  - Medications (i.e. valproic acid, anti-retrovirals)

Consumption of more than 21 standard drinks/week in men and more than 14 standard drinks/week in women over a two-year period preceding baseline liver histology is considered significant; one standard drink contains 14 g ethanol [1]. The European Association for the Study of the Liver defines significant alcohol consumption as daily alcohol consumption of 30 g or more for men and 20 g or more for women [2]. The term NAFLD encompasses the entire spectrum of disease ranging from uncomplicated simple hepatic steatosis (NAFL) to non-alcoholic steatohepatitis (NASH) and cirrhosis. NASH is a histologic diagnosis and differentiating NASH from NAFL requires a liver biopsy. At the current time, NASH cannot be diagnosed accurately with imaging or blood work. NASH is characterized by the presence of 5% or more hepatic steatosis with inflammation and hepatocyte ballooning, with or without fibrosis. The presence of NASH is associated with progression to advanced fibrosis, cirrhosis and its complications, whereas the risk of developing advanced fibrosis is minimal in NAFLD [1]. Although most patients with NAFLD have an elevated body mass index (BMI), 10–15% of patients with NAFLD have normal BMI; this is defined as lean NAFLD, which appears to be more prevalent in patients of Asian descent. Recently, the term metabolic dysfunction-associated fatty liver disease (MAFLD) has been proposed to replace NAFLD, to more appropriately reflect the association with metabolic disease and move away from NAFLD as a diagnosis of exclusion, and to remove alcohol from the definition. New "positive" criteria have been proposed for the diagnosis of MAFLD and include evidence of hepatic steatosis in addition to one of the following three criteria: elevated BMI/obesity, T2DM, or evidence of metabolic dysregulation [3].

Epidemiology

The global prevalence of NAFLD is estimated to be approximately 25% [4]. Prevalence is higher in Asia Pacific, Latin America, and the Middle East. The lowest prevalence is observed in Africa. The prevalence is also increased in high-risk groups (i.e. those with metabolic syndrome), as will be discussed later. Lean NAFLD is more common in Asian populations, where its prevalence has been reported at 19% [5]. Estimates on the prevalence of NASH are limited by the requirement of a liver biopsy for diagnosis. From the available data, the prevalence is estimated to be 1.5–6.45% in the general population. The prevalence of NASH in the NAFLD population ranges from 7% to 30% [4, 6]. In Canada, the prevalence of NAFLD is projected to increase by 20% between the year 2019 and 2030, with an even greater increase in cases of advanced fibrosis and the associated liver-related complications including hepatocellular cancer [7].

Pathophysiology

The liver plays a central role in human metabolism and the disposal or storage of excess metabolic energy. NAFLD is thought to reflect the hepatic manifestation of the metabolic syndrome. Visceral adipose tissue makes up a small percentage of total body fat, but is highly metabolically active, and plays a significant role in free fatty acid delivery to the liver. The accumulation of fatty acids in hepatocytes is the hallmark of NAFLD. This results from multiple interacting pathways involving genetics, comorbidities, microbiome, and lifestyle (nutrition/behavior), but a key contributing factor is insulin resistance. The accumulation of free fatty acids in the liver leads to hepatocyte stress and inflammation, which activates stellate cells and leads to progressive fibrosis. Interestingly, as fibrosis worsens in NAFLD, biopsy features of steatosis and hepatitis often improve, and this is referred to as "burned out" NAFLD.

Risk Factors

Over the years, multiple risk factors for the development and progression of NAFLD have been identified. Perhaps the biggest risk factors are elevated intra-abdominal or visceral fat and metabolic syndrome (three or more of: waist circumference ≥ 89 cm in women, 102 cm in men; high-density lipoprotein < 1.3 mmol/l in women, 1.04 mmol/l in men; triglycerides ≥ 1.7 mmol/l; blood pressure ≥ 130/85 mmHg; fasting blood glucose ≥ 5.6 mmol/l). Studies have demonstrated that approximately 75% of patients who are overweight and 90–95% of patients with morbid obesity have NAFLD [8]. Likewise, 50% of patients with NAFLD and 90% of patients with NASH are likely to have metabolic syndrome [9].

BMI is a simple calculation and is commonly used in clinical practice to assess for obesity. A BMI ≥ 25 kg/m^2 or > 23 kg/m^2 in Asian populations is considered overweight, and a BMI > 30 kg/m^2 or > 27 kg/m^2 in Asian populations is diagnostic of obesity. However, this metric does not perform well at the extremes of height and in those with a high muscle mass. It also does not distinguish between subcutaneous and visceral fat. Waist circumference is considered a better indicator of intra-abdominal or visceral fat, and has a greater association with metabolic disease than BMI. The UK National Institute for Health and Care Excellence suggests that men with a waist circumference greater than 94 cm and women with a waist circumference 85 cm or greater are at increased risk of comorbidity. The presence of the metabolic syndrome has been demonstrated to increase the likelihood of histologically confirmed NASH by 40% and is independently associated with increased overall mortality among patients with NAFLD [8, 9].

Lifestyle and diet play an important role in obesity. The consumption of a high-calorie diet with elevated amounts of fructose, refined carbohydrates, and saturated fats, coupled with a sedentary lifestyle, has been associated with higher rates of NAFLD. Given the role of insulin resistance in the pathogenesis of NAFLD and metabolic syndrome, it is not surprising that T2DM is a risk factor for the development and progression of NAFLD, and insulin resistance is almost universal in patients with NASH. In regard to the other constituents of metabolic syndrome, hypertension and dyslipidemia (hypertriglyceridemia and low high-density lipoprotein in particular) are associated with an increased risk of NAFLD [8, 10]. Age and sex also appear to be risk factors for NAFLD. The prevalence of NAFLD and stage of liver disease increases with age. Epidemiologic studies have demonstrated a higher prevalence of NAFLD in men than women, and advanced disease tends to present later in life in women, suggesting a potentially protective role for sex hormones. As noted above, there is a variability in the prevalence of NAFLD based on ethnicity/geographic region (i.e. Asia Pacific, Latin America, and the Middle East) and these differences are thought to be related to the frequency of specific gene alleles, such as *PNPLA3*. Alcohol-related liver disease is another common cause of hepatic steatosis, but it is a separate diagnosis and is not discussed here. However, NAFLD and alcohol-related liver disease are not mutually exclusive and are often present concurrently. Other conditions that have been associated with NAFLD are hypothyroidism, obstructive sleep apnea, polycystic ovarian syndrome, vitamin D deficiency, hypogonadism, hypopituitarism, osteoporosis, and psoriasis [8].

Natural History/Prognosis

Patients with NAFLD have an increased overall mortality compared with patients without NAFLD. Cardiovascular disease is the primary cause of death in patients with NAFLD without advanced fibrosis, followed by cancer. Liver-specific mortality increases with progressive fibrosis and is highest in those with NASH and advanced fibrosis [6].

The extent of underlying hepatic fibrosis, not steatosis, is the most important predictor of prognosis and liver-related morbidity and mortality in patients with NAFLD. As noted above, NASH is typically associated with progression of liver fibrosis. Patients with NAFLD and no fibrosis at baseline generally progress to stage 1 fibrosis over approximately 14 years, whereas patients with NASH and no fibrosis at baseline progress to stage 1 fibrosis over around 7 years. Previous data suggested that around 20% of patients with NAFLD also have NASH; however, recent studies suggest that this may be an underestimate [11]. Prospective studies have revealed progression from simple steatosis to NASH in 23–44% of patients over

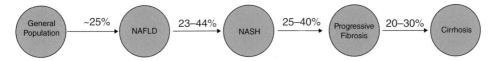

Figure 17.1 Prevalence and progression of non-alcoholic fatty liver disease. NAFLD, non-alcoholic fatty liver disease; NASH, non-alcoholic steatohepatitis.

a period of 2.2–6.6 years [12]. Other evidence suggests that NASH is a dynamic process with fluctuating progression and resolution [11]. It is estimated that approximately 25–40% of patients with NASH will develop progressive liver fibrosis and that 11% of patients with NASH will progress to cirrhosis [13]. The typical progression of NAFLD is illustrated in Figure 17.1.

NAFLD, including lean NAFLD, is an independent risk factor for cardiovascular disease. Studies have demonstrated that patients with NAFLD have an approximately 65% increased risk of cardiovascular disease and are more likely to die from cardiovascular disease than liver disease in those without advanced fibrosis [14]. Thus, counseling on risk factors for cardiovascular disease, including smoking and metabolic disease, is essential to the general care of patients with NAFLD.

Obesity is commonly associated with an increased risk of malignancy. Recent evidence suggests that NAFLD may potentiate the risk of cancer in patients with obesity, and may also be an independent risk factor. Hepatocellular carcinoma (HCC) is the most common malignancy in patients with NAFLD, but increased rates of uterine, gastric, pancreatic, and colonic cancer have also been observed [15]. Aside from HCC screening in patients with NASH cirrhosis, cancer screening guidelines are not different in patients with NAFLD compared with the general population. However, given the increased risk of malignancy, strong adherence to age-related cancer screening guidelines is recommended.

End-stage liver disease due to NAFLD is currently the second most common indication for liver transplant and is expected to become the leading cause for liver transplant in the near future. Patients with cirrhosis of any etiology have an increased risk of HCC, approximately 3–5% per year, and this is also applicable to those with NAFLD. There is recent evidence suggesting that NAFLD and metabolic syndrome may be risk factors for HCC, independent of cirrhosis, but screening and surveillance of NAFLD patients without cirrhosis for HCC is not currently recommended. Comorbid conditions, such as cardiovascular disease and morbid obesity or other end-organ injury from T2DM, such as chronic kidney disease, often limits eligibility for liver transplantation due to increased peri- and postoperative morbidity.

Clinical Features and Diagnosis

The vast majority of patients with NAFLD are asymptomatic and the only clinical finding suggesting the presence of underlying NAFLD is an elevated BMI or central adiposity. It is not typically until the development of cirrhosis and the appearance of stigmata of chronic liver disease (i.e. spider telangiectasias, splenomegaly, and ascites) that the presence of underlying liver disease is evident on clinical examination. NAFLD is typically diagnosed during the evaluation of elevated liver enzymes or after the incidental identification of hepatic steatosis on abdominal imaging.

Liver enzymes such as aspartate amino transferase (AST) and alanine amino transferase (ALT) are inconsistently elevated in patients with NAFLD, and there is no association between the degree of elevation of liver enzymes and the severity of underlying disease; the entire histologic spectrum of NAFLD can be seen in individuals with normal ALT values. In general, amino transferases (ALT and AST) are not elevated above four times the upper limit of normal and the AST : ALT ratio is <1. Higher aminotransferase levels should prompt the consideration of alternative or concomitant etiologies as well as advanced liver disease. AST : ALT > 1 suggests alcohol-related liver disease or advanced fibrosis. Cholestatic liver enzymes alkaline phosphatase (ALP) and gamma-glutamyl transferase can also be elevated in patients with NAFLD (approximately one third of patients with NAFLD have an elevated ALP), but is not typical and evaluation for cholestatic disease is recommended. Additionally, there are multiple extrahepatic factors that must be considered when analyzing a panel of liver enzymes(Table 17.1).

Ultrasound and computed tomography (CT) detect hepatic steatosis when there is greater than 20–30% macrovesicular fat. Thus, the absence of steatosis on imaging does not rule out the possibility of NAFLD (only 5% steatosis is required for the diagnosis of NAFLD).

As noted above, NAFLD is defined as hepatic steatosis, as evidenced by radiologic or histologic examination, in the absence of secondary causes of hepatic fat accumulation. Thus, to make a diagnosis of NAFLD, other etiologies of chronic liver disease must be ruled out, especially those that are associated with hepatic steatosis. Alcohol misuse is the most common competing cause of steatosis, and a detailed alcohol consumption history must be obtained. Other conditions associated with hepatic steatosis are listed in Box 17.1. In addition, it is prudent to rule out any concomitant liver disease, such as viral hepatitis or alpha-1-antitrypsin deficiency, which may accelerate the progression of liver damage.

Table 17.1 Extrahepatic factors affecting alanine amino transferase (ALT) and aspartate amino transferase (AST) levels.

Factor	AST	ALT
Time of day	No effect	45% variation (highest in afternoon, lowest overnight)
Day to day	5–10%	10–30% variation
Race/sex	15% higher in African Americans	No effect
Body mass index (BMI)	40–50% higher with increased BMI	40–50% higher with increased BMI
Exercise	Threefold increase with strenuous exercise	20% lower with regular exercise
Hemolysis	Significant increase	Moderate increase
Meals	No effect	No effect

The results of investigations must be considered carefully and in the context of NAFLD. Ferritin levels are often elevated in patients with NAFLD, owing to underlying inflammation and the role of ferritin as an acute-phase reactant. Thus, it is important to get a complete set of iron indices and to determine whether any risk factors for iron overload are present. Autoantibodies, such as antinuclear antibody (ANA) and anti-smooth muscle antibody (ASMA) commonly return mildly positive (i.e. ANA <1:100, ASMA <1:40) in patients with NAFLD and must be considered in the clinical context (i.e. serum immuno-globulin G level and risk factors for autoimmune disease).

Although liver biopsy is the gold standard for the diagnosis of NAFLD and is required for the diagnosis of NASH, it is not routinely obtained due to the associated morbidity and mortality, as well as the limited availability of resources and expertise required for the procedure. In addition, assessment of hepatic fibrosis in patients with NAFLD is affected by sampling error and interobserver variability. Thus, it is important to look at the entire clinical picture when reviewing biopsy results. Liver biopsy is typically reserved for patients with NAFLD who are at increased risk of having NASH and or advanced fibrosis, or to rule out competing etiologies of liver disease.

Non-Invasive Assessment

Steatosis Assessment

There are currently several non-invasive tests available to assess for underlying hepatic steatosis and fibrosis. Blood tests to estimate steatosis have limited clinical utility. Liver ultrasound is often the initial test ordered to evaluate for fatty liver disease. Hepatic steatosis typically presents as hepatomegaly with increased echogenicity and intrahepatic vascular blurring. As noted above, it can detect steatosis when greater than 20% of hepatocytes contain histologically visible fat droplets and has a sensitivity of approximately 80% with a specificity of 86%. Non-enhanced CT of the liver are more specific than ultrasound for detecting steatosis. Hepatic steatosis manifests as reduced attenuation in the liver parenchyma. Unenhanced CT can detect $\geq 30\%$ macrovesicular steatosis with a sensitivity of 100% and a specificity of 95% at a cutoff of 58 HU. Both ultrasound and CT are poor at detecting mild hepatic steatosis. The lack of reported steatosis should not exclude NAFLD from the differential diagnosis in the right clinical context [16]. The controlled attenuation parameter is a relatively new measurement that is obtained with the same device used for vibration-controlled transient elastography (VCTE; FibroScan®, Echosens, Boston, MA), which is becoming more commonplace in medical units. Studies have demonstrated that the controlled attenuation parameter is good at diagnosing steatosis at stage 1 and above, but is potentially disease specific and is less effective at differentiating between higher levels of steatosis. Performance of this test also decreases with increasing BMI, making it less useful in the NAFLD patient population. Magnetic resonance imaging (MRI) with proton density fat fraction estimation (PDFF) is the best non-invasive modality for characterizing and quantifying steatosis. MRI has a sensitivity of 76.7–90.0% and a specificity of 87.1–91% for detecting histologically confirmed steatosis ($\geq 5\%$). However, MRI-PDFF is not routinely available outside academic or tertiary referral centers. While some studies suggest that the degree of steatosis may predict the severity of histological features [17], quantification of hepatic steatosis in the patient with obesity is generally of little clinical value and rarely changes management.

Fibrosis Assessment

Having determined that the patient is obese and has steatosis and NAFLD, determining the degree of underlying hepatic fibrosis is important in risk stratification and prognostication. While liver biopsy is considered the gold standard, it has many limitations, as noted above. Several non-invasive tests have been developed and validated to estimate fibrosis stage over the years. The two most validated simple blood-based tests scores in patients with NAFLD are the Fibrosis-4 Index for Liver Fibrosis (FIB-4) score and NAFLD fibrosis score (NFS). These scores are easily calculated with standard blood work and clinical information (i.e. AST, ALT, platelets, BMI, albumin, diagnosis of insulin resistance/diabetes), and can be calculated in the primary care setting with easily accessible digital applications. Both tests are sensitive at ruling out advanced fibrosis (F3–F4). Optimal cutoff points have been evaluated in multiple studies and a FIB-4 cutoff of less than 1.30 (sensitivity 74%, specificity 71%) and a NFS cutoff of less than minus 1.455 (sensitivity 90%, specificity 60%) are typically used to identify patients at low risk for advanced fibrosis [1]. It should be noted that these scores may have reduced accuracy in elderly patients, and that the FIB-4 score performs better than NFS in patients with obesity and or diabetes. In addition, these scores lack specificity and yield indeterminate values in one third of patients, which limits their use as a single test. Other more complex scores using proprietary biomarkers are available in some but not all countries (FibroSure™, eviCore Healthcare, Bluffton, SC; ELF™ test, Siemens Healthcare, Tarrytown, NY: FibroMeter™, Echosens, Boston, MA). However, these scores are costly and generally outside of the scope of practice of primary care providers. To improve specificity for F3–4, a secondary test such as ultrasound elastography is required for patients with indeterminate values on FIB-4 or NFS. This sequential testing approach is important in low F3–4 prevalence cohorts such as primary care to reduce the referral burden on specialist centers.

Another modality commonly used to assess hepatic fibrosis is elastography. This can be assessed by multiple ultrasound-based methods, such as VCTE, shear-wave elastography, or magnetic resonance elastography (MRE). It should be noted that the liver stiffness measurement obtained by different elastography techniques are not directly comparable (i.e. MRE results cannot be directly compared with VCTE results). MRE is the most accurate method to assess the entire hepatic field; it is operator independent, and is not affected by body habitus; however, it is not readily available outside academic tertiary centers, and use is often limited to research studies.

VCTE is the most commonly used ultrasound elastography method. Unlike MRE, VCTE requires minimal time and resources, and is available as a point-of-care test at many centers globally. Quality measures have also been established (i.e. > 10 validated measurements, interquartile range < 30%) to ensure accuracy and reproducibility of results. Studies have looked at the optimal cutoff point for detecting advanced fibrosis in patients with NAFLD. A level between 6 and 11 kPa is typically considered for secondary assessment of advanced fibrosis [8, 18]. The results of VCTE must be considered in the context of the underlying disease process, as optimal liver stiffness thresholds vary depending on the underlying disease etiology. Additionally, there are multiple confounding variables that may affect measurements, resulting in false positive elevated liver stiffness, and include hepatic congestion, active hepatitis, increase hepatic blood flow (i.e. after eating, exercise), infiltrative disease (i.e. amyloidosis), and cholestasis.

As one would expect, using different modalities sequentially to assess for underlying fibrosis increases the accuracy of the assessment. At this time, there are no validated non-invasive tools available to differentiate NASH from NAFLD, or to accurately assess for disease progression. However, this is an active area of research and may become important in the future to determine the subset of patients that will respond to lifestyle management or therapeutic intervention.

Treatment

At this time, the mainstay in the management of NAFLD is lifestyle intervention and treatment of underlying metabolic diseases. Weight loss has the greatest impact, and in general, targeted weight loss of more than 5% total body weight has been shown to improve hepatic steatosis, more than 7% improves steatohepatitis, and more than 10% improves hepatic fibrosis in patients without advanced liver disease [1].

Diet is the biggest contributor to weight loss. There are multiple popular commercial diets, such as the low carbohydrate diet, ketogenic diet, intermittent fasting diet, and paleolithic diet; however, there is currently no strong evidence to support any of these diets in patients with NAFLD. The Mediterranean diet, which is high in vegetables, olive oil, nuts, and fish, has the most evidence for benefit in the NAFLD population. The Mediterranean diet has demonstrated an impact on hepatic steatosis and insulin sensitivity, and lowers the risk of cardiovascular disease and the development of diabetes, both of which are prominent in the NAFLD patient population. However, in general, the best diet for any patient is a diet that is palatable to the individual and can be maintained as part of a healthy lifestyle in the long term.

General advice for patients without advanced liver disease is to follow a hypocaloric (500–1000 kcal reduction/day), high protein (ideally plant protein), low carbohydrate/fructose, and low saturated/trans-fat diet. A high protein and low glycemic index diet can be helpful in maintaining weight loss. The management of cirrhosis is outside of the scope of this chapter; however, patients with cirrhosis are typically in a catabolic state an require more calories and protein (1.2–1.5 g/kg of protein per day) than those without cirrhosis. Thus, maintaining muscle mass and avoiding significant weight loss should be the goal. Dieticians and nutritionists are great resources and can be an invaluable member of a patient's care team, especially in the setting of advanced liver disease and cirrhosis.

Regular physical activity and exercise is important in achieving a negative calorie balance and weight loss, but has benefits even in the absence of weight loss, including improvements in mental health, increased lean body mass, decreased visceral fat, decreased insulin resistance, and increased cardiorespiratory fitness. Thus, physical activity is also an important intervention in patients with lean NAFLD. Both aerobic and anaerobic exercise appear to be beneficial. A general recommendation is for more than

150 minutes of moderate intensity exercise/week or 30–60 minutes most days of the week [1]. Regular low-impact resistance activity should be considered for patients with musculoskeletal concerns.

Multiple dietary supplements have been studied in patients with NAFLD. Consuming three to four cups of coffee/day has been associated with decreased liver enzymes, reduced progression of fibrosis, decreased mortality in patients with cirrhosis, and decreased risk of HCC. Vitamin E at a dose of 800 iu/day has been shown to improve liver enzymes and steatohepatitis in patients with biopsy confirmed NASH, but does not have a significant effect on fibrosis. It has not been adequately studied in patients with diabetes or cirrhosis and is not recommended in these patient populations. It has also been associated with an increased risk of prostate cancer, hemorrhagic stroke, and all-cause mortality; and these issues should be considered when prescribing vitamin E. There is currently not enough data to support the use of other anti-oxidants, such as vitamin C, resveratrol, anthocyanin, and bayberries. Probiotics/prebiotics have shown some benefits in patients with NAFLD, with no significant adverse effects, and can be considered, but are not part of most guidelines. Omega-3 fatty acids have demonstrated some utility in reducing hepatic steatosis and liver enzymes, but the optimal dose is unclear and further data is required before a formal recommendation can be made for their use in patients with NAFLD. However, they remain a therapeutic option for hypertriglyceridemia and may have an added benefit in patients with concomitant NAFLD. Weight loss supplements are often tempting to patients, but are generally not recommended, as many of these are not regulated and may contain impurities and potential hepatotoxins that can potentiate liver injury.

Most major guidelines do not recommend strict abstinence from alcohol in patients with NAFLD without cirrhosis. Although, a "safe" amount of alcohol consumption in patients with NAFLD has not been studied. Patients with mild/moderate alcohol consumption may have decreased improvement in steatosis or resolution of NASH. Thus, efforts should be made to minimize alcohol consumption to the lowest level possible.

Currently, there are no licensed medications specifically for the treatment of NAFLD. There are multiple clinical trials in progress, evaluating existing medications used for other metabolic disease, as well as novel agents. In the past, metformin was considered as a potential therapeutic agent due to improvement in insulin resistance; however, multiple studies have failed to demonstrate any significant benefit in multiple NAFLD endpoints and metformin is not recommend for treating NASH in recent guidelines [1]. There is growing interest in the use of glucagon-like peptide-1 (GLP-1) agonists, such as liraglutide, semaglutide, and exenatide, in patients with NAFLD. These agents are associated with improved insulin sensitivity, satiety, weight loss, and histological improvement in NASH with less progression of fibrosis. GLP-1 agonists currently do not have a primary indication for NAFLD but provide a good option for weight loss in patients with diabetes and NAFLD. Peroxisome proliferator-activated receptor (PPAR) agonists are another class of medication that is being evaluated in clinical trials. The PPAR-γ agonist, pioglitazone, has been extensively evaluated and has improved histology in patients with biopsy confirmed NASH with and without diabetes. Thus, it may be considered in patients with NASH; however, similar to GLP-1 agonists, pioglitazone is not indicated for use beyond diabetes, and has the undesired adverse effect of weight gain. Sodium–glucose cotransporter-2 (SGLT-2) inhibitors, such as empagliflozin, promote renal glucose wasting and weight loss. The use of empagliflozin has demonstrated reductions in hepatic steatosis and ALT, but available data are still limited and there is currently no indication for the use of SGLT-2 inhibitors in NAFLD.

In the past, the use of statins was limited in patients with liver disease, because of concerns over hepatotoxicity. However, recent evidence suggests that statins are safe to use in NAFLD and have a potential benefit in steatosis, steatohepatitis, fibrosis, and HCC risk. As a result, the use of statins is encouraged if indicated for treatment of dyslipidemia or increased cardiovascular risk. Farnesoid X receptor agonists, such as obeticholic acid (OCA), are the most promising class of medication and OCA is currently in phase three trials and under review by regulatory agencies. OCA has been shown to reverse fibrosis in a dose-dependent manner, but its use is complicated by adverse effects of pruritus and elevated low-density lipoprotein.

Bariatric or weight loss clinics may be helpful for obese patients who are unable to lose weight or maintain weight loss. These clinics often have more expertise in adjuvant pharmacotherapy for weight loss. Pharmacologic options include orlistat (decreased lipid digestion), naltrexone–bupropion combination (decreased hunger and cravings), and liraglutide [19]. Naltrexone–bupropion should be used with caution in patients with hepatic dysfunction.

Bariatric surgery is an option for patients with morbid obesity ($BMI \geq 40\,kg/m^2$ or $BMI \geq 35\,kg/m^2$ with one or more obesity-related disease) that fail alternative weight loss methods and meet regional criteria. Bariatric surgery is effective at causing sustained weight loss, treating metabolic disease, and decreasing NASH and hepatic fibrosis. The decision regarding the type of surgery should be made by a multidisciplinary team.

The increasing global prevalence of NAFLD is posing a significant and increasing burden on the healthcare system. Thus, managing and triaging patients to the appropriate level of care (primary care or specialist gastroenterology/hepatology) is essential to prevent overwhelming the healthcare system. Many different care pathways have been proposed over the past five years, and an example of this is illustrated in Figure 17.2. The core concept of these pathways is risk stratification using established risk factors (i.e. age, obesity, metabolic disease) and non-invasive fibrosis tests. Patients meeting criteria for low risk of advanced fibrosis can be monitored in the primary care setting with reassessment for advancing disease at regular intervals (three to five years), whereas patients who fall into intermediate or high-risk categories should be referred to specialists for further assessment and care.

Conclusion

In summary, NAFLD is an increasingly recognized consequence of metabolic disease with systemic manifestations, silent presentation, and growing footprint across the globe. Increasing awareness of the disease, identifying those at risk, initiating early lifestyle intervention to reduce progression to advanced disease, using available tools to identify patients with advanced disease for triaging patients to the appropriate care setting are essential in preventing the inevitable overburdening of the healthcare system. NAFLD is a currently an active area of research and better assessment tools for risk stratification, referral care pathways, and targeted treatments are likely to be available in the near future.

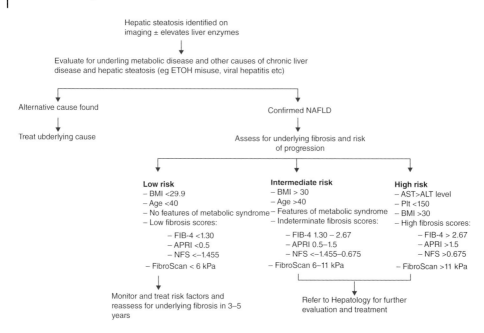

Figure 17.2 Risk stratification and referral pathway for advanced non-alcoholic fatty liver disease. APRI, AST to Platelet Ratio Index; BMI, body mass index; ETOH, ethyl alcohol; FIB-4, Fibrosis-4 Index for Liver Fibrosis; NAFLD, non-alcoholic fatty liver disease; NFS, NAFLD Fibrosis Score; Plt, platelets.

References

1. Chalasani, N., Younossi, Z., Lavine, J.E. et al. (2018). The diagnosis and management of nonalcoholic fatty liver disease: practice guidance from the American Association for the Study of Liver Diseases. *Hepatology* 67: 328–357.
2. European Association for the Study of the Liver, European Association for the Study of Diabetes, and European Association for the Study of Obesity (2016). EASL-EASD-EASO clinical practice guidelines for the management of non-alcoholic fatty liver disease. *J. Hepatol.* 64: 1388–1402.
3. Eslam, M., Newsome, P.N., Sarin, S.K. et al. (2020). A new definition for metabolic dysfunction-associated fatty liver disease: an international expert consensus statement. *J. Hepatol.* 73: 202–209.
4. Younossi, Z.M., Koenig, A.B., Abdelatif, D. et al. (2016). Global epidemiology of nonalcoholic fatty liver disease-meta-analytic assessment of prevalence, incidence, and outcomes. *Hepatology* 64: 73–84.
5. Mitra, S. and De Chowdhury, A. (2020). Epidemiology of non-alcoholic and alcoholic fatty liver diseases. *Transl. Gastroenterol. Hepatol.* (5): 16.

6. Younossi, Z., Tacke, F., Arrese, M. et al. (2019). Global perspectives on nonalcoholic fatty liver disease and nonalcoholic steatohepatitis. *Hepatology* 69: 2672–2682.

7. Swain, M.G., Ramji, A., Patel, K. et al. (2020). Burden of nonalcoholic fatty liver disease in Canada, 2019-2030: a modelling study. *CMAJ Open* 8: E429-E436.

8. Cotter, T.G. and Rinella, M. (2020). Nonalcoholic fatty liver disease 2020: the state of the disease. *Gastroenterology* 158: 1851–1864.

9. Marchesini, G., Bugianesi, E., Forlani, G. et al. (2003). Nonalcoholic fatty liver, steatohepatitis, and the metabolic syndrome. *Hepatology* 37: 917–923.

10. Byrne, C.D. and Targher, G. (2015). NAFLD: a multisystem disease. *J. Hepatol.* 62: S47–S64.

11. Kleiner, D.E., Brunt, E.M., Wilson, L.A. et al. (2019). Association of histologic disease activity with progression of nonalcoholic fatty liver disease. *JAMA Netw. Open* 2: e1912565.

12. AJ, L.C.C.M. (2018). The natural history of nonalcoholic fatty liver disease-an evolving view. *Clin. Liver Dis.* 22: 11–21.

13. Dyson, J.K., Anstee, Q.M., and Mcpherson, S. (2014). Non-alcoholic fatty liver disease: a practical approach to diagnosis and staging. *Frontline Gastroenterol.* 5: 211–218.

14. Kasper, P., Martin, A., Lang, S. et al. (2020). NAFLD and cardiovascular diseases: a clinical review. *Clin. Res. Cardiol.* 110: 921–937.

15. Kumar, R., Priyadarshi, R.N., and Anand, U. (2020). Non-alcoholic fatty liver disease: growing burden, adverse outcomes and associations. *J. Clin. Transl. Hepatol.* 8: 76–86.

16. Li, Q., Dhyani, M., Grajo, J.R. et al. (2018). Current status of imaging in nonalcoholic fatty liver disease. *World J. Hepatol.* 10: 530–542.

17. Chalasani, N., Wilson, L., Kleiner, D.E. et al. (2008). Relationship of steatosis grade and zonal location to histological features of steatohepatitis in adult patients with non-alcoholic fatty liver disease. *J. Hepatol.* 48: 829–834.

18. Siddiqui, M.S., Vuppalanchi, R., Van Natta, M.L. et al. (2019). Vibration-controlled transient elastography to assess fibrosis and steatosis in patients with nonalcoholic fatty liver disease. *Clin. Gastroenterol. Hepatol.* 17 (156–163.e2).

19. Wharton, S., DCW, L., Vallis, M. et al. (2020). Obesity in adults: a clinical practice guideline. *CMAJ* 192: E875–E891.

Section 4

Practical Issues in Patients with Liver Abnormalities

18

Prescribing in Patients with Abnormal Liver Tests or Liver Disease: A Pragmatic Approach

Paul Selby

Cambridge University Hospitals NHS Foundation Trust, Cambridge, UK

KEY POINTS

- Prescribing in patients with abnormal liver function tests (LFTs) or liver disease is challenging.
- Many patients with liver disease present with comorbidities.
- Balancing therapeutic benefit and minimizing harm is key goal of prescribing in liver disease.
- Analysis of LFT trends can be helpful in assessing progression or resolution of liver disease.
- LFTs multiple times above the normal range should prompt guidance/advice from specialists.
- The degree of liver impairment and complications from liver disease must be established to prescribe safely.

Introduction

Prescribing in patients with abnormal liver tests can be difficult, with no means to measure precisely the remaining metabolic or excretory capacity of the liver. However, patients with liver disease commonly have other comorbidities and complications that require treatment. As the principal site of metabolism and detoxification of drugs in the body, liver impairment will affect the majority of drugs used in practice, and therapy should be carefully selected.

In patients with liver disease, the consideration of changes within the liver physiology adds to the complexity of prescribing decisions. The underlying physiology provides only a partial guide for prescribing adjustments, as the hepatic reserve prevents direct attribution of liver function from a specific level of liver injury. As many clinical trials exclude patients with pre-existing liver disease, there is often a lack of clear prescribing information on dosing for these patients. Similarly, interpreting information on the safe prescribing of drugs based on abnormal liver blood tests alone is difficult.

This chapter takes you through guiding principles to consider when prescribing for patients with abnormal liver tests or liver disease. An understanding of the patient's liver health and the specifics of the liver blood tests is central to designing a management plan. Licensing information and first principles of drug handling help to identify considerations

The Liver in Systemic Disease: A Clinician's Guide to Abnormal Liver Tests, First Edition.
Edited by Gideon M. Hirschfield, Paramjit Gill, and James Neuberger.

for safety. Generalists and specialists should use their existing knowledge of the therapeutic drugs they are planning to prescribe to help support prescribing in these patients.

The terms "hepatic impairment" and "liver impairment" are often used in regulatory or published literature, and reflect a broad range of conditions resulting from damage to the liver. It is important to ascertain the cause and extent of liver impairment when prescribing as this will help with assessing the overall risks for an individual patient.

The goal of prescribing in liver disease is to provide therapeutic benefit, while minimizing adverse effects of the drug, preserving any remaining liver function and avoiding exacerbating complications and stigmata of liver disease.

Abnormal Liver Tests

In the context of prescribing, liver blood tests are useful in establishing an overall picture of the patient's liver health. The finding of abnormal liver tests does not preclude prescribing new medicines outright; they can be used in assessing the specifics of underlying disease and therefore the risks associated with prescribing medicines. LFTs multiple times greater than the upper limit of normal should prompt further advice and guidance from specialist services.

Dividing LFTs into those that show acute or continuing damage and those that represent functional impairment is helpful to understand the overall presentation. In particular, interpretation of blood tests that suggest functional impairment influences prescribing advice in liver impairment. Serum bilirubin is an important marker when prescribing in liver disease; very high levels represent a significant disease burden. It is also an indicator for cholestasis, alongside elevations in alkaline phosphatase (ALP) and gamma-glutamyl transferase (GGT). This reflects a reduction in biliary excretion and requires consideration when prescribing medicines excreted via the biliary tract. Table 18.1 presents some information on liver blood tests and their use in identifying types of liver disease.

Looking at trends in liver blood tests can also be helpful in identifying progression or resolution of liver disease. Caution is warranted in patients whose disease is progressing to avoid exacerbating or potentiating further liver damage. Repeated monitoring should be continued in patients with abnormal liver tests when starting or increasing doses of medication, including those that are perceived to be relatively safe in liver disease.

In certain circumstances, bilirubin levels alone are used to guide recommendations on dose reductions for extensively biliary-excreted medicines. This is often an approach taken in the dosing for cytotoxic chemotherapy where local protocols should be followed.

In the presence of significantly raised transaminases, prescribing should be avoided where the need is not immediately required. To maintain existing function and support recovery of the liver, the cause of the dysfunction should be investigated, and, ideally, evidence of resolution of transaminases resolved before new medicines are initiated.

When assessing liver impairment, some liver blood tests will suggest severe impairment. Investigation for causes should be undertaken and careful consideration should be made for prescribing, with dose reductions considered in patients with:

- prothrombin time greater than 130% of normal
- platelets less than 150×10^9/l

Table 18.1 Simple interpretations and considerations for prescribing from abnormal liver function tests.

Liver blood test	Simple interpretation	Notes for prescribing
ALT	Continuing hepatocyte inflammation/injury	Increased levels may suggest a DILI after newly started medication
	Acute rises often seen in acute liver injury	
	More specific of hepatic injury	
ALP	Continuing hepatocyte inflammation/injury	Consider alongside bilirubin if obstructed bile ducts suspected
	Elevated in cholestasis	
AST	Continuing hepatocyte inflammation/injury	
GGT	Continuing hepatocyte inflammation/injury	Interpret alongside ALP for hepatic origin of elevated ALP
	Elevated in cholestasis	
Bilirubin (total bilirubin)	Marker of hepatocellular function	Elevated levels may indicate impairment in biliary excretion with implications for drugs excreted in bile
	Elevated in chronic and acute liver disease	
Albumin	Reduced levels indicate impairment of synthetic function over a long period of time	If abnormal consider chronic cirrhosis
		Poor prognostic value in acute liver failure
		Sarcopenia may indicate further dose reductions for low body weight
Prothrombin time/international normalized ratio	Raised levels indicate impairment of synthetic function and may reflect an acute derangement in liver function	If abnormal consider chronic cirrhosis
Platelet count	Thrombocytopenia suggests pancreatic involvement in disease and functional impairment of portal flow	If abnormal consider chronic cirrhosis; consider long-term trend

ALP, alkaline phosphatase; ALT, alanine amino transaminase; AST, Aspartate amino transaminase; DILI, drug-induced liver injury; GGT, gamma-glutamyl transferase.

- bilirubin greater than 100 µmol/l (> 5.8 mg/dl)
- hyponatremia.

Liver blood tests are important in monitoring adverse reactions in response to prescribed medicines. The monitoring of liver blood tests is often recommended in prescription medicines to detect any liver insult at an early stage. Many drugs known to cause idiosyncratic drug-induced liver injury (DILI) require monitoring with specific guidance on dosing adjustments should liver blood tests become abnormal. Liver blood tests for monitoring continuing drug therapy should include those discussed above.

Drug Licensing for Patients with Liver Disease and Prescribing Guidance

Prescribing in line with licensed information is the simplest and most convenient way to prescribe specific drugs in liver disease. Where this information exists, it will be present in the manufacturer's licensing submission, such as the summary of product characteristics or prescribing information associated with the drug. National formularies will also contain similar advice, where they exist. The term or section on "hepatic impairment" is most commonly used in licensing information when giving advice.

Caution and contraindication in licensing may be listed because there is a lack of evidence to support a recommendation, or based on theoretical concerns. This merits further consideration, as the cause of a warning can help to guide the risk of prescribing the drug.

Where evidence or advice is reported in manufacturers' literature for patients with liver disease it is common to divide patients in to mild, moderate, and severe liver disease categories. Often, no indication is provided as to what these categories represent. Some studies or product information consider Child–Pugh scoring (Table 18.2) as a surrogate marker for such categories, and will direct prescribing advice for patients with either Child–Pugh class A, B, or C cirrhosis. Using these surrogate markers for the terms mild, moderate, and severe impairment, respectively, can be helpful, and is a reasonable strategy if used cautiously in conjunction with signs and symptoms present in the patient.

Liver disease staging is important in establishing the presence of cirrhosis, as patients without cirrhosis generally require no dose adjustments as they are unlikely to have functional impairment. However, the involvement of the biliary system should be considered for drugs that are known to have significant biliary excretion. Although rarely discussed directly in the licensing, information on the clinical pharmacology and pharmacological properties is usually presented. Caution should be used when prescribing drugs reported to have significant hepatic excretion due to a risk of accumulation.

Where prescribing information is unavailable, assessing "first principles" of how the drug is handled by the body can be used to assess the likelihood of a specific drug to be

Table 18.2 Child–Pugh score.

Clinical and biochemical measurements	Points scored for increasing abnormality		
	1	2	3
Bilirubin (µmol/l)	< 35	35–50	> 50
Albumin (g/dl)	> 35	28–35	< 28
Ascites	Absent	Slight	Moderate or severe
Encephalopathy (grade)	None	1–2	3–4
International normalized ratio	< 1.7	1.7–2.2	> 2.2
Total points: 5–6 = class A; 7–9 = class B 10–15 = class C			

affected by liver disease. Pharmacological parameters are commonly included in prescribing information and available through medicines information departments based in primary or secondary care institutions, and pharmaceutical companies.

Prescribing Hepatotoxic Medication and Drug-Induced Liver Injury

There are situations when medicines known to cause DILI are required to be prescribed in patients with liver impairment or abnormal liver blood tests. Although DILI is an uncommon complication of drug therapy, it is a common cause of liver dysfunction and any changes to liver blood tests or liver function should arouse suspicions of a DILI. Idiosyncratic DILI can occur from hours to weeks after initiation of medicines and requires careful observation.

As the number of medications prescribed increases so does the risk of DILI. Reducing and preventing polypharmacy is an important consideration when prescribing for patients with liver injury.

Idiosyncratic Drug-Induced Liver Injury

When prescribing a drug that causes idiosyncratic liver injury in patients with pre-existing liver test abnormalities, careful consideration should be given to whether treatment can be delayed until the cause is investigated and liver blood tests have resolved.

When prescribing a drug that causes idiosyncratic liver injury in patients with existing cirrhosis and functional impairment, consideration should be given to the risks and benefits of individual drugs, and investigation of alternative options. For drugs which cause idiosyncratic DILI, existing liver disease is not related to an increased risk of liver injury, but should liver injury develop, the clinical consequences are likely to be more severe.

Dose-Dependent Drug-Induced Liver Injury

When prescribing drugs that cause a dose-dependent liver injury, the benefit and risks must be carefully considered and, as a general rule, such drugs should be avoided. However, understanding the mechanism of action will help to support the decision-making process and the prescriber should use their knowledge of the drugs they are prescribing to identify risk and benefit. Dose-dependent liver injury can be caused by cumulative use (such as steatosis caused by methotrexate) or by an individual event of high dosing (such as the hepatic insult seen in acute paracetamol overdose).

In the case of paracetamol, toxicity is known to be associated with high doses and a reduction in the dose or frequency it is given to patients may be sufficient to prevent DILI occurring. Induction of cytochrome P450 (CYP) enzymes can increase toxicity in paracetamol overdose, and therefore cautions in the prescribing of paracetamol with CYP inducers such as rifampicin, carbamazepine, or phenytoin exist.

Having considered the risks of DILI, it is sensible to make a management plan, which may include monitoring of liver blood tests and explanation of complications that may arise so that patients can monitor for adverse events.

"First Principles" to Consider in Prescribing for Patients with Liver Disease

Interpreting the principles of pharmacokinetics and pharmacodynamics, combined with an understanding of the extent of liver dysfunction allows assessment of safety when prescribing. These principles are covered in greater detail elsewhere, but an understanding of the underlying principles can enable a safety profile and assessment to be made to make prescribing decisions. Pharmacokinetics govern the relationship between drug dosing and drug concentration in the body; all the associated pharmacokinetic processes can be affected by liver impairment.

Absorption

Absorption of drugs from the gastrointestinal tract is affected by a number of patient and drug-specific factors. Following passive or active uptake in the gut, the flow of blood through the liver allows first-pass metabolism and clearance to occur before the drug has a systemic therapeutic effect.

Clearance of a drug by the liver is assessed using the hepatic extraction ratio, which is dependent on the intrinsic ability of the liver to metabolize the drug (intrinsic clearance) and the unbound fraction of the drug. Drugs with a high hepatic extraction ratio are more dependent on the rate of blood flow to the liver to increase clearance.

Drugs which undergo extensive first-pass metabolism will have low bioavailability due to the metabolism of the drug before reaching systemic circulation. A reduction of blood flow to the liver (as seen in portal hypertension or portosystemic shunts) can decrease the extent of first-pass metabolism, resulting in an increase in bioavailability.

Some drugs are administered as pro-drugs, which require modification into active metabolites, and this is also often completed during first-pass metabolism. Where first-pass metabolism is impaired, the expected concentrations of the active drug will be reduced, and therapy is less likely to be successful.

Complications from liver disease can affect the extent to which absorption takes place through changes to the gut. Fat-soluble (lipophilic) drugs require bile salts to aid their absorption, and in the setting of cholestasis, a lack of bile flow into the gut may cause reduced absorption. The presence of ascites can decrease absorption of drugs. Drugs which undergo enterohepatic recycling may have reduced reabsorption with respective lower systemic levels.

Distribution

Distribution reflects the extent to which a drug distributes into tissues and is dependent on lipid solubility, plasma protein binding, and tissue binding of a drug. Albumin performs a significant role in binding drugs in plasma rather than as a free (active) fraction. In liver disease, a reduction in albumin can result in an increased free fraction of highly protein-bound drugs (such as sodium valproate or phenytoin). This results in a higher concentration of the drug in the serum. Drugs that are highly protein-bound should therefore be used cautiously. Bilirubin may displace other drugs from albumin, further causing increased levels of the drug where bilirubin is raised.

Elevation of plasma volume and ascites can increase the volume of distribution (Vd; the proportion of the drug in the body compared to the measurable concentration in the blood) with complications for drugs with a high Vd. The increase in Vd results in slower elimination and a longer half-life.

Elimination

The liver plays an important role in the elimination of drugs, particularly those reliant on significant metabolism in their elimination pathway, or drugs eliminated through secretion into bile. Drugs eliminated by conjugation to glucuronides, glutathione, or sulfates are also largely eliminated from excretion into bile. Elimination of these compounds will be decreased in the presence of cholestasis.

It is also important to consider the presence of active metabolites in the elimination pathway, as this may also affect the safety profile of a medicine. An active metabolite excreted in bile may be increased when the parent drug is not.

Metabolism

Metabolism can affect the bioavailability and elimination of a drug, and as the liver is the predominant site of drug metabolism, this is significantly affected in liver disease. Metabolism is usually considered to occur in two phases.

Phase I typically results in a metabolite that is more reactive, allowing phase II metabolism to occur successfully. The process is usually completed enzymatically. Phase II typically results in conjugation of the metabolite, with conjugates being more water soluble that are easily excreted.

In patients with liver impairment, phase I metabolism is significantly more impaired than phase II, with impairment of CYP expression and activity correlating to the severity of the liver disease [1]. The etiology may also play a part in overall effects on enzyme expression.

Pharmacodynamics govern the effect of the drug on receptors and the physiological effect of a drug. In liver impairment, altered receptor sensitivity is unclear, but should be considered for individual drugs. Drugs with a narrow therapeutic index (that is where there is a small difference between therapeutic dose and toxic dose) may have altered pharmacokinetics, with increased adverse effects and should be used with caution. Drugs with cumulative pharmacological effects either from direct or indirect drug–drug interactions should also be used cautiously.

A number of pharmacodynamic changes have been noted in liver impairment and should be considered when prescribing drugs affecting these sites of action. Increased effects from drugs acting on the central nervous system should be expected, including when prescribing opiates, anxiolytics, and sedatives. The blood–brain barrier is more permeable, with its association with encephalopathy and patients have increased risk from adverse effects. Opiates are associated with increased respiratory depression in liver disease.

Other reported complications include reduced betablocker effect, reduced diuresis and increased risk of infections from proton-pump inhibitor or histamine type 2 receptor antagonist use [1]. Transjugular intrahepatic portosystemic shunt is reported to increase baseline QT interval prolongation, increasing risks for drugs known to prolong the QT interval.

The factors above highlight the complexity of assessing the "safe" use of drugs when prescribing in liver disease. Drugs with minimal metabolism, good oral bioavailability, renal elimination, and few pharmacodynamic and pharmacokinetic interactions are likely to represent favorable characteristics.

Prescribing in the Context of Liver Disease

To prescribe safely in patients with liver disease, it is important to establish the stage of liver disease, underlying pathology, and complications resulting from the patients' liver disease. Understanding the stage of liver disease will help to suggest changes to the patient's metabolic or excretory capacity, and therefore how the drug will be handled by the patient. Understanding the pathology can guide specific recommendations relating to how individual drugs are excreted or metabolized. Understanding the complications will guide the safety of drugs which may worsen or exacerbate symptoms already existing from the liver disease. Figure 18.1 presents a flowchart of how to approach the prescribing decision.

As described above, optimizing dosing to avoid accumulation of drugs in liver disease can be achieved through assessing the pharmacokinetic and pharmacodynamic particulars of a drug. Drugs with large therapeutic indices are best suited, as dose reductions are unlikely to prevent the drug from being sub-therapeutic, while ensuring toxicity does not become a problem.

Establishing the extent of the patient's liver impairment and the pharmacokinetic and pharmacodynamic actions of the drug to be prescribed are the backbone to making safe prescribing decisions. This is helpful in identifying drugs which are likely to be problematic, and those which might require dose adjustment or monitoring.

Liver Fibrosis

Patients with mild fibrosis can be treated in the same way as the general population; where risk factors exist for the development of continuing fibrosis is present, regular blood tests should be completed.

In patients with moderate fibrosis without cirrhosis the choice of drug and decision to prescribe needs to consider potential hepatotoxicity, particularly long-term damage, as prevention of further liver damage, and preservation of the existing liver is important in improving prognosis for the patient. Adjustments to dosing is unlikely to be required, but the prescriber should consider any licensing requirements.

Cholestatic Liver Disease

When prescribing for patients with cholestatic liver disease, the prescriber should ensure that the elimination profile of the drug is considered to prevent accumulation of biliary-excreted drugs.

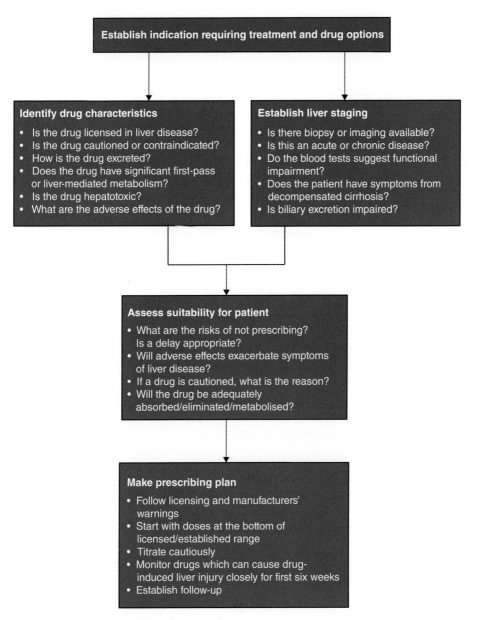

Figure 18.1 Prescribing flowchart.

Compensated Cirrhosis

For patients with cirrhosis, the clinical condition of the patient should guide prescribing decisions, including both symptoms and staging of liver disease, particularly in those with decompensated cirrhosis. Regular monitoring of liver function should be completed prior to and on starting prescribed medication. This is particularly important for chronically prescribed treatments as liver disease can fluctuate over time. Child–Pugh and MELD

(Model for End-stage Liver Disease) scores can be useful in establishing a prognosis and therefore the likely severity of disease. However, when prescribing drugs without specific recommendations, patients with cirrhosis should be considered to have a degree of liver impairment.

Decompensated Cirrhosis

In patients with decompensated cirrhosis, the need for a drug should be established as being essential to control the disease. An assessment should be made to establish that the overall goals of the patient's care is met with relation to overall prognosis. An overarching assessment of all prescribed medicines should be completed, to avoid any pharmacodynamic or pharmacokinetic interactions. It may that be an alternative drug with a safer profile in liver disease should be selected in preference to those more commonly used.

The symptoms and complications of liver disease present should be taken into account for the individual patient and the individual drug prescribed. In particular, consideration should be made of:

- ascites
- hypoalbuminemia
- impaired clotting.

These may affect the decision to start treatment where complications could be worsened by drug treatment.

Where a drug is identified as essential and there is no licensing or prescribing advice to support its use, the drug should be started cautiously, with a dose reduction considered. Dose reductions should be made for drugs with:

- low oral bioavailability due to high first-pass extraction
- drugs with high liver extraction or significant biliary excretion
- drugs cleared principally through phase I hepatic metabolism
- drugs with a narrow therapeutic index
- drugs with a long half-life
- drugs that are highly protein-bound.

Generally, the oral route of administration is preferred, and intramuscular injections are best avoided, particularly in patients with impaired clotting.

Cytochrome P450 Enzyme System

With a reduction in function of CYP enzymes expected in decompensated cirrhosis, consideration of drugs that undergo extensive metabolism via these routes should be made in this population (Table 18.3). This is particularly important in patients co-prescribed drugs that cause CYP inhibition or induction. The effect of CYP inhibition in addition to existing reduced function could cause a significant increase in the levels of the substrate. Specific examples of complications requiring caution when prescribing are shown in Box 18.1.

Table 18.3 Cytochrome P450 (CYP) isoforms involved in phase I metabolism and the effect of liver disease on activity.

P450 isoform	Substrates	Effect of liver disease on P450 activity
CYP1A2	Clozapine, theophylline	↓↓↓
CYP2A6	Halothane, methoxyflurane	↓↓
CYP2C9	Diclofenac, losartan, warfarin	↓
CYP2C19	Citalopram, diazepam, omeprazole	↓↓↓
CYP2D6	Codeine, haloperidol, metoprolol, nortriptyline	↔
CYP2E1	Enflurane, halothane, paracetamol	↓
CYP3A4	Amiodarone, carbamazepine, ciclosporin, tacrolimus, diltiazem	↓↓

Source: Pirmohamed [1]/with permission of Elsevier.

Box 18.1   Examples of Complications of Drugs that Require Caution when Prescribing for Patients with Symptoms of Liver Disease

- Ascites:
  - Can be affected by drugs that promote salt and water retention, such as non-steroidal anti-inflammatory drugs (NSAIDs), corticosteroids.
  - The sodium content of prescribed products should be considered (e.g. soluble/effervescent preparations).
- Coagulopathies:
  - Careful consideration of further anticoagulation is required.
  - Drugs known to cause gastrointestinal irritation and ulceration should also be carefully considered (e.g. corticosteroids, NSAIDs, selective serotonin reuptake inhibitors). Special consideration is required in the presence of esophageal varices or other gastric bleeding.
- Encephalopathy:
  - Associated with increased sensitivity to central nervous system depressants and hypnotics, and which can mask encephalopathic symptoms.
  - Drugs that cause constipation (e.g. antimuscarinics, opiates) may increase ammonia absorption; additional or increased doses of laxatives may be required to maintain two to three loose stools per day.

Preserving Renal Function

A final consideration should be the prescribing of drugs that are known to cause damage to the kidneys, as the development of renal failure in addition to liver impairment is associated with a poor prognosis. Reducing elimination from the kidneys also has the potential to affect existing drug therapy risking additional adverse events.

Summary

Prescribing must consider the stage of liver disease, current liver tests, and complications present in the patient. The rate of deterioration can further guide the risks of prescribing. In patients with decompensated liver disease, sedatives and drugs that constipate may worsen or mask encephalopathy and should be prescribed with caution.

Careful consideration should be given to the pharmacokinetic characteristics of prescribed medication to predict how liver impairment may affect the normal handling of the drug in the body. Pharmacodynamic actions of the drug should be considered to ensure that complications from concomitant treatment are reduced. Drugs with low oral bioavailability, high hepatic extraction, narrow therapeutic indices, and long half-lives present the greatest risk.

An assessment of the likelihood of the prescribed drugs to cause hepatotoxicity should be made to ensure that treatments are unlikely to worsen existing liver injury. Where idiosyncratic liver injury is a known adverse effect, careful and close monitoring should be considered. As described above, some general considerations in prescribing can help to reduce the risk of adverse effects, such as reducing polypharmacy and avoiding drugs susceptible to pharmacokinetic or pharmacodynamic interactions.

Where licensing information does not exist, using a low starting dose and/or reducing the frequency remain a sensible approach to starting a new treatment. Titration should be made slowly with careful observation both shortly and after starting treatment and throughout, as late onset toxicity may present.

Obtaining the information to give the prescriber sufficient information to prescribe safely can be difficult, and information is often limited. Specialist resources such as medicines information departments are often useful in supporting such decisions and should be approached where available.

Reference

1. Pirmohamed, M. (2019). Prescribing in liver disease. *Medicine* 47 (11): 718–722. https://doi.org/10.1016/j.mpmed.2019.08.012.

Further Reading

Johnson TN, Thomson AH. Pharmacokinetics of drugs in liver disease. In: North-Lewis P (Ed.) Drugs and the Liver, 103–135. London: Pharmaceutical Press; 2008.

Knighton, S. (2015). Liver impairment: ensuring medicines safety. *Pharm. J.* 294 (7854/5): 346–350.

Lewis, J.H. and Stine, J.G. (2013). Review article: prescribing medications in patients with cirrhosis: a practical guide. *Aliment. Pharmacol. Ther.* 37 (12): 1132–1156. https://doi.org/10.1111/apt.12324.

Verbeeck, R.K. (2008). Pharmacokinetics and dosage adjustment in patients with hepatic dysfunction. *Eur. J. Clin. Pharmacol.* 64 (12): 1147–1161.

Wilcock, A., Charlesworth, S., Prentice, W. et al. (2019). Prescribing in chronic severe hepatic impairment. *J. Pain Symptom Manage.* 58 (3): 515–537.

19

Invasive Procedures in Patients with Liver Disease

Will Lester

University Hospitals Birmingham, Birmingham, UK

KEY POINTS

- Many patients with liver disease have changes in pro- and anticoagulant factors and in platelet numbers and function, resulting in a rebalancing of hemostasis.
- While the prothrombin time and platelet count have been historically used to determine the safety and management of invasive procedures, these parameters do not accurately reflect the risk of bleeding or the need for prophylactic transfusion of blood products.
- For low-risk procedures (such as therapeutic paracentesis or endoscopy), clinicians should not routinely correct thrombocytopenia and coagulopathy.
- For higher-risk procedures (such as liver biopsy), thresholds of hematocrit $\geq 25\%$, platelet count $> 50 \times 10^9/l$, and fibrinogen $> 1.2\,g/l$ may be used as guide to the risk of bleeding associated with invasive procedures pending further evidence.
- The role of fresh frozen plasma (FFP) and of platelet transfusions is unclear; FFP may increase the risk of bleeding and complications from invasive procedures.
- Thrombopoietin receptor agonists (TPO-RA) are now licensed for preprocedure use in patients with thrombocytopenia associated with liver disease but may be associated with an increased risk of thrombosis.
- Clinicians should seek expert advice before undertaking invasive procedures in patients with acute on chronic decompensated liver disease.

Introduction

Historically, it was assumed that the raised prothrombin time (the ratio commonly expressed as an international normalized ratio, INR) seen in liver disease reflected a bleeding risk and that correction with plasma products, specifically FFP, would reduce/correct this hemostatic failure. However, more recent studies have shown quite the reverse; there is often a prothrombotic state and transfusion of FFP is usually unnecessary, ineffective, and potentially hazardous. Published cohort studies of patients with liver disease undergoing invasive procedures demonstrate low bleeding risks.

The Liver in Systemic Disease: A Clinician's Guide to Abnormal Liver Tests, First Edition.
Edited by Gideon M. Hirschfield, Paramjit Gill, and James Neuberger.
© 2023 John Wiley & Sons Ltd. Published 2023 by John Wiley & Sons Ltd.

Coagulation Testing in Patients with Liver Disease

In patients with chronic liver disease, the use of the INR to predict bleeding risk following invasive procedures in liver patients is not supported by clinical evidence. Although there is reduced synthesis/consumption of many procoagulant proteins and reduced numbers of platelets, there is an increase in factor VIII and von Willebrand factor, and a reduction in natural anticoagulants. Hemostasis in chronic stable liver disease is often referred to as "rebalanced," with a net effect of normal hemostasis or even a procoagulant state. The INR is sensitive only for fibrinogen, FII, FV, FVII, and FX, and does not test the hemostatic balance in a patient with liver disease. Therefore, an INR of 2.0 in a patient with chronic liver disease is not comparable to the same result in a patient taking warfarin. There appears to be a similar rebalancing in acute liver disease.

The INR is, however, a surrogate marker of liver fibrosis and portal hypertension, which is the likely explanation for the weak association of a higher INR with an increased bleeding risk from liver biopsy. Consistent with this understanding that the INR is not representing a bleeding diathesis, preprocedural FFP, and/or platelet transfusions prior to transcutaneous liver biopsy, have not been shown to have a significant effect on hemorrhagic complication rates, and will just serve to increase intravascular volume and portal pressure, which is likely to be counterproductive.

More global assays of coagulation in patients with liver disease have been used to assess hemostasis; a few studies have examined their use to predict bleeding prior to invasive procedures. In one study of thrombin generation in patients with cirrhosis, FFP only slightly improved coagulation test values in a limited number of patients and even appeared to worsen them in one third of cases.

Viscoelastic testing (thromboelastography or rotational thromboelastometry) is generally normal, or at least near normal, in patients with chronic liver disease, including in the presence of a prolonged INR, and limited studies have used them to reduce blood product usage compared with transfusion triggers using standard assays of coagulation and platelets. However, there is still insufficient evidence to show that global tests of coagulation can be used routinely to predict bleeding prior to invasive procedures in patients with liver disease.

Platelet Count in Patients with Liver Disease

There is limited evidence for a platelet threshold above which invasive procedures can be safely performed. Table 19.1 gives an indication of platelet thresholds for various invasive procedures. Although not specific for patients with liver disease, these thresholds give some indication of typical target values. For high-risk procedures, preoperative platelet testing should be undertaken. It is traditionally considered that a platelet count less than 50×10^9/l requires intervention prior to invasive procedures with a significant risk of bleeding.

Table 19.1 Recommended platelet threshold for patients undergoing invasive procedures.

Procedure	Platelet threshold × 10^9/l	Level of evidence
Venous central lines (tunnelled and untunnelled), inserted by experienced staff using ultrasound guidance techniques	≥ 20	1B
Lumbar puncture	≥ 40	2C
Major surgery	≥ 50	1C
Minor surgery	≥ 30	1C
Insertion/removal of epidural catheter	≥ 80	2C
Neurosurgery or ophthalmic surgery involving the posterior segment of the eye	≥ 100	1C
Percutaneous liver biopsy	≥ 50	2B

Source: Adapted from Escourt et al. [1] and Hogshire et al. [2].

Which Patients with Liver Disease are at Increased Risk of Bleeding?

Decompensated liver disease, typically with acute on chronic liver failure, can be associated with a progressive consumptive coagulopathy and hypofibrinogenemia, often with hyperfibrinolysis. Spontaneous mucocutaneous and other bleeding manifestations may become evident at this stage. In one study, a platelet count less than 30×10^9/l, fibrinogen level less than 0.6 g/l, and activated partial thromboplastin time values above 100 seconds were the strongest independent predictors for new onset of major bleeding. All but the most essential invasive procedures should be avoided under these circumstances. Bacterial infection and renal impairment can increase bleeding risk in liver patients, so invasive procedures may be associated with a transient increased bleeding risk. If procedures in patients with a high bleeding risk cannot be delayed, blood product support may be indicated and alternative procedures may be an option (e.g. transjugular rather than percutaneous liver biopsy).

Use of Blood Products in Patients with Liver Disease Requiring Invasive Procedures

Systematic reviews of the limited studies looking at invasive procedures in cirrhotic patients have found that there was generally a low risk of bleeding with or without blood product replacement. FFP is often given at subtherapeutic doses and rarely impacts significantly on the INR, with failure of correction in almost all patients.

Updated guidelines (e.g. from the American Gastroenterological Association) are now recommending that clinicians should not routinely correct thrombocytopenia and coagulopathy before low-risk therapeutic paracentesis, thoracentesis, and routine upper endoscopy for variceal ligation in patients with hepatic synthetic dysfunction-induced coagulation abnormalities. For higher-risk procedures, they recommend thresholds of hematocrit 25% of greater, platelet count greater than 50×10^9/l, and fibrinogen > 1.2 g/l.

In view of the paucity of evidence for the use of FFP and the large volumes required, four-factor prothrombin complex concentrates have been considered as an alternative; however, they do not correct the fibrinogen, and dosage, efficacy, and safety remain unclear, so specialist advice would be required in the absence of more robust clinical data.

Additional Treatments Used to Reduce Procedural Bleeding in Patients with Liver Disease

For correction of thrombocytopenia, platelet transfusion would traditionally be considered prior to invasive procedures, but the response can be unpredictable in patients with liver disease, which is often associated with portal hypertension and hypersplenism. An alternative option is the use of TPO-RA, of which a number are now licensed for preprocedure use in patients with thrombocytopenia associated with liver disease. In some studies, TPO-RAs have been associated with an increased risk of thrombosis, including portal vein thrombosis, so should be used with caution in patients considered to be at higher risk of thrombosis.

In addition to blood products, use of antifibrinolytic agents (e.g. tranexamic acid) may be considered, although more recent data on their use in acute gastrointestinal bleeding has indicated a thrombotic signal in patients with liver disease.

Treatment with intravenous vitamin K should be considered in patients with an increased INR, which may in part reflect vitamin K deficiency; particularly in patients in intensive care, with malnutrition, in patients using antibiotics and in patients with cholestatic liver disease.

Medication History

Just as with patients without liver disease, a medication history must be taken prior to invasive procedures associated with a risk of bleeding. Patients with liver disease commonly have a thrombotic history requiring treatment. In patients taking antiplatelet agents and/or anticoagulants, the decision to pause will be determined by the risk of bleeding if continuing against the risk of thromboembolism from pausing treatment and should be included in the patient consent process. Table 19.2 gives some guidance on pausing antiplatelet agents and anticoagulants.

Learning Points

- Hemostasis in chronic stable liver disease is often referred to as "rebalanced" with a net effect of normal hemostasis or even a procoagulant state.
- The risk of bleeding from procedures in patients with stable liver disease is low.

Table 19.2 Management of antiplatelet drugs and anticoagulants prior to invasive procedures.

Drug	Elective	Urgent	Notes
Aspirin	Continue unless very high bleeding risk	Continue	Expected to correct within 4 days of stopping
Clopidogrel	Stop 5–7 days	If cannot delay, consider stopping for 24 hours; platelet transfusion may be considered	Patients on dual antiplatelet platelet therapy, prasugrel, or ticagrelor should be discussed with a cardiologist
Prasugrel	Stop 7 days		
Ticagrelor	Stop 3–5 days		
Dipyridamole	Omit on day of procedure		Reversible weak platelet inhibitor
Low molecular weight heparin	Prophylactic dose stop > 12 hours pre-procedure		
	Higher than prophylactic dose stop > 24 hours pre-procedure		
Unfractionated heparin	Stop 4–6 hours	Consider protamine only if very urgent	
Parenteral direct thrombin inhibitors (argatroban or bivalirudin)	≥ 4 hours	No reversal agent	
Fondaparinux	Stop 1–2 days after prophylactic dose and ≥ 3 days after therapeutic dose	No reversal agent	Half-life is approximately 17 hours
Warfarin	Stop 5 days	Consider reversal with IV vitamin K if ≥ 24 hours with four-factor prothrombin complex if < 24 hours	IV vitamin K will approximately halve INR after approximately 6 hours
Direct oral anticoagulants	Omit for 2 days before procedure unless low bleeding risk	Discuss with hematologist	Omit for > 2 days for patients on dabigatran if impaired renal function. Idarucizumab can be used to reverse dabigatran prior to urgent procedures

INR, international normalized ratio; IV, intravenous.

- The INR is poorly predictive of bleeding and there is no evidence that transfusion of FFP before invasive procedures is effective and may even increase the risk of complications.
- Global tests of hemostasis are not yet fully validated for use in predicting bleeding risk prior to invasive procedures in patients with liver disease.
- Alternatives to transfusion (e.g. TPO-RA) can be used prior to invasive procedures.
- A drug history should always be taken prior to invasive procedures and consideration given to pausing medications which may increase the risk of bleeding.

References

1. Escourt, L.J., Birchall, J., Allard, S. et al. (2017). Guidelines for the use of platelet transfusions. *Br J Haematol* 176: 365–394.
2. Hogshire, L.C., Patel, M.S., Rivera, E., and Carson, J.L. (2013). Evidence review: periprocedural use of blood products. *J Hosp Med* 8: 647–652.

Further Reading

Neuberger, J., Patel, J., Caldwell, H. et al. (2020). Guidelines on the use of liver biopsy in clinical practice from the British Society of Gastroenterology, the Royal College of Radiologists and the Royal College of Pathology. *Gut* 69: 1382–1403.
O'Leary, J.G., Greenberg, C.S., Patton, H.M., and Caldwell, S.H. (2019). AGA clinical practice update: coagulation in cirrhosis. *Gastroenterology* 157: 34–43.e1.

20

Diagnosing Drug-Induced Liver Injury

Guruprasad P. Aithal[1,2]

[1]*Nottingham University Hospitals NHS Trust, Nottingham, UK*
[2]*University of Nottingham, Nottingham, UK*

KEY POINTS

- The diagnosis of drug-induced liver injury (DILI) remains a challenge in many cases: the risk of unnecessary discontinuation must be balanced against the risks of continuing treatment.
- DILI may be caused by prescribed medications, over-the-counter medications, herbal remedies, and natural remedies, so a full history should be obtained.
- DILI should always be considered in cases of unexplained abnormal liver tests.
- While some drugs have a characteristic pattern of liver damage, the spectrum associated with any one drug may be broad.
- Causality assessment tools such as the Roussel Uclaf Causality Assessment Method (RUCAM) may help in attributing causality to a drug.
- The diagnosis of DILI includes one of the three criteria: alanine transaminase elevation five-fold or more above the upper limit of normal (ULN), alkaline phosphatase twofold or more above ULN or alanine amino transferase (ALT) threefold or more above ULN with elevation of bilirubin twofold or more above ULN.
- Evaluation should include a search for evidence of hypersensitivity (such as fever, rash, and peripheral blood eosinophilia); liver histology and genetic tests may also aid diagnosis.
- Before making a diagnosis of DILI, other causes for liver damage should be considered.

Acute onset of liver injury attributable to the exposure to a drug taken in its therapeutic dose is referred to as DILI. The term "drug" includes non-prescription medicinal products, herbal remedies, and dietary supplements unless specified. Overdoses, whether intentional or inadvertent, are not discussed in this chapter. Distinction between intrinsic and idiosyncratic is hypothetical, as a subtle dose relationship (within the therapeutic range) exists in relation to DILI secondary to a number of drugs.

The Liver in Systemic Disease: A Clinician's Guide to Abnormal Liver Tests, First Edition.
Edited by Gideon M. Hirschfield, Paramjit Gill, and James Neuberger.
© 2023 John Wiley & Sons Ltd. Published 2023 by John Wiley & Sons Ltd.

Challenges in the Diagnostic Approach

Identifying a particular drug as the etiology of an acute liver injury early is of critical importance, as its prompt withdrawal can reduce the risk of serious consequences. On the other hand, interruption of antituberculosis, antiepileptic, or antineoplastic agents may reduce the effectiveness of the treatment regimen. The general approach to diagnosis in clinical practice, as with other conditions, involves pattern recognition, assessing the pretest probabilities, and performing suitable tests to support or refute the diagnosis. However, confident diagnosis of DILI has remained a challenge because of a number of factors. First, over 650 medicinal products have been associated with adverse liver reactions; medications that accounted for DILI in consecutive patients enrolled into a cohort study are listed in Table 20.1. Polypharmacy has risen with the prevalence of multimorbidity. Truly distinct "signature patterns" of liver injury attributable to a particular drug or group of drugs are exceptions than a rule. Although lack of specific tests is highlighted as a barrier, specialist tests such as liver biopsy and genetic tests are underused.

We make rapid decisions, deemed necessary while managing medical emergencies or when evaluating many patients in a time-limited manner. Our approach is aided by "heuristics," strategies that provide short cuts to quick decisions, which in turn are pitfalls in diagnosis. In a large European study involving over 10 000 patients presenting with jaundice, doctors had an overall diagnostic accuracy of 77% at the time of initial assessment compared with the final diagnosis. However, diagnostic accuracy was 49% for DILI and it was ranked 15th of 18 categories of diagnoses considered in the study. Systematic evaluation would be able to overcome some of these limitations.

Be Aware of the Base Rates

Knowledge of how frequently particular condition occurs in different clinical contexts informs the pretest probability of a diagnosis. Considering DILI as a differential diagnosis in all acute presentation of liver injury is the first step in the systematic evaluation.

Raised Liver Enzymes

An international expert working group established the threshold for defining DILI, which includes any one of the three criteria: alanine transaminase elevation fivefold or more above the ULN, alkaline phosphatase twofold or more above ULN or ALT threefold or more above ULN with elevation of bilirubin twofold or more above ULN [1]. Aspartate amino transaminase (AST) is a substituted for ALT when the latter is not a part of the available panel of tests. Unexplained elevation of ALT five or more times ULN unrelated to the drug exposure have been observed in 0.3–0.4% of large population monitored regularly over one year. In a recent study involving 3155 patients on standard regimen of antituberculosis treatment, 218 (6.9%) developed ALT elevation between three and five times ULN [2]; of these, 193/218 (88.5%) resolved without significant (more than seven days) interruption in the treatment, while none of the 25/218 (11.5%) who developed DILI (ALT ≥ fivefold ULN) in this group progressed to acute liver failure. Lower thresholds of ALT elevation may be

Table 20.1 Etiological agents of consecutive 78 cases of drug-induced liver injury (DILI) presenting to secondary care hospitals in the UK.

Drug group	Drug	Cases (*n*)	Total DILI (%)	Pattern of DILI
Antimicrobial	Co-amoxiclav	13	16.46	Eight hepatocellular; three mixed; two cholestatic
	Flucloxacillin	12	15.19	Five hepatocellular; five mixed; two cholestatic
	Nitrofurantoin	4	5.06	Three hepatocellular; one cholestatic
	Doxycycline	2	2.53	Two cholestatic
	Pivmecillinam	1	1.27	Hepatocellular
	Isoniazid	1	1.27	Hepatocellular
	Total	33	41.77	
Immune checkpoint inhibitors	Ipilimumab/nivolumab	11	13.92	All hepatocellular
	Nivolumab	1	1.27	Mixed
	Total	12	15.19	
Statin	Atorvastatin	9	11.39	Four hepatocellular; five cholestatic
Antimetabolites	Azathioprine	3	3.80	Two mixed; one cholestatic
	Methotrexate	2	2.53	Hepatocellular
	Gemcitabine	1	1.27	Cholestatic
	Total	6	7.59	
Antineoplastic	Asparaginase	2	2.53	One hepatocellular; one mixed
	Temozolomide	1	1.27	Hepatocellular
	Docetaxel	1	1.27	Mixed
	Total	4	5.06	
Biologics	Infliximab	2	2.53	Hepatocellular
	Vedolizumab	1	1.27	Hepatocellular
	Total	3	3.80	
Tyrosine kinase inhibitor	Zanubrutinib	1	1.27	Hepatocellular
	Panzopanib	1	1.27	Hepatocellular
	Total	2	2.53	Hepatocellular
NSAIDS	Ibuprofen	1	1.27	Hepatocellular
	Naproxen	1	1.27	Hepatocellular
	Total	2	2.53	
Angiotensin ii receptor antagonists	Irbesartan	1	1.27	Cholestatic
Anesthetics	Propofol	1	1.27	Hepatocellular
Anabolic steroids	SD matrix	1	1.27	Cholestatic
	DNP (2,4-dinitrophenol)	1	1.27	Hepatocellular
Estrogens	Tibolone	1	1.27	Hepatocellular
Antispasmodics	Alverine citrate	1	1.27	Hepatocellular
	Promethazine/ dextromethorphan (supplement)	1	1.27	Hepatocellular

suitable for monitoring adverse liver reactions in clinical trials, where knowledge about the efficacy and safety of a medication is yet to be confirmed. However, unexplained elevation of ALT between above threefold ULN has been observed in 0.26% of people per year in the placebo group of a clinical trial and most were not explained by diagnosable liver disease. However, six of these who had raised bilirubin greater than twofold ULN all had liver disease requiring hospitalization. In a group of patients with atrial fibrillation attending routine outpatient care, 0.2% had new persistent elevation of ALT greater than twofold ALT. Cohort studies describing etiology underlying ALT/AST elevation of greater than 10-fold ULN or greater than 20-fold ULN have found 9% of these are due to DILI [3, 4].

The threshold for investigating raised alkaline phosphatase (when bony origins of the enzyme is ruled out) has been set low as the marker has prognostic significance. In a recent study, higher initial alkaline phosphatase (ALP) at DILI onset was associated with a 43% longer recovery time [5].

Jaundice

Of 2080 consecutive patients attending a rapid-access jaundice clinic over a 14-year period, biliary obstruction was found in 1199 (58%). Among the remaining 881 patients (grouped under medical jaundice), DILI was the underlying etiology in 15%, making it the second most common cause of hepatocellular jaundice after decompensated alcoholic liver disease, which accounted for 25% of cases (Figure 20.1) [6].

Acute Liver Failure

Idiosyncratic DILI contributes to 7–22% of cases of acute liver failure worldwide, highlighting the potentially serious consequences of this adverse reaction.

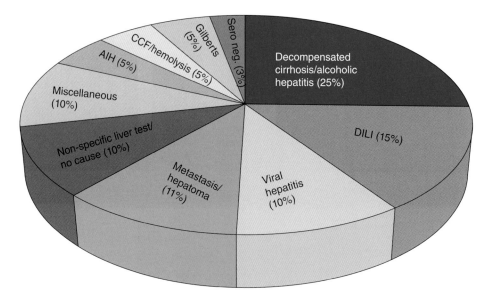

Figure 20.1 Etiology of jaundice in 881 consecutive patients where biliary obstruction is ruled out. Modified from [6].

Consider Drug-Induced Liver Injury

Considering that DILI may underlie a particular clinical manifestation is an important first step in the diagnosis. In a secondary care inpatient service, diagnosis of DILI increased 12-fold through a proactive approach, which involved all elevated liver enzymes beyond a predetermined threshold. A designated biochemist and a designated hepatologist reviewed all individual patients to identify the underlying diagnosis [7].

Probe for Information on Medications

Assessment of the temporal relationship between an acute event and exposure to one or more medications is the next step in the diagnosis. A list of all medications that individual was taking at the time of first manifestation and the duration of exposure to each is desirable. However, there is a wide range of drugs associated with the adverse reaction and polypharmacy. Therefore, focus should be on the drugs (or dose changes) that were introduced within three months of the first manifestation of the event. Majority of DILI occur 2–90 days of onset of the particular drug treatment. After the first year of exposure, incidence of DILI is substantially lower; in patients taking methotrexate or leflunomide regularly, the incidence of DILI falls from 3.9/1000 and 5/1000 person-years, respectively, for the first year to 1/1000 and 1.7/1000 person-years after the first year [8]. DILI secondary to statins has also been reported after the first year of exposure, but dose escalation appears to be the trigger in a proportion of these events. A higher daily dose of the drug (within its therapeutic range) increases the risk of DILI [9].

It is uncommon for DILI to manifest after the discontinuation of the drug, but these have been well described in relation with antibiotics, co-amoxiclav, and flucloxacillin. It is therefore important to inquire about recent (in addition to concurrent) medications as well as recent changes in the dose for long-term prescriptions. Patients may not consider over-the-counter products, traditional/herbal remedies, dietary/nutritional supplements as medications, and only on probing can such crucial information be extracted during clinical evaluation.

Look for Features of Hypersensitivity

Among DILI cohorts, 20–25% have typical features of hypersensitivity reactions, including fever, rash, and peripheral blood eosinophilia. In a meta-analysis of 570 case reports of DILI due to specific drugs (co-amoxiclav, carbamazepine, diclofenac, disulfiram, erythromycin, flucloxacillin, halothane, isoniazid, phenytoin, sulindac, and co-trimoxazole), 34% had peripheral eosinophilia [10]. Therefore, in the context of acute liver injury and a potential drug etiology, eosinophilia favors the diagnosis of DILI.

Identify the Pattern of Liver Injury

The approach to abnormal liver biochemistry starts with the recognition of acute liver injury as defined by the threshold set by the international expert working group (as summarized above). When the temporal relationship with the introduction of the drug and the onset of injury is clear and certain, then withdrawal of the drug would be associated with a prompt resolution of the liver injury.

However, when the diagnosis is not secure, the pattern of liver injury will guide further investigations. At first, ALT activity (ALT*) and ALP activity (ALP*) are determined by calculating how many times above the ULN the patient's liver enzymes are elevated [11]. If the ALT alone is elevated fivefold or more above ULN or the ratio (R value) of ALT*/ALP* is ≥ 5, it is classified as hepatocellular pattern, while ALP alone is elevated twofold or more above ULN or R is ≤ 2, the pattern is classified as cholestatic; mixed pattern is when R is greater than two and less than five. These patterns indicate whether exclusion of biliary obstruction or parenchymal liver disease should be prioritized during further investigations.

Consider Alternative Explanations

Hypoxic Hepatitis

This condition is also referred to as "ischemic hepatitis;" it manifests in individuals with heart failure, chronic obstructive lung disease, and chronic renal failure. A systematic review found that while a prior hypotension or syncope was documented in 53% of patients, in 68% evidence of liver injury followed an episode of hypoxia; hence, the term hypoxic hepatitis is preferred [12]. This syndrome is among the key diagnoses incorrectly attributed to DILI; it accounts for 50% of cases where AST is greater than 400 iu/l [3] and 61% of cases when ALT is greater than 1000 iu/l [4].

Observational studies have described acute hepatocellular pattern of injury associated with "ischemic hepatitis" and rise in ALP and gamma-glutamyl transferase in association with "congestive hepatopathy." Detailed history and careful physical examination should lead to confident diagnosis in either of these scenarios. In relation to hypoxic hepatitis, ALT elevation peaks on the day of the event with a rapid fall within two days of the event, while the course of DILI spans weeks (Figure 20.2).

Rule Out Biliary Obstruction

In the vast majority of patients with acute liver injury, exclusion of biliary obstruction using an imaging modality (such as ultrasound of the abdomen) is necessary. A group of patients with clearly hepatocellular pattern of liver injury of 5–24% were found to have underlying pancreaticobiliary etiology [3, 4]. Overall, 4% of those with common bile duct stones (confirmed on endoscopic retrograde cholangiopancreatography) have ALT or AST greater than 400 iu/l in the absence of cholangitis. These have been referred to as "gallstone hepatitis"; 97.5% of the latter group have moderate to severe pain compared with 37% of those with common bile duct stones, but without a rise in transaminases [13]. This group is more than 40-fold more likely to have abdominal pain and to have moderate or severe pain (compared to those with common bile duct stones without a rise in transaminase.

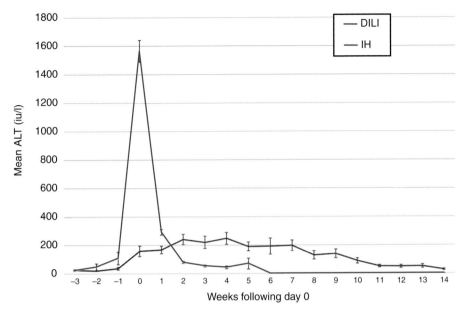

Figure 20.2 Pattern of rise and fall of alanine amino transferase in patients with hypoxic hepatitis compared with drug-induced liver injury.

When the index of suspicion for acute biliary obstruction is high, as in patients who present with moderate to severe right upper-quadrant pain, further imaging with computed tomography or magnetic resonance imaging is justified.

Evaluate Causality Systematically

Causality assessment tools have been developed for formal pharmacovigilance and facilitate rigorous evaluation of cases in research projects. RUCAM and the Clinical Diagnostic Scale are two such tools, both designed to quantify the strength of association between a liver injury and the medication implicated as a potential cause of liver injury. These tools have specific domains of assessment and input of information from the suspected DILI event results in a weighted score [11, 14]. The total score from all the domains is used to classify the suspected DILI event as definite, highly probable, probable, possible, unlikely, or excluded.

RUCAM is the most widely used tool internationally in research studies. Causality assessment tools provide a checklist to consider during clinical evaluation of acute liver injury where DILI is a differential diagnosis (Table 20.2). However, a complete data set requires extensive investigation in each case and application of these tools still demands expertise. Therefore, if and when the initial steps of assessment do not lead to a firm conclusion, then a specialist should lead the systematic evaluation.

Table 20.2 Domains for evaluation included in the causality assessment methods.

Domain	CIOMS/RUCAM	Clinical diagnostic scale
Exposure to medication to onset of DILI	✓	✓
Course after withdrawal of medication	✓	✓
Exclusion of alternative diagnosis	✓	✓
Re-challenge (previous or inadvertent)	✓	✓
Previous reports of DILI	✓	✓
Host risk factors	✓	
Concomitant medications	✓	
Extrahepatic manifestations		✓

CIOMS, Council for International Organizations of Medical Sciences; DILI, drug-induced liver injury; RUCAM, Roussel Uclaf Causality Assessment Method.

RUCAM is currently being updated based on contemporary literature and iterative modeling with an intention to make it user friendly and widely accessible. The hope is that a revised electronic tool will be widely used to improve consistency in the assessment of patients with suspected DILI and accuracy of the diagnosis.

Perform Liver Biopsy

Distinguishing DILI from other competing diagnoses can be assisted by histological examination of the liver. One such scenario is when autoimmune hepatitis is a differential diagnosis; in a cohort of cases of autoimmune hepatitis, 9% were deemed to have been triggered by exposure to particular drugs [15]. Conversely, in cohorts of DILI 9% are classified as drug-induced autoimmune hepatitis (AIH) due to overlapping features [16]; these have been described with a number of drugs including nitrofurantoin, minocycline, diclofenac, statins, and anti-tumor necrosis factor α agents.

It is of paramount importance to secure a diagnosis in both these groups of patients, as missing drug etiology would commit an individual to potentially lifelong immunosuppressive therapy. Evidence of canalicular cholestasis in liver biopsy would favor a diagnosis of DILI (or drug-induced AIH) while the presence of fibrosis supports the diagnosis of idiopathic AIH. Liver biopsy may add certainty to the diagnosis when a suspected DILI has atypical features. With the emergence of immune checkpoint inhibitor therapy targeting a wide range of cancers, the occurrence of DILI due to this group of drugs is increasing. These patients are currently being treated with heavy doses of immunosuppressant drugs, which may not be necessary nor effective in a proportion of cases. Therefore, a full characterization of DILI, including liver biopsy, would be informative in decision making in relation to checkpoint inhibitor-induced liver injury. Finally, in patients where the course of suspected DILI is too rapid (leading to listing for transplantation), or when there is failure of DILI to resolve, liver histology may strengthen the diagnosis (excluding rare conditions such as micrometastasis presenting with acute liver failure) as well as prognosis (such as identifying features of ductopenia).

Use Genetic Tests

An accurate and confident diagnosis of DILI is vital. Common causative agents are antibiotics (co-amoxiclav and flucloxacillin), biologicals (infliximab), and antiepileptics (carbamazepine) are highly effective. The continued use of these drugs is important for individual patients care as well as for clinical practice. DILI from more than 15 currently used drugs has been associated with human leukocyte antigen (HLA) genotype or haplotype [17]. Performance characteristics of these tests when used selectively are comparable or better than some routinely used blood tests (Table 20.3). Single gene testing (as employed for *HLA-B*57:01* to avoid skin reaction from abacavir) is affordable and adds value compared with liver autoantibody panel, which is used widely (arguably indiscriminately).

HLA genotyping can be an adjunct in differentiating DILI from AIH; carriage of the *HLA-DRB1*0301* or *DRB1*0401* allele is associated with idiopathic AIH and is a part of international AIH diagnostic criteria. Among individuals developing DILI secondary to flucloxacillin, 85% carry *HLA-B*5701* allele compared with 6% of the general population. Testing for *HLA-B*57:01* can thus be used to support or refute a diagnosis of flucloxacillin-induced DILI. In acute liver injury with a history of exposure to co-amoxiclav, testing for *HLA-DRB1*1501* can help to differentiate DILI from seronegative hepatitis by providing supportive (although not conclusive) evidence for the diagnosis of DILI.

Importance of the Diagnosis

Timely diagnosis of DILI permits prompt withdrawal of the causative agent, which leads to the resolution of liver injury, but DILI leads to death in 7.6% [18]. In addition, higher liver enzymes (ALP) at diagnosis are associated with persistent liver injury in the long term (one year) with lower quality of life [19]. Inaccurate diagnosis can lead to inappropriate withdrawal of an effective medication (such as antimicrobials, anticonvulsants) or a missed

Table 20.3 Performance characteristics of liver autoantibody profile compared with those of specific human leukocyte antigen alleles associated with drug-induced liver injury secondary to antibiotics.

Test	Positive in AIH (%)	Positive in normal (%)
ANA 1:60	68–75%	15 (<40 female)–24 (>40 female)
Anti-SMA	52–59	≤43
IgG >1600 mg/dl	86	5
Anti-LKM	4–20	1
Human leukocyte antigens:		
DRB1*1501	57–67 (amoxicillin-clavulanate)	15–20
B*5701	84–87 (flucloxacillin)	6
B*3502	16 (minocycline)	0.6

ANA, anti-nuclear antibodies; IgG, immunoglobulin G; LKM, liver–kidney microsomal antibody; SMA, smooth muscle antibody.

alternative diagnosis (such as autoimmune hepatitis or choledocholithiasis) that merits prompt treatment.

When patients with DILI caused by a particular drug are re-exposed to the same medication, 11–55% develop recurrent DILI [20]. Re-exposure is often inadvertent and may be a consequence of previously unrecognized DILI. Compared with the initial event, DILI after re-challenge occurs more rapidly (generally after days or weeks) than after initial exposure. DILI on re-challenge leads to jaundice in 64%, hospitalization in 52%, and mortality in 13% of cases; all of these can be considered preventable.

References

1. Aithal, G.P., Watkins, P.B., Andrade, R.J. et al. (2011). Case definition and phenotype standardization in drug-induced liver injury (DILI). *Clin. Pharmacol. Ther.* 89 (6): 806–815.
2. Jiang, F., Yan, H., Liang, L. et al. (2021). Incidence and risk factors of anti-tuberculosis drug induced liver injury (DILI): large cohort study involving 4652 Chinese adult tuberculosis patients. *Liver Int.* 41 (7): 1565–1575.
3. Whitehead, M.W., Hawkes, N.D., Hainsworth, I., and Kingham, J.G.C. (1999). A prospective study of the causes of notably raised aspartate aminotransferase of liver origin. *Gut* 45: 129–133.
4. Galvin, Z., McDonough, A., Ryan, J., and Stewart, S. (2015). Blood alanine aminotransferase levels >1,000 IU/l – causes and outcomes. *Clin. Med.* 15 (3): 244–247.
5. Ashby, K., Zhuang, W., González-Jimenez, A. et al. (2021). Elevated bilirubin, alkaline phosphatase at onset, and drug metabolism are associated with prolonged recovery from DILI. *J. Hepatol.* 75 (2): 333–341.
6. Donaghy, L., Barry, F.J., Hunter, J.G. et al. (2013). Clinical and laboratory features and natural history of seronegative hepatitis in a nontransplant centre. *Eur. J. Gastroenterol. Hepatol.* 25 (10): 1159–1164.
7. M'Kada, H., Perazzo, H., Munteanu, M. et al. (2012). Real time identification of drug-induced liver injury (DILI) through daily screening of ALT results: a prospective pilot cohort study. *PLoS One* 7 (8): e42418.
8. Nakafero, G., Grainge, M.J., Card, T. et al. (2021). What is the incidence of methotrexate or leflunomide discontinuation related to cytopenia, liver enzyme elevation or kidney function decline? *Rheumatology (Oxford)* 60: 5785–5794.
9. Lammert, C., Einarsson, S., Saha, C. et al. (2008). Relationship between daily dose of oral medications and idiosyncratic drug-induced liver injury: search for signals. *Hepatology* 47 (6): 2003–2009.
10. Björnsson, E., Kalaitzakis, E., and Olsson, R. (2007). The impact of eosinophilia and hepatic necrosis on prognosis in patients with drug-induced liver injury. *Aliment. Pharmacol. Ther.* 25: 1411–1421.
11. Danan, G. and Benichou, C. (1993). Causality assessment of adverse reactions to drugs–I. A novel method based on the conclusions of international consensus meetings: application to drug-induced liver injuries. *J. Clin. Epidemiol.* 46 (11): 1323–1330.
12. Tapper, E.B., Sengupta, N., and Bonder, A. (2015). The incidence and outcomes of ischemic hepatitis: a systematic review with meta-analysis. *Am. J. Med.* 128: 1314–1321.

13. Huh, C.W., Jang, S.I., Lim, B.J. et al. (2016). Clinicopathological features of choledocholithiasis patients with high aminotransferase levels without cholangitis: prospective comparative study. *Medicine (Baltimore)* 95 (42): e5176.

14. Maria, V.A. and Victorino, R.M. (1997). Development and validation of a clinical scale for the diagnosis of drug-induced hepatitis. *Hepatology* 26 (3): 664–669.

15. Björnsson, E., Talwalkar, J., Treeprasertsuk, S. et al. (2010). Drug-induced autoimmune hepatitis: clinical characteristics and prognosis. *Hepatology* 51 (6): 2040–2048.

16. Licata, A., Maida, M., Cabibi, D. et al. (2014). Clinical features and outcomes of patients with drug-induced autoimmune hepatitis: a retrospective cohort study. *Dig. Liver Dis.* 46 (12): 1116–1120.

17. Kaliyaperumal, K., Grove, J.I., Delahay, R.M. et al. (2018). Pharmacogenomics of drug-induced liver injury (DILI): molecular biology to clinical applications. *J. Hepatol.* 69 (4): 948–957.

18. Hayashi, P.H., Rockey, D.C., Fontana, R.J. et al. (2017). Death and liver transplantation within 2 years of onset of drug-induced liver injury. *Hepatology* 66 (4): 1275–1285.

19. Fontana, R.J., Hayashi, P.H., Barnhart, H. et al. (2015). Persistent liver biochemistry abnormalities are more common in older patients and those with cholestatic drug induced liver injury. *Am. J. Gastroenterol.* 110 (10): 1450–1459.

20. Hunt, C.M., Papay, J.I., Stanulovic, V., and Regev, A. (2017). Drug rechallenge following drug-induced liver injury. *Hepatology* 66 (2): 646–654.

Index

Page locators in **bold** indicate tables. Page locators in *italics* indicate figures. This index uses letter-by-letter alphabetization.

a

AAT *see* alpha 1-antitrypsin
absorption   230, 236
ACE2 *see* angiotensin-converting enzyme 2
activated partial thromboplastin time   239
acute fatty liver of pregnancy (AFLP)   90–91, **92**
acute heart failure   115
acute kidney injury (AKI)   145–146, 147–158, **147–148**, *149*, *151–153*, **153**, **159**
acute liver failure (ALF)
  diagnosing drug-induced liver injury   246
  immunosuppression   66
  intensive care   52
  mental health and neurology   202
  renal medicine   146, 156
acute liver injury   52, 53
acute on chronic liver failure   239
acute porphyrias   207
acute tubular necrosis (ATN)   147, 150, 158
acute viral hepatitis   56–58, 63

Addison's disease   108
adenoma   179
ADME principles   230–232, 236
ADPKD *see* autosomal dominant polycystic kidney disease
adrenal diseases of the liver   108
AF *see* atrial fibrillation
AFLP *see* acute fatty liver of pregnancy
AFP *see* alpha-fetoprotein
AIH *see* autoimmune hepatitis
AKI *see* acute kidney injury
Alagille syndrome   161
alanine amino transferase (ALT)
  cardiac disease   112, 115
  dermatology   172
  diagnosing drug-induced liver injury   244–246, 248
  endocrinology and metabolic diseases   101, 104
  gastroenterology   136–137, 140–141
  global perspective   31, 33–37, 39, 42–45
  hematology   192
  immunosuppression   65–70
  intensive care   53, *55*
  liver function tests   4–5, 6–7

The Liver in Systemic Disease: A Clinician's Guide to Abnormal Liver Tests, First Edition.
Edited by Gideon M. Hirschfield, Paramjit Gill, and James Neuberger.
© 2023 John Wiley & Sons Ltd. Published 2023 by John Wiley & Sons Ltd.

alanine amino transferase (ALT) (*cont'd*)
 mental health and neurology   201,
  203–205
 non-alcoholic fatty liver
  disease   214, **214**
 oncologic diseases   181, 184, 186, 188
 postoperative patient   76, 79, 82
 pregnancy   91, 95
 prescribing   226
 primary care   22–24
 respiratory disease   122–123
albumin
 endocrinology and metabolic
  diseases   101
 intensive care   60
 liver function tests   4–6
 mental health and neurology   201
 postoperative patient   82
 prescribing   231
alcohol-related liver disease (ARLD)
 cardiac disease   117–118
 dermatology   174–175
 global perspective   37
 hematology   193
 non-alcoholic fatty liver disease   212
alcohol use
 endocrinology and metabolic
  diseases   103
 global perspective   43
 immunosuppression   66
 liver function tests   16
 mental health and
  neurology   205, 206
 non-alcoholic fatty liver disease   210,
  214, 218
 primary care   23
ALF *see* acute liver failure
alkaline phosphatase (ALP)
 cardiac disease   115
 dermatology   174
 diagnosing drug-induced liver
  injury   246, 248, 251–252
 endocrinology and metabolic diseases
  101, 104, 106–107

gastroenterology   135–136
global perspective   31, 33, 38–40, 42
immunosuppression   72
intensive care   *55*, 58–59
liver function tests   4, 7–8
mental health and neurology   201
non-alcoholic fatty liver disease   214
oncologic diseases   180–181, 184, 188
postoperative patient   77, 79, 81
pregnancy   88, *89*, 90, 95
prescribing   226
primary care   22
respiratory disease   122, 129
ALP *see* alkaline phosphatase
alpha 1-antitrypsin (AAT)
  deficiency   12, 126, *127*
alpha-fetoprotein (AFP)   12
ALSPAC *see* Avon Longitudinal Study of
  Parents and Children
ALT *see* alanine amino transferase
AMA *see* anti-mitochondrial antibody
ammonia   60
amoxicillin–clavulanate   76
amyloidosis   117
ANA *see* antinuclear antibody
analbuminemia   6
anemia   11
angiotensin-converting enzyme 2 (ACE2)
  receptors   69
anorexia nervosa   204–205
anticoagulants   59–60, 240, **241**
antidepressants   202–204, **203**
antifibrinolytic agents   240
antifungal therapy   173
anti-mitochondrial antibody
  (AMA)   13, 38
antineoplastic drugs   180, **181**, 182–184
antinuclear antibody (ANA)   13, 215
antiplatelet agents   240, **241**
antipsychotics   204–205, **204**
anti-smooth muscle antibody
  (ASMA)   215
ARLD *see* alcohol-related liver disease
arterial hypoxemia   121–123, *122*

arteriovenous malformations (AVM)
127–128
ascites
dermatology 172
postoperative patient 78
prescribing 235
renal medicine 154, 163–164
respiratory disease 122, 125, *125*, 128
ASMA *see* anti-smooth muscle antibody
aspartate amino transferase (AST)
cardiac disease 112, 115
diagnosing drug-induced liver
injury 244–246, 248
gastroenterology 140–141
global perspective 31, 33, 37, 42–45
hematology 192
immunosuppression 67–68, 70
intensive care 53, *55*
liver function tests 4, 6–7
mental health and
neurology 201, 205
non-alcoholic fatty liver
disease 214, **214**
oncologic diseases 181, 184, 188
postoperative patient 76–77, 79, 82
pregnancy 91, 95
prescribing 226
primary care 22–24
respiratory disease 122–123
Aspergillus spp. 73
AST *see* aspartate amino transferase
ATN *see* acute tubular necrosis
ATP7B gene 38–39, 205
atrial fibrillation (AF) 115
autoantibodies
global perspective 38
liver function tests 5
markers of malignancy 13
non-alcoholic fatty liver disease 215
autoimmune hepatitis (AIH)
diagnosing drug-induced liver injury
250–251, **251**
endocrinology and metabolic diseases
100, 101–103, *103*

global perspective 38
hematology 193
postoperative patient 79
pregnancy 95
respiratory disease 123–124
autosomal dominant polycystic kidney
disease (ADPKD) 159–161
AVM *see* arteriovenous malformations
Avon Longitudinal Study of Parents and
Children (ALSPAC) 23
azathioprine 172

b
bariatric surgery 219
benign liver lesions 179
bile acids *55*
biliary disease 8
biliary drainage system *135*
biliary injury 78
biliary obstruction 248–249
biliary strictures 78
biliary tract necrosis 127–128
bilirubin
cardiac disease 115
dermatology 175
diagnosing drug-induced liver
injury 244–246
endocrinology and metabolic
diseases 101
gastroenterology 135
global perspective 31, 33, 39
immunosuppression 65, 67
intensive care *55*, 58–59
liver function tests 9–11, *9*
mental health and neurology 201
oncologic diseases 181, 184
postoperative patient 76–77, 79, 82
prescribing 226–227, 231
respiratory disease 122–123
biomarkers 155
Blastomycosis spp. 73
bleeding/hemorrhage
gastroenterology 139
invasive procedures 237–242

bleeding/hemorrhage (*cont'd*)
  postoperative patient 79
  pregnancy 94
  renal medicine 150
blood-transmitted viral infection 77
body mass index (BMI) 210, 211–214
  see also obesity and overweight
Borrelia burgdorferi 71
Brucella spp. 70
Budd–Chiari syndrome
  hematology 193–196
  intensive care 58
  pregnancy 95
bulimia nervosa 204–205

c

CALI *see* chemotherapy-associated
  liver injury
Candida spp. 72–73, 166
cardiac disease 111–119
  acute heart failure 115
  atrial fibrillation 115
  causes of abnormal
    LFTs 111–112, **112**
  cirrhotic cardiomyopathy 113
  drug-induced liver
    injury 118–119, **118**
  heart and liver disease caused by
    common disorder 116–118, **116**, **118**
  heart disease causing liver
    disease 113–116, **113**
  left ventricular assist and cardiac
    support devices 115
  liver disease causing cardiac
    disease 112–113
  liver disease in congenital heart
    disease 115–116
  liver disease unrelated to heart
    disease 119
  respiratory disease 127–128
  right-sided heart failure and hepatic
    congestion 114
cardiac failure 77

cardiac output 150
cardiac support devices 115
CASH *see* chemotherapy-associated
  steatohepatitis
causality assessment 42, 249–250, **250**
CCM *see* cirrhotic cardiomyopathy
celiac disease
  dermatology 175
  gastroenterology 138–139
  markers of malignancy 13
ceruloplasmin 12
CF *see* cystic fibrosis
chemotherapy-associated liver injury
  (CALI) 182, 183–184
chemotherapy-associated steatohepatitis
  (CASH) 182
chest X-ray *124–125*, *127*
Child–Pugh score 17
  prescribing 228–229, **228**, 233–234
  respiratory disease 123
Chinese herbal medications 174
choledocholithiasis 78, 136–137
cholestatic liver injury
  endocrinology and metabolic
    diseases 100
  gastroenterology 134
  global perspective 39
  intensive care 58–59
  postoperative patient 75, 77–78
  prescribing 232
  primary care 26–27
chronic hepatic failure 66
chronic kidney disease (CKD)
  global perspective 40
  renal medicine 145–146, 154–163,
    160, **160**
chronic viral hepatitis
  gastroenterology 142–144
  global perspective 34, 37, 41
  hematology 194
  immunosuppression 66–67
  oncologic diseases 180
  primary care 24–25

cirrhosis
  cardiac disease   112–113
  dermatology   172
  endocrinology and metabolic
    diseases   104, 108
  gastroenterology   139
  global perspective   37, 44
  hematology   193
  immunosuppression   67
  non-alcoholic fatty liver
    disease   210, 217–218
  oncologic diseases   180, 182, 187
  postoperative patient   78–79, **78**
  pregnancy   93–94
  prescribing   228, 233–234
  primary care   22–23
  renal medicine   145–156, **147–148**,
    149, 151–153, **153**
  respiratory disease   122–123, *122*,
    126, 128, *130*
cirrhotic cardiomyopathy (CCM)   113
CKD *see* chronic kidney disease
CMV *see* cytomegalovirus
coagulation testing   238
compensated cirrhosis   233–234
computed tomography (CT)
  gastroenterology   135, 138
  immunosuppression   71
  non-alcoholic fatty liver disease   214
  postoperative patient   81
  respiratory disease   126–127, *130*
congenital heart disease   115–116
conjugated hyperbilirubinemia
    26–27
contrast-enhanced transthoracic
    echocardiography   122–123
corticosteroids   41, 184
coumarin therapy   59
COVID-19/SARS-CoV-2   69
Coxiella burnetti   70–71
Crigler–Najjar syndrome   11, 26
cryoglobulinemia   152, *152*
Cryptococcus spp.   73–74

CT *see* computed tomography
CTNS gene   161
Cushing's syndrome   108
cutaneous cryoglobulinemic
    vasculitis   152, *152*
cyclosporin   173
CYP450 *see* cytochrome P450
cystic fibrosis (CF)   128
cystinosis   161
cytochrome P450 (CYP450) enzymes
  endocrinology and metabolic
    diseases   203
  prescribing   229, 231, 234, **235**
cytomegalovirus (CMV)
  hematology   192
  immunosuppression   68
  intensive care   56–58
  postoperative patient   77
  pregnancy   96
  renal medicine   166

d
DAA *see* direct-acting antiviral agents
decompensated cirrhosis   234
delirium   205, 207
Dengue fever   67–68, 117
dermatitis herpetiformis   175
dermatology   169–177
  dermatological drugs and LFTs
    169–174, **171**
  investigation and management of
    abnormal LFTs   169, *170*
  liver disease associated with
    dermatological disease   175–176
  liver disease that mimics
    dermatological disease   174
  unexplained abnormal LFTs and
    known dermatological disease   176
dermatomyositis   176
dialysis   161–163
diet and nutrition   217–218
dietary supplements   42
DILI *see* drug-induced liver injury

direct-acting antiviral agents
(DAA) 163, 165
distribution 230–231, 236
dose-dependent drug-induced liver
injury 229–230
drain fluid analysis 78, **78**
drug-induced acute hepatocyte necrosis
54–56, *57*
drug-induced autoimmune hepatitis
250–251, **251**
drug-induced liver injury (DILI)
acute liver failure 246
base rates 244–246, *246*
biliary obstruction 248–249
cardiac disease 118–119, **118**
causality assessment 249–250, **250**
challenges in diagnostic approach
244, **245**
considering alternative explanations
248–249
considering DILI in diagnosis 247
diagnosing drug-induced liver injury
243–253
endocrinology and metabolic
diseases 101, **102**, 108
gastroenterology 134, 142–144, **142**
genetic tests 251, **251**
global perspective 39, 42
hypersensitivity reactions 247
immunosuppression 66
importance of the diagnosis 251–252
intensive care 58–59
ischemic hepatitis 248, *249*
jaundice 246, *246*
liver biopsy 250
mental health and
neurology 202–205, **203–204**
oncologic diseases 180–181, **181**
pattern of liver injury 247–248
postoperative patient 76
pregnancy 95
prescribing 227, 229–230
probing for information on
medications 247

raised liver enzymes 244–246
renal medicine 164
drug licensing 228–229, **228**, 236
Dubin–Johnson syndrome 27
dyslipidemia 100, 107–108

e
EBV *see* Epstein–Barr virus
Echinococcus histolytica 44
echocardiography
cardiac disease 113
intensive care 54
respiratory disease 122–123
eclampsia 91–92
eGFR *see* estimated glomerular
filtration rate
EHPVO *see* extrahepatic portal venous
obstruction
electrocardiography 54
elimination 231, 235–236
ELISA *see* enzyme-linked
immunosorbent assay
emphysema 126, *127*
endocrinology and metabolic diseases
99–109
cardiac disease 117–118
mental health and
neurology 204, 206–207
non-alcoholic fatty liver
disease 210–212, 217–219
nutrient homeostasis and the liver 100
oncologic diseases 182
patients with known endocrinology
disease 103–108
referral to liver specialist 108
role of liver and impact of endocrine
disorders 99–100
unexplained abnormal
LFTs 100–101, **102**
workup for excluding alternative
causes 101–103
endoscopic retrograde
cholangiopancreatography
(ERCP) 137, 140

end-stage kidney disease
(ESKD) 159, 161–163
end-stage liver disease
dermatology 172
endocrinology and metabolic
diseases 100
pregnancy 94
see also Model for End-stage
Liver Disease
Entamoeba histolytica 166
enteric fever 69
enzyme-linked immunosorbent assay
(ELISA) 67, 70
epistasis 127
Epstein–Barr virus (EBV)
hematology 192
immunosuppression 68
intensive care 56–58
postoperative patient 77
pregnancy 96
ERCP *see* endoscopic retrograde
cholangiopancreatography
ESKD *see* end-stage kidney disease
estimated glomerular filtration rate
(eGFR) 146
exercise/physical activity 217–218
external compression 78
extracorporeal liver support
devices 154
extrahepatic biliary
obstruction 134–139
extrahepatic cholestasis 78
extrahepatic portal venous obstruction
(EHPVO) 39
extrapyramidal dysfunction 204, 206
extravascular loss 6

f
factor VIII 238
farnesoid X receptor agonists 219
ferritin 12–13, 192, 215
FFP *see* fresh frozen plasma
fibrates 107–108
fibrinogen 239–240

fibrosis
dermatology 172
endocrinology and metabolic diseases
104–105, 108
gastroenterology 137
invasive procedures 238
liver function tests 15
mental health and
neurology 206–207
non-alcoholic fatty liver disease 210,
215, 216–217, 219
oncologic diseases 182, 187
prescribing 232
respiratory disease 128, 129
focal nodular hyperplasia 179
Fontan's physiology 115–116
fresh frozen plasma (FFP)
237–240, 242
fulminant hepatic failure 66
fulminant liver disease 90, 202
functional tests of liver function 17

g
gallbladder disease 94
gallbladder surgery 78
gallstones 27
gamma-glutamyl transferase (GGT)
cardiac disease 112
dermatology 174
endocrinology and metabolic
diseases 104, 106
gastroenterology 135–136
global perspective 31, 33, 42, 45
hematology 192
immunosuppression 70
intensive care 58–59
liver function tests 4, 8–9
mental health and neurology 201
non-alcoholic fatty liver disease 214
oncologic diseases 188
postoperative patient 81
prescribing 226
primary care 22–24
respiratory disease 129

gastroenterology 133–144
   abnormal LFTs in gastroenterological
      disease 133–139, **134**
   causes of biliary obstruction: bile duct
      wall 136
   hepatology as subspeciality of 133
   liver diseases associated with
      gastroenterological diseases 141
   liver diseases mimicking
      gastroenterological
      diseases 139–140, **140**
   luminal conditions 138–139
   monitoring LFTs in gastroenterology
      143, 144
   pancreatobiliary
      conditions 134–138, *135*
   unexplained abnormal LFTs and
      known gastroenterological
      disease 141–144, **142**
general practitioners (GP) 21–22
genetic tests 251, **251**
GFR *see* glomerular filtration rate
GGT *see* gamma-glutamyl transferase
Gilbert's syndrome
   global perspective 40
   liver function tests 10–11
   primary care 26
global perspective 31–47
   Africa 42–45
   Far East 41–42, **41**
   India *32*, 33–41, **34–36**
glomerular filtration rate (GFR) 146
glomerulonephritis 145, 147, **148**,
      150, 155
glucagon-like peptide-1 (GLP-1)
      agonists 218
glucose and glycemic control 100
GP *see* general practitioners
graft-versus-host disease (GVHD)
      191, 196–197
gut loss 6
GVHD *see* graft-versus-host disease

h
HAV *see* hepatitis A virus
HBV *see* hepatitis B virus
HCC *see* hepatocellular carcinoma
HCV *see* hepatitis C virus
HDV *see* hepatitis D virus
heart transplants 118
HELLP syndrome 91–92, **92**, 193
hemangioma 179
hematology 191–199
   hematologic analytes 11–12
   investigation and management of
      abnormal LFTs 191–192
   liver diseases associated with
      hematologic diseases **194**
   liver diseases that mimic hematologic
      diseases **193**
   unexplained abnormal LFTs and
      hematologic disease 192–199, *195*,
      196–197, *198*
hematopoietic stem-cell transplantation
      (HSCT) 191, 196–197, **197**
hemochromatosis 40, 117, 174
hemodialysis 7
hemolysis 11
hemophagocytic
      lymphohistiocytosis 194
hemophagocytic syndrome 194
hepatic congestion 114
hepatic encephalopathy 79, 205–206
hepatic granuloma 175
hepatic hydrothorax 125
hepatic infarction 77
hepatic sinusoidal injury 182–183
hepatitis A virus (HAV)
   global perspective 33–34, **34**
   hematology 192
   immunosuppression 63, 65
   intensive care 56–58
   liver function tests 14
   postoperative patient 77
   pregnancy 96

hepatitis B virus (HBV)
  cardiac disease   118
  dermatology   171–172
  gastroenterology   142–144
  global perspective   34–36, **35**, 41, **41**
  hematology   192, 196, **196**
  immunosuppression   63, 66
  intensive care   56–58
  liver function tests   14–15, **14**
  oncologic diseases   180, 185–187, **186**
  postoperative patient   77
  pregnancy   96
  primary care   24–25
  renal medicine   145, 158, 162–163, 165
hepatitis C virus (HCV)
  cardiac disease   118
  dermatology   174–175
  global perspective   36, **36**
  hematology   192, 194
  immunosuppression   63, 66–67
  liver function tests   15
  oncologic diseases   180, 186–187
  postoperative patient   77
  pregnancy   96
  primary care   24–25
  renal medicine   145, 152, *152*, 155,
    158, 162–165
hepatitis D virus (HDV)   36
hepatitis E virus (HEV)
  global perspective   36–37
  hematology   192
  immunosuppression   63, 65–66
  intensive care   56–58
  liver function tests   15
  postoperative patient   77
  pregnancy   96
  renal medicine   163, 165–166
hepatocellular carcinoma (HCC)
  dermatology   172
  endocrinology and metabolic
    diseases   104
  immunosuppression   67

non-alcoholic fatty liver disease   213
oncology   180
hepatocellular liver injury
  intensive care   53–58, *55–57*
  postoperative patient   75, 76–77
hepatocellular necrosis   54
hepatopulmonary syndrome
    (HPS)   121–123, *122*, 124
hepatorenal syndrome (HRS)   145,
    149–156, *149*, *151–153*, **153**
hepatotoxicity
  endocrinology and metabolic diseases
    107–108
  gastroenterology   134, 142–144, **142**
  global perspective   42, 44–45
  intensive care   54–56, *57*, 58
  mental health and
    neurology   203–204
  non-alcoholic fatty liver
    disease   218–219
  oncologic diseases   184
  prescribing   229–230, 236
herbal remedies   42, 174
hereditary hemochromatosis   95
hereditary hemorrhagic telangiectasia
    (HHT)   127–128
herpes simplex virus (HSV)
  immunosuppression   69
  intensive care   56–58
  postoperative patient   77
  pregnancy   96
  renal medicine   166
HEV *see* hepatitis E virus
HG *see* hyperemesis gravidarum
HHT *see* hereditary hemorrhagic
    telangiectasia
high-output heart failure   127–128
Histoplasma spp.   73
HIV/AIDS
  cardiac disease   117
  global perspective   44
  immunosuppression   68, 70–71, 73

HLA *see* human leukocyte antigen
HPS *see* hepatopulmonary syndrome
HRS *see* hepatorenal syndrome
HSCT *see* hematopoietic stem-cell
   transplantation
HSV *see* herpes simplex virus
human leukocyte antigen
   (HLA)   251, **251**
hyperbilirubinemia
   dermatology   173
   gastroenterology   137
   liver function tests   9, *9*
   primary care   25–28
hyperemesis gravidarum (HG)   89–90
hyperglycemia   58–59
hypersensitivity reactions   247
hypersplenism   11
hyperthyroidism   107
hypoalbuminemia   175
hypofibrinogenemia   239
hypoglycemia   91
hypothyroidism   106
hypoxic hepatitis *see* ischemic hepatitis

i

IBD *see* inflammatory bowel disease
IBS *see* irritable bowel syndrome
ICI *see* immune checkpoint inhibitors
ICP *see* intrahepatic cholestasis of
   pregnancy
idiopathic pulmonary fibrosis (IPF)   129
idiosyncratic drug-induced liver
   injury   229
IG *see* immunoglobulins
ILD *see* interstitial lung disease
immune checkpoint inhibitors
   (ICI)   184, 250
immune-mediated hepatitis   184
immunization   36, 162
immunoglobulin A (IgA)
   nephropathy   155
immunoglobulin IgG4-related
   disease   137, 139

immunoglobulins (IG)
   immunosuppression   65–67, 70
   markers of malignancy   13
immunologic disease   128–130, *130*
immunology screen   150, 152, *152*, **153**
immunosuppression
   bacterial and parasitic
      infections   69–72
   cardiac disease   118
   diagnosing drug-induced liver
      injury   250
   fungal infections   72–73
   gastroenterology   142–144
   global perspective   41
   hematology   195–197, **196**
   immunocompetent versus
      immunocompromised
      patients   63, **64**
   infections affecting the liver   63–74
   intensive care   56–58
   renal medicine   164, 166
   systemic and non-hepatotropic
      organisms   63–65, *65*
   viral infections   63, 65–69
infiltrative disease   77
inflammatory bowel disease (IBD)
   101–103, 138–142
inflammatory disease
   cardiac disease   117
   endocrinology and metabolic
      diseases   103–104
   respiratory disease   128–130, *130*
   systemic inflammation   58–59
INR *see* international normalized ratio
insulin resistance   211, 217
intensive care   51–62
   approach to supportive care   61–62
   assessment of severity of liver
      injury   59–60
   cholestatic pattern of liver
      injury   58–59
   classification and
      prevalence   51–53, *52*

discussion with specialist
 liver unit   62
hepatocellular pattern of liver injury
 53–58, *55–57*
patterns of liver test abnormalities
 53–59, *55–57*
sequential clinical assessment   61
international normalized ratio
 (INR)   59–60
endocrinology and metabolic
 diseases   101
hematology   192
invasive procedures   237–238,
 240–242
mental health and neurology   201
oncologic diseases   181
postoperative patient   82
respiratory disease   123
interstitial lung disease
 (ILD)   129–130, *130*
intrahepatic biliary
 obstruction   134–139
intrahepatic cholestasis   77–78, 134
intrahepatic cholestasis of pregnancy
 (ICP)   86, 93
intrapulmonary vascular dilation (IPVD)
 122–123, *122*
invasive procedures   237–242
 coagulation testing   238
 liver disease patients' risk of
  bleeding   239
 medication history   240, **241**
 platelet count   238, **239**
 reducing procedural bleeding   240
 use of blood products in liver
  disease   239–240
IPF *see* idiopathic pulmonary fibrosis
IPVD *see* intrapulmonary vascular
 dilation
iron overload   117
irritable bowel syndrome (IBS)   139, 141
ischemic hepatitis
 cardiac disease   114

diagnosing drug-induced liver
 injury   248, *249*
intensive care   54, *55–56*
postoperative patient   76–77
pregnancy   93
isolated raised alkaline phosphatase   40
itraconazole   173

j
JAG1 gene   161
jaundice
 diagnosing drug-induced liver injury
  246, *246*
 gastroenterology   137, 140–141
 liver function tests   9–11, *9*
 primary care   25–28

k
Kawasaki disease   176
kidney blood tests   11
kidney disease *see* renal medicine
kidney transplantation   163–167
Korsakoff syndrome   206

l
lactate   60
left ventricular assist devices
 (LVAD)   115
Leptospira spp.   70
leukopenia   11
LFT *see* liver function tests
lichen planus   175
lifestyle management   182, 217–218
liver biopsy   17
 dermatology   172
 diagnosing drug-induced liver
  injury   250
 invasive procedures   238
 non-alcoholic fatty liver disease   215
liver function tests (LFT)   3–18
 alcohol use   16
 bilirubin   9–11, *9*
 characteristics   4

liver function tests (LFT) (*cont'd*)
  functional tests of liver function   17
  global perspective   31–47
  guidelines for management of
    abnormal liver tests   5
  hepatic fibrosis   15
  hepatic steatosis   15–16
  liver biopsy   17
  models assessing prognosis in liver
    disease   16
  other analytes in liver disease   11–15
  primary care   21–29
  prothrombin time   11
  reference range   3–4
  standard liver function tests   4–9
  see also individual diseases;
    individual tests
liver transplantation
  hematology   199
  pregnancy   94
  renal medicine   145, 155–158, **157**
luminal conditions   138–139
lung-brain perfusion
    scanning   122–123, *122*
LVAD *see* left ventricular assist devices
Lyme disease   71
lymphoma   194
lysosomal storage disorders   161

m
MAFLD *see* metabolic dysfunction-
    associated fatty liver disease
magnetic resonance
    cholangiopancreatography
    (MRCP)   81, 135, 137
magnetic resonance elastography
    (MRE)   216
magnetic resonance imaging
    (MRI)   215–216
malaria   72, 117
malignancies *see oncologic diseases*
malignant obstruction   135, 137–138
malnutrition   204–205

MAOI *see* monoamine oxidase inhibitors
mAST *see* mitochondrial aspartate amino
    transferase
mastocytosis   175–176
Mediterranean diet   217
MELD *see* Model for End-stage
    Liver Disease
mental health and neurology   201–208
  antidepressants   202–204, **203**
  antipsychotics   204–205, **204**
  investigation and management of
    abnormal LFTs   201–202
  liver diseases associated with
    psychiatric disease   206–207
  liver diseases that mimic psychiatric
    disease   205–206
  unexplained abnormal LFTs and
    known psychiatric
    disease   207–208
  unexplained abnormal LFTs in mental
    health and
    neurology   202–205, **203–204**
metabolic dysfunction-associated fatty
    liver disease (MAFLD)   210
metabolic liver disease   79
metabolic syndrome
  cardiac disease   112
  mental health and
    neurology   204, 206
  non-alcoholic fatty liver disease   211
  patients with known endocrinology
    disease   103–106, 108
metabolism   231–232, 236
methotrexate   170–173
mitochondrial aspartate amino
    transferase (mAST)   7
Model for End-stage Liver Disease
    (MELD)   17
  prescribing   233–234
  renal medicine   155
  respiratory disease   123
monoamine oxidase inhibitors
    (MAOI)   202

MRCP *see* magnetic resonance cholangiopancreatography
MRE *see* magnetic resonance elastography
MRI *see* magnetic resonance imaging
Mycobacterium spp.   167

n
N-acetyl cysteine (NAC)   55–56
NAFLD *see* non-alcoholic fatty liver disease
NASH *see* non-alcoholic steatohepatitis
neonatal jaundice   27–28
nephrogenic ascites   163–164
neurofibromatosis   176
neurology *see* mental health and neurology
nodular regenerative hyperplasia (NRH)   182, 183–184
non-alcoholic fatty liver disease (NAFLD)   209–221
  cardiac disease   112
  clinical features and diagnosis 213–215, **214**
  concepts and definitions   209–210
  dermatology   175
  endocrinology and metabolic diseases 100–101, *103*
  epidemiology   211
  global perspective   37, 41
  liver function tests   8–9, 13, 15
  markers of malignancy   13
  mental health and neurology   206–207
  natural history/ prognosis   212–213, *213*
  non-invasive assessment   215–217
  oncologic diseases   182
  pathophysiology   211
  patients with known endocrinology disease   103–108
  postoperative patient   79
  pregnancy   93
  primary care   22–24
  renal medicine   145, 155, 162, 164
  risk factors   211–212
  treatment   217–219, *220*
non-alcoholic steatohepatitis (NASH)
  clinical features and diagnosis   214–215
  concepts and definitions   210
  epidemiology   211
  global perspective   37
  non-alcoholic fatty liver disease   212–213, *213*
  non-invasive assessment   215–217
  oncologic diseases   182
  patients with known endocrinology disease   103–106
  primary care   22–23
  risk factors   212
  treatment   218–219
NOTCH2 gene   161
NRH *see* nodular regenerative hyperplasia
nutrient homeostasis   100
nutritional deficiency   6

o
obesity and overweight
  cardiac disease   117
  endocrinology and metabolic diseases 100, 104
  non-alcoholic fatty liver disease   210, 211–214, 217–219
obstructive jaundice   137
occult hepatitis B virus   41, **41**
oncologic diseases   179–190
  chemotherapy-associated steatohepatitis   182
  dermatology   176
  drug-induced liver injury   180–181, **181**
  gastroenterology   135, 137–138
  global perspective   43
  hepatic sinusoidal injury   182–183

oncologic diseases (*cont'd*)
  hepatitis B virus
    reactivation   185–186, **186**
  immune-mediated hepatitis   184
  liver diseases associated with
    oncologic diseases   180–186
  liver diseases that mimic oncologic
    diseases   179
  liver enzyme elevations   180–181
  markers of malignancy   12–13
  nodular regenerative
    hyperplasia   182, 183–184
  radiation-induced liver
    injury   184–185
  unexplained abnormal LFTs and
    known oncologic
    disease   186–188, *187*
  see also individual malignancies

p
PAH *see* pulmonary artery hypertension
pancreatitis   137
pancreatobiliary
    conditions   134–138, *135*
paracetamol toxicity   54–56, 58
paraneoplastic syndromes   180
parenteral nutrition   58–59, 77
pathological jaundice   28
PAVM *see* pulmonary arteriovenous
    malformations
PBC *see* primary biliary cholangitis
PCR *see* polymerase chain reaction
PDFF *see* proton density fat fraction
    estimation
peripheral edema   78
peroxisome proliferator-activated
    receptor (PPAR) agonists   218
PH *see* primary hyperoxaluria
physiological jaundice   27–28
Plasmodium spp.   72
platelet count   101, 238–239, **239**
platelet transfusions   238
pleural effusions   124–125, *125*

PNPLA3 gene   212
poisoning   43
polycystic kidney disease   159–161
polymerase chain reaction (PCR)   70
POPH *see* portopulmonary hypertension
porphyria cutanea tarda   174
portal biliopathy   39
portal hypertension
  dermatology   172, 175
  gastroenterology   139
  hematology   193
  invasive procedures   238
  oncologic diseases   183–184
  postoperative patient   79
  pregnancy   94
  renal medicine   149–150, 161
  respiratory disease   122–124, *124*, 128
portopulmonary hypertension
    (POPH)   123–124, *124*
postoperative patient   75–83
  approach to abnormal
    LFTs   79–82, *80*
  common causes of liver
    injury   75–76, *76*
  predominantly cholestatic
    injury   77–78
  predominantly hepatocellular
    injury   76–77
  underlying chronic liver
    conditions   78–79, **78**
PPAR *see* peroxisome proliferator-
    activated receptor
prebiotics   218
pre-eclampsia   86, 91–92
pregnancy   85–97
  acquired non-pregnancy related
    disease   95–96, **96**
  acute fatty liver of
    pregnancy   90–91, **92**
  alkaline phosphatase in normal
    pregnancy   88, *89*
  autoimmune hepatitis   95
  Budd–Chiari syndrome   95

cirrhosis 93–94
drug-induced liver injury 95
gall bladder disease 94
HELLP syndrome 91–92, **92**
hereditary hemochromatosis 95
history and overlapping
    symptoms 86–87, **87**
hyperemesis gravidarum 89–90
hypertensive disorders of
    pregnancy 91–92
intrahepatic cholestasis of
    pregnancy 86, 93
investigations 86, **88**, 89
ischemic hepatitis 93
liver transplant 94
non-alcoholic fatty liver disease 93
normal pregnancy 86–88, **87–88**
pre-existing liver disease 93–95
pregnancy-related liver disease
    88–93, **90, 92**
primary biliary cholangitis 94–95
primary sclerosing cholangitis
    94–95
viral hepatitis 96, **96**
Wilson's disease 95
prescribing 225–236
    abnormal liver tests 226–227, **227**
    ADME principles for liver disease
        patients 230–232, 236
    assessing and monitoring liver
        impairment 226–227
    concepts and definitions 225–226
    decision-making for liver
        disease 232–236, *233*, **235**
    drug licensing and prescribing
        guidance 228–229, **228**, 236
    hepatotoxic medication and drug-
        induced liver injury 229–230
primary biliary cholangitis (PBC)
    dermatology 174–175
    endocrinology and metabolic
        diseases 100, 101–103, 108
    gastroenterology 134, 139

global perspective 38
pregnancy 94–95
respiratory disease 124, *124*, 130
primary care 21–29
    chronic infections of the liver 24–25
    global perspective 42
    hyperbilirubinemia and jaundice
        25–28
    isolated raised AST/ALT in healthy
        individuals 22
    liver disease in the UK 22
    non-alcoholic fatty liver
        disease 22–24
primary hyperoxaluria (PH) 161
primary myelofibrosis 192
primary sclerosing cholangitis (PSC)
    endocrinology and metabolic
        diseases 100, 101–103
    gastroenterology 134, 139–141
    global perspective 39
    pregnancy 94–95
    respiratory disease 124, 129
probiotics 218
progressive consumptive
        coagulopathy 239
prolonged jaundice 27–28
prothrombin time
    gastroenterology 135
    hematology 192
    invasive procedures 237
    liver function tests 11
prothrombotic vascular occlusion 77
proton density fat fraction estimation
        (PDFF) 215–216
PSC *see* primary sclerosing cholangitis
psoriasis 175
psychiatric disease *see* mental health and
        neurology
psychosis 205, 207
pulmonary arteriovenous malformations
        (PAVM) 127–128
pulmonary artery hypertension
        (PAH) 121, 123–124, *124*

pulmonary venous hypertension
(PVH)   123
pyogenic liver abscesses   166

q
Q fever   71

r
radiation-induced liver injury
(RILD)   184–185
radionuclide imaging   81
recurrent pyogenic cholangitis   42
refeeding   205
renal biopsy   150–151
renal cell carcinoma   180
renal coagulopathies   235
renal encephalopathy   235
renal loss   6
renal medicine   145–167
abnormal LFTs in acute kidney injury
158, **159**
abnormal LFTs in chronic kidney
disease   158–161, *160*, **160**
acute kidney injury in patients with
cirrhosis   147–155, **147–148**, *149*,
151–153, **153**
chronic kidney disease in patients
with cirrhosis   155–156
dialysis   161–163
kidney disease and abnormal LFTs
145–146, 158–167, **159–160**, *160*
liver disease in kidney transplant
recipients   163–164
measurement of renal function in
patients with cirrhosis   146
prescribing   235
renal impairment in acute liver failure
patients   156
renal impairment in liver transplant
recipients   156–158, **157**
renal impairment in patients with liver
disease   146–158
viral hepatitis in kidney transplant
patients   164–167

renal replacement therapy
(RRT)   154–156
respiratory disease   121–132
arterial hypoxemia   121–123, *122*
further diagnostic tests   **131**
genetic lung abnormalities
126–128, *127*
immunologic/inflammatory lung
disorders with liver
manifestations   128–130, *130*
liver–lung problems with systemic
presentation   126–130, **131**
lung problems due to unexpected liver
issues   121–125, **131**
pleural effusions   124–125, *125*
pulmonary hypertension   121,
123–124, *124*
retinoids   172
Rickettsia rickettsii   71
right-sided heart failure   114
RILD *see* radiation-induced liver injury
Rocky Mountain spotted fever   71
rotational thromboelastometry   238
Roussel Uclaf Causality Assessment
Method (RUCAM)   42,
249–250, **250**
RRT *see* renal replacement therapy
RUCAM *see* Roussel Uclaf Causality
Assessment Method

s
Salmonella typhi   69
sarcoidosis   117, 128–129, 175
SCA *see* sickle-cell anemia
Schistosoma spp.   71–72
SCr *see* serum creatinine
secondary biliary cirrhosis   141
secondary sclerosing
cholangitis   137, 141
selective serotonin reuptake inhibitors
(SSRI)   202
sepsis
cardiac disease   117

intensive care   58–59, 62
postoperative patient   77
renal medicine   150
serotonin noradrenaline reuptake
   inhibitors (SNRI)   202
serum creatinine (SCr)   146
SGLT-2 *see* sodium–glucose
   cotransporter-2
short telomere syndromes (STS)   129, *130*
sickle-cell anemia (SCA)   191,
   197–199, *198*
sinusoidal obstruction syndrome
   (SOS)   182–183, 191, 195–197
skin telangiectasis   127
SLE *see* systemic lupus erythematosus
SNRI *see* serotonin noradrenaline
   reuptake inhibitors
sodium–glucose cotransporter-2
   (SGLT-2) inhibitors   218–219
SOS *see* sinusoidal obstruction syndrome
SSRI *see* selective serotonin reuptake
   inhibitors
statins   107–108, 219
Stauffer syndrome   180
steatosis
   endocrinology and metabolic diseases
      103–104
   liver function tests   15–16
   mental health and neurology   205
   non-alcoholic fatty liver disease
      209–210, 214–219
steroid-responsive
   cholangiopathies   137
stool analysis   44
STS *see* short telomere syndromes
Swansea criteria   91
syphilis   70
systemic lupus erythematosus
   (SLE)   117

t
T2DM *see* type 2 diabetes mellitus
TB *see* tuberculosis

TBA *see* total bile acids
TE *see* transient elastography
telomere disorders   129, *130*
terbinafine   173
thoracentesis   124–125
thrombocytopenia   12
thromboelastography   60, 238
thrombopoietin receptor agonists
   (TPO-RA)   237, 240, 242
thyroid disease   99, 106–107
thyrotoxicosis   107
TIPS *see* transjugular intrahepatic
   portosystemic shunt
total bile acids (TBA)   86
toxic epidermal necrolysis   176
TPO-RA *see* thrombopoietin receptor
   agonists
traditional medicines   44, 174
transferritin   192
transient elastography (TE)
   dermatology   172, 173
   hepatic fibrosis   15, *16*
transjugular intrahepatic portosystemic
   shunt (TIPS)   154, 232
Treponema pallidum   70
tuberculosis (TB)
   global perspective   39, 40
   immunosuppression   71
   renal medicine   167
tumor markers   138
type 2 diabetes mellitus (T2DM)
   cardiac disease   117
   non-alcoholic fatty liver
      disease   212–213
   patients with known endocrinology
      disease   103–106
   role of liver and impact of endocrine
      disorders   99–100
   unexplained abnormal LFTs   100

u
UDCA *see* ursodeoxycholic acid
UGT1A1 gene   10, 40

ultrasound
  hepatic fibrosis   15, *16*
  non-alcoholic fatty liver disease   214
  postoperative patient   81
  renal medicine   150
unconjugated hyperbilirubinemia   26
upper gastrointestinal
  bleeding   139, 150
urinalysis   44, 150
urine microscopy   150, *151*
ursodeoxycholic acid (UDCA)   93

v

varicella zoster virus (VZV)   166
vascular liver injury   76–77
vibration-controlled transient
  elastography (VCTE)   215,
  216–217
visceral obesity   100
vitamin D deficiency   40
vitamin K deficiency
  intensive care   59
  invasive procedures   240
  postoperative patient   82

vitamin K-dependent clotting factor
  deficiency   135
vitamin supplementation   218
von Willebrand factor   238
VZV *see* varicella zoster virus

w

warfarin   238
Wernicke's encephalopathy   206
Wilson's disease
  global perspective   38–39
  hematology   193
  markers of malignancy   12
  mental health and neurology   205
  pregnancy   95
withdrawal effects   205

x

xanthelasmas   174

y

yellow fever   67

z

zoonotic disease   70–71